Springer Japan KK

Eiichi Tahara (Ed.)

Molecular Pathology of Gastroenterological Cancer

Application to Clinical Practice

With 80 Figures, Including 8 in Color

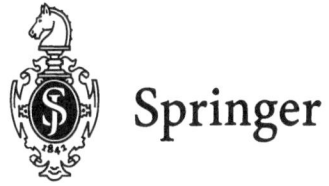

Springer

Eiichi Tahara, M.D., Ph.D.
Director, Faculty of Medicine
Professor and Chairman, First Department of Pathology
Hiroshima University School of Medicine
1-2-3 Kasumi, Minami-ku
Hiroshima 734, Japan

ISBN 978-4-431-65917-4   ISBN 978-4-431-65915-0 (eBook)
DOI 10.1007/978-4-431-65915-0

Library of Congress Cataloging-in-Publication Data

Molecular pathology of gastroenterological cancer: application to
    clinical practice / Eiichi Tahara, ed.
        p. cm.
    Includes bibliographical references and indexes.

    1. Gastrointestinal system—Cancer—Molecular aspects.
    I. Tahara, Eiichi, 1936– .
    [DNLM: 1. Digestive System Neoplasms—pathology. 2. Digestive
System Neoplasms—etiology. 3. Digestive System Neoplasms—
diagnosis. WI 149 M718 1997]
    RC280.D5M65   1997
    616.99′433—dc21
    DNLM/DLC
    for Library of Congress   97-4383

Printed on acid-free paper

© Springer Japan 1997
Originally published by Springer-Verlag Tokyo in 1997
Softcover reprint of the hardcover 1st edition 1997

Typesetting: Best-set Typesetter Ltd., Hong Kong

SPIN: 10570188

Preface

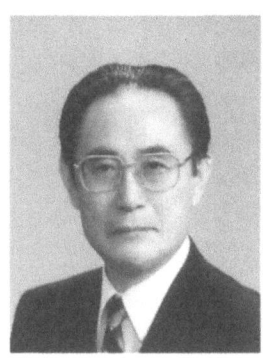

Twenty years have passed since I became a professor in the First Department of Pathology, Hiroshima University School of Medicine. It is my great pleasure that *Molecular Pathology of Gastroenterological Cancer—Application to Clinical Practice* has been published by Springer-Verlag Tokyo to commemorate the 20th anniversary of my professorship.

Seeing the academic achievements of our department during these 20 years, I am confident that we could establish a department of oncology to research the pathogenesis of human cancer through systemic application of a variety of molecular techniques. We have demonstrated that the development and progression of esophageal, gastric, and colon cancer require multiple alterations affecting DNA mismatch repair genes, oncogenes, and tumorsuppressor genes, and that common and uncommon genetic changes exist for esophageal, gastric, and colorectal carcinomas. In addition to these genetic changes, the majority of gastrointestinal cancers express telomerase activity, with overexpression of telomerase RNA, indicating a powerful additional tool for early detection of gastrointestinal cancer.

By transferring these basic observations to the clinic, we now are able to make accurate cancer diagnoses, thus determing the grade of malignancy and patient prognosis. We also can identify patients at high risk for developing cancer and create new therapeutic approaches. In fact, we have routinely implemented a new molecular diagnosis strategy at the Hiroshima City Medical Association Clinical Laboratory since August 1993.

This book presents the latest information about molecular diagnosis strategy and gastroenterological cancers. The contributors, some of them my colleagues, are highly renowned researchers from abroad and from Japan. Among them are Professors Sugimura, Nakamura, McGee, Lotan, Tarin, Ide, and Fidler, who have worked with us for these many years. I must express my sincere gratitude to them and to my sons for their valuable contributions to this book and for our collaborative studies.

It is hoped that *Molecular Pathology of Gastroenterological Cancer* will be of use not only in cancer research but also in the prevention, diagnosis, and therapy of gastrointestinal cancers as the twenty-first century approaches.

I would like to take this opportunity to express again my appreciation to the scientists and colleagues who contributed their work to this book and for their willingness to provide readers with insight into molecular pathology. Finally, I gratefully acknowledge the dedicated work of the staff of Springer-Verlag Tokyo.

December 1996

EIICHI TAHARA

Contents

Experimental Stomach Carcinogenesis

Hiroko Ohgaki[1] and Takashi Sugimura[2]

Summary. Sugimura and Fujimura first succeeded in selective induction of gastric carcinomas in rats by putting N-methyl-N'-nitro-N-nitrosoguanidine (MNNG) in their drinking water in 1967. Since then, similar models have been established for the induction of stomach carcinomas in other species using MNNG and its ethyl derivative N-ethyl-N'-nitro-N-nitrosoguanidine (ENNG). N-Methyl-N-nitrosourea (MNU) has also been demonstrated to induce a high incidence of gastric adenocarcinomas in rats and mice when given in their drinking water. Susceptibility to gastric carcinogenesis and the histologic types of gastric carcinomas depend on the mode of treatment, species, strain, and sex. The organ specificity of MNNG correlates well with the level of DNA methylation in target and nontarget tissues following oral administration in rats. The high concentration of methylated DNA bases in the glandular stomach appears to result from thiol-mediated acceleration of the decomposition of MNNG. Experimental gastric carcinogenesis is greatly modified by various factors and agents, indicating that both host and environmental factors contribute significantly. Although possible gastric carcinogens in humans have not been clearly identified, results in experimental animals suggest that avoidance of factors that enhance stomach carcinogenesis, especially those that enhance cell proliferation in the gastric mucosa, could help prevent gastric carcinogenesis in humans.

Experimental Models of Gastric Cancer

Rats

Generally, young adult male rats are given N-methyl-N'-nitro-N-nitrosoguanidine (MNNG) ad libitum in their drinking water at concentrations of 50–83 µg/ml for 4–8 months. After several months of additional observation, 60–100% of rats develop gastric adenocarcinomas (Table 1) [4–9]. Most tumors induced by MNNG in the drinking water are located in the pyloric region of the glandular stomach, but tumors are also induced in the fundic region, duodenum, and jejunum at a lesser frequency. Histologically, most gastric tumors are adenomas or adenocarcinomas, although sarcomas also develop. Most adenocarcinomas developed in rats are well differentiated, although rare poorly differentiated adenocarcinomas and signet ring cell carcinomas are seen. Gastric adenocarcinomas frequently invade the muscle layers or serosa, but metastasis of gastric adenocarcinomas are rare.

Female rats are generally less susceptible to gastric carcinogenesis induced by MNNG than male rats [10]. Castration or injection of estradiol in male rats reduces the incidence of gastric adenocarcinomas induced by MNNG [11, 12]. The age at which rats are treated with MNNG is also an important factor determining susceptibility to gastric carcinogenesis. Young rats are more susceptible than old animals [13].

There is a remarkable strain difference in susceptibility to MNNG in rats [9, 10, 14]. The incidences of gastric adenocarcinomas in randombred Wistar, inbred Wistar-May-Furth, and inbred Buffalo rats were 73%, 10%, and 0%, respectively, after administration of MNNG (83 µg/ml) for 52 weeks [14]. Treatment with MNNG in susceptible ACI rats, resistant Buffalo rats, and their F_1 and F_2 offspring demonstrated that susceptibility to MNNG was genetically

[1] Unit of Molecular Pathology, International Agency for Research on Cancer, 150 cours Albert Thomas, 69372 Lyon, France
[2] National Cancer Center Research Institute, 1-1 Tsukiji, 5-chome, Chuo-ku, Tokyo 104, Japan

Table 1. Induction of experimental gastric tumors

Species/strain	Treatment	Experimental period[a]	Gastric tumor incidence (%)
Rats			
Wistar	MNNG 50 µg/ml for 4 months	10 months	70
Wistar	MNNG 84 µg/ml for 7 months	16 months	57
Wistar	MNNG 167 µg/ml for 7 months	16 months	70
BN	MNNG 83 µg/ml for 7 months	18 months	92
BDIX	MNNG 83 µg/ml for 7 months	18 months	75
ACI	MNNG 83 µg/ml for 8 months	17 months	80
Buffalo	MNNG 83 µg/ml for 8 months	17 months	18
F344	MNU 100 ppm for 42 weeks	42 weeks	24
F344	MNU 400 ppm for 25 weeks	45 weeks	100
F344	MNU 400 ppm for 15 weeks	35 weeks	38
F344	MNU 100 ppm for 15 weeks	40 weeks	76
Mice			
C3H	MNU 120 ppm for 30 weeks	42 weeks	44
Dogs			
	ENNG 100 µg/ml for 5–6 months	13–37 months	100
	ENNG 100 µg/ml for 8–9 months	17–49 months	100
	ENNG 150 µg/ml for 5–6 months	20–40 months	100
	ENNG 150 µg/ml for 9 months	15–22 months	100

MNNG, N-methyl-N'-nitro-N-nitrosoguanidine; MNU, N-methyl-N-nitrosourea; ENNG, N-ethyl-N'-nitro-N-nitrosoguanidine.
Modified from [8].
[a] Total period of experiment including the treatment period.

determined, and resistance to MNNG in the Buffalo strain was a dominant trait [10]. Interestingly, gastric mucosa in these Buffalo rats showed less proliferative response during MNNG treatment than did that in susceptible ACI rats, which may constitute a key factor determining the susceptibility to MNNG-induced gastric carcinogenesis in these two rat strains [15]. Linkage analysis studies in F_2 offspring of ACI and Buffalo strains are ongoing to identify the genes that control cell proliferation responding to MNNG and to determine susceptibility to gastric cancer [16].

A single intragastric dose of MNNG (50–250 mg/body weight) given to ACI or Wistar rats produced a high incidence of forestomach tumors but only a few adenocarcinomas in the glandular stomach [17, 18]. For the development of glandular stomach carcinomas, continuous administration of MNNG appears to be essential.

Maekawa et al. [19] reported that gastric adenocarcinomas developed in 24% of F344 rats exposed to N-methyl-N-nitrosourea (MNU) in their drinking water (100 ppm) for 42 weeks. These animals also developed simultaneously a high incidence of tumors in the brain and spinal cord. F344 rats given MNU (200 ppm) in their drinking water developed, in addition to brain tumors, a high incidence of squamous cell carcinomas in the oral cavity and esophageal papillomas and carcinomas, but adenocarcinoma in the glandular stomach was rare [19]. In ACI rats given MNU (200 ppm) in their drinking water, renal pelvis papillomas developed frequently in addition to brain tumors, but gastric carcinomas were rare [19]. Hirota et al. [2] reported that invasive gastric adenocarcinomas were selectively induced in 100% of rats given MNU (400 ppm) in distilled water for 25 weeks and then maintained without a carcinogen for another 20 weeks. No neoplastic lesions were found in the esophagus, forestomach, or duodenum [2]. Later it was found that administration of MNU (100 ppm) for 15 weeks was an optimal condition for the selective induction of gastric adenocarcinomas in F344 rats [20].

Mice

Mice have been considered to be resistant to gastric carcinogenesis, as several efforts to induce gastric adenocarcinomas by MNNG, ENNG, or catechol in various strains of mice have been unsuccessful [5, 21, 22]. In contrast, BALB/c mice given 10 weekly administrations of MNU by intragastric intubation (0.5 mg/mouse) developed carcinomas in both forestomach and glandular stomach at high incidences [23]. Tatematsu et al. [3] reported that C3H mice given MNU ad libitum in the drinking water at 30–120 ppm for 30 weeks selectively developed adenocarcinomas in the glandular stomach. Adenocarcinomas developed in a dose-dependent manner and were histologically well-differentiated, poorly differentiated, and signet ring cell carcinomas.

Using C3H, BALB/c, and their chimeric mice, Tatematsu et al. [24] analyzed the clonality of gastric carcinomas. Mice were given MNU (0.5 mg/mice) once a week for a total of 10 weeks by intragastric intubation and observed until week 50. In normal gastric mucosa of the chimeras, each gland was composed entirely of C3H strain-specific antigen-positive or antigen-negative cells; no mixed glands were observed. Cells of all adenomatous hyperplasias and adenocarcinomas in chimeric mice were, in each case, homogeneous for one or other of the parental types. Thus it was clearly shown that individual carcinomas are derived from single cells with multipotential activities and that cellular differentiation of gastric cancer cells occurs secondarily [24].

Dogs

Mongrel and beagle dogs given MNNG (50–83 µg/ml) ad libitum in their drinking water developed a high incidence of gastric adenocarcinomas [25]. The most common type of gastric carcinoma in dogs given MNNG was well differentiated adenocarcinoma of the fundic region [26]. However, MNNG concurrently induced sarcomas in the small intestine, which caused early death of the dogs [27].

It has been found that administration of N-ethyl-N'-nitro-N-nitrosoguanidine (ENNG), either mixed with a pellet diet or given ad libitum in the drinking water (100–150 µg/ml for 3–9 months), produced a high incidence of gastric carcinomas in mongrel and beagle dogs without development of small-intestinel tumors [7, 28, 29]. The preferential sites for the induction of carcinomas in dogs were the angulus and antrum, but carcinomas also developed in the corpus. With concentrations of ENNG higher than 150 µg/ml,

esophageal squamous cell carcinomas also developed frequently [30].

Histologically, the gastric carcinomas in dogs were well- or poorly differentiated adenocarcinomas and signet ring cell carcinomas. Different histologic types of carcinomas often develop in the same stomach [29]. Only signet ring cell carcinomas and poorly differentiated adenocarcinomas developed in the antrum in 50% of the dogs treated with ENNG for 3 months (total dose per dog was 6 g). After treatment for 6 and 9 months (total dose per dog was 12–18 g), well differentiated adenocarcinomas developed in addition to poorly differentiated adenocarcinomas or signet ring cell carcinomas (or both) in 90% of dogs [31]. Thus the concentration of ENNG and duration of treatment appear to affect the incidence, histological type, and location of gastric carcinomas [29, 31]. Metastases of gastric adenocarcinomas to regional lymph nodes, liver, and other organs are frequent [30, 32–34]. The process of gastric carcinogenesis and the effect of treatment were successfully confirmed by radiographic examination and endoscopy in stomach cancer in these dogs [33].

Monkeys

Two cynomolgus monkeys given ENNG (100 µg/ml) ad libitum in the drinking water for 10 months and two rhesus monkeys given MNNG (83 µg/ml) for 10 months did not develop gastric carcinomas after 54–104 months of observation [35]. Rhesus and cynomolgus monkeys given ENNG at a concentration of 200 or 300 µg/ml in their drinking water for 11–26 months developed gastric adenocarcinomas after 11–38 months of observation [35]. All the tumors were located in the pyloric region. Histologically, they were poorly differentiated adenocarcinomas and signet ring cell carcinomas, with a few moderately to well-differentiated adenocarcinomas. The histological appearance of these carcinomas was similar to that in human cancers for the respective histological types. Metastasis was not found in any of the monkeys. One cynomolgus monkey given ENNG for 26 months was examined sequentially by endoscopy and biopsy. A tumor was first detected in the angulus of the stomach at the 31st month and was diagnosed as signet ring cell carcinoma. At autopsy in the 109th experimental month, this tumor was found to be still in the early (intramucosal) stage [36].

O^6-Alkylguanine-DNA alkyltransferase was measured in the gastric mucosa of 15 *Macaca fascicularis* monkeys before and during chronic oral exposure to ENNG in order to investigate possible causes of interindividual differences in susceptibility to its gastrocarcinogenic effect. A wide range of O^6-alkylguanine-DNA alkyltransferase activity (307–1903 fmol/mg protein) was found before treatment, which decreased significantly during the first year of exposure [37]. It remains to be clarified whether the level of O^6-alkylguanine-DNA alkyltransferase and its decrease during ENNG treatment correlate with susceptibility to ENNG-induced gastric carcinogenesis in monkeys.

Ferrets

Ferrets have *Helicobacter mustelae*, which naturally colonizes in their stomachs and causes chronic gastritis. A ferret infected with *H. mustelae* developed a spontaneous adenocarcinoma in the pyloric region of the stomach [38]. Ferrets infected with *H. mustelae* were given a single dose of MNNG (50–100 mg/kg). Nine of ten ferrets developed adenocarcinomas 29–55 months after the treatment [39]. Ferrets would be a good model for studies on the role of *Helicobacter* during the development of gastric cancer [39–41].

Possible Mechanisms of Experimental Gastric Carcinogenesis

MNNG-Induced Gastric Carcinogenesis

A direct-acting mutagenic and carcinogenic compound, MNNG, causes methylation of nucleic acids and protein without requiring metabolic activation [42–44]. On the other hand, nonenzymatic decomposition of MNNG, which is accelerated by SH compounds (L-cysteine and reduced glutathione), is necessary for its macromolecular binding [43]. The major methylated base caused by exposure to MNNG is 7-methylguanine, but 3-methyladenine, 1-methyladenine, 3-methylcytosine, and O^6-methylguanine are also produced at smaller amounts [42, 43]. Of these, O^6-methylguanine is considered to be the most critical adduct leading to mutation.

MNNG was first found to be carcinogenic by Sugimura et al. [45] and Schoental [46], who in-

duced fibrosarcomas in rats by subcutaneous injection. It was unexpected that rats treated with MNNG in their drinking water developed adenocarcinomas selectively in the glandular stomach without developing tumors in the upper digestive tract. The organ specificity of MNNG correlates well with the level of DNA methylation following oral administration of MNNG in rats (Table 2). After a single oral dose in rats, the concentration of methylpurines in the glandular stomach was 9 times higher than in the forestomach and 20 times higher than in the esophagus [47]. Similarly, during chronic administration of MNNG (80 μg/ml in the drinking water) to inbred Wistar rats, the amounts of O^6-methylguanine in the pylorus were about 3 times higher than in the fundus and in the duodenum [48]. These regional differences in DNA methylation correlate with the concentrations of cellular thiols, which enhance the decomposition of MNNG and the extent of its macromolecular binding (Table 2) [47]. Under the acidic conditions of gastric juice, MNNG is rapidly converted to *N*-methyl-*N'*-nitroguanidine, which is not mutagenic or carcinogenic [49]. This conversion may explain the low tumor incidence in the small and large intestine despite the high thiol concentration in these tissues. The amount of O^6-methylguanine DNA methyltransferase, which repairs O^6-methylguanine, has been reported to be low in rat glandular stomach (about 15% of the amount in the forestomach and 2% of that in the liver) [50]. The low repair capacity for O^6-methylguanine may also play a role in selective induction of adenocarcinomas in the glandular stomach by MNNG.

The distribution of cells highly exposed to MNNG were identified in the surface epithelium of fundus and pylorus of the glandular stomach in rats [15, 48]. Most superficial pyloric epithelial cells are postmitotic and rapidly desquamate into the gastric lumen; they are therefore considered not susceptible to the initiation of malignant transformation. The proliferating cell zone is located deeper in the pyloric glands, where the level of exposure to MNNG is much lower. Owing to this difference in the location of highly exposed cells and proliferating cells within the mucosa, the mutation frequency is predicted to be low when normal gastric mucosa is exposed to MNNG. However, during MNNG treatment the number of proliferating cells increases and the range of the proliferative cell zone extends greatly [15, 51, 52].

Table 2. Concentrations of free thiols and DNA methylation in rat tissues after treatment with MNNG or MNU

Organ	Thiols[a] (μmol/g wet tissue)	MNNG[b] 7-meG (mol/mol G)	MNU[c] O⁶meG (μmol/mol G)
Esophagus	0.279	9.9	124
Forestomach	0.119	22.2	185
Glandular stomach	1.249	196.8	98
Duodenum	2.149	155.0	109
Jejunum	2.659	16.0	ND
Colon	ND	ND	59
Liver	5.003	5.7	29
Brain	ND	ND	228

ND, not determined.

[a] From Wiestler et al. [47].

[b] Wistar rats were treated with a single dose of MNNG (80 ppm; 2.5 mg/kg body weight) in the drinking water [47].

[c] F344 rats were treated with MNU in the drinking water (400 ppm) for 2 weeks [55].

With this condition, the gastric mucosa is considered to be much more susceptible to additional MNNG exposure, which may explain the need for continuous MNNG treatment for induction of glandular stomach carcinomas.

Little is known about the molecular mechanisms of MNNG-induced gastric carcinogenesis in experimental animals. c-Ha-*ras* p21 immunoreactivity was detected in 3 of 17 carcinomas but in none of 10 adenomas that developed in rats given MNNG [53]. Immunoreactivity to transforming growth factor alpha (TGF-α) monoclonal antibody was confined to the differentiated compartment of the mucosa, whereas MNNG caused a significant increase in the intensity of TGF-α expression after 16 weeks of treatment in Wistar rats [54]. TGF-α expression was perinuclear in adenocarcinomas [54].

MNU-Induced Gastric Carcinogenesis

A multipotent carcinogen, MNU, induces tumors in various tissues depending on the route of administration. In contrast to MNNG treatment, chronic administration of MNU produced the highest levels of O⁶-methylguanosine in the brain and significant amounts of O⁶-methylguanosine in all the digestive tract tissues measured (i.e. esophagus, forestomach, pylorus and fundus of the glandular stomach, duodenum, and colon) in F344 rats given MNU (400 ppm) in the drinking water for 2 weeks [55]. There was no clear correlation between target organ specificity and the extent of methylation (Table 2). It was also found that the distribution of cells exposed to MNU was not restricted to the surface epithelium, but whole gastric mucosal cells were equally exposed [55]. In contrast to MNNG, MNU is stable under the acidic condition of the intragastric environment, and its decomposition to a methylating intermediate (i.e. methyldiazonium hydroxide) is not affected by intracellular thiols. Thus it is likely that gastric mucosa is exposed to MNU from the gastric lumen and from the bloodstream when rats are given this carcinogen in the drinking water.

Mutations in the *ras* and *neu* genes were not found in MNU-induced gastric carcinomas in rats [56].

Preneoplastic and Related Lesions During Gastric Carcinogenesis Induced by MNNG

Biochemical Changes

Expression of Pg1, which is one of three pepsinogen isozymes normally present in the pyloric mucosa, decreases beginning 1 week after the start of MNNG treatment [57, 58]. The decrease or disappearance of Pg1 is also consistently observed in gastric adenocarcinomas [59]. Thus the decrease in Pg1 expression is a good biochemical marker for preneoplastic or neoplastic lesions. Tatematsu et al. [60] analyzed methylation patterns in CCGG and GCGC sites of the Pg1 gene in gastric adenocarcinomas and adenomatous hyperplasias induced by MNNG. The Pg1 gene was more methylated in adenocarcinoma or adenomatous hyperplasia than in nontreated pyloric mucosa.

Preneoplastic Lesions

Erosion, regenerative hyperplasia at the margin of erosions (until 21 weeks), adenomatous hyperplasia (21–30 weeks), and adenocarcinoma (31–60 weeks) were sequentially observed in male Wistar rats given MNNG in their drinking water at 167 μg/ml for 40 weeks and then 84 μg/ml until the end of the experiment [61]. Ohgaki et al. [52] compared the sequential histologic changes during MNNG-induced gastric carcinogenesis in susceptible ACI rats and resistant Buffalo rats given MNNG (83 μg/ml) in the drinking water. In ACI rats sequential histologic changes were similar to those observed in Wistar rats. In Buffalo rats the major histologic changes following MNNG treatment were consistent erosions and hyperplasia of pyloric glands at the margin of erosions, but no atypical changes were observed. After cessation of MNNG treatment, glandular hyperplasia of pyloric glands subsided followed by atrophy of these glands [52]. The weak gastric carcinogen N-propyl-N'-nitro-N-nitrosoguanidine (PNNG) was found to induce gastric carcinomas in male Wistar rats without previous ulceration or regenerative changes [62]. It is suggested that the first histologically detectable changes that eventually lead to adenocarcinomas are atypical glands or adenomatous hyperplasia. Erosions and regenerative hyperplasia are not directly related to gastric carcinogenesis in rats.

Intestinal Metaplasia

Because a close relation has been found between intestinal metaplasia and human gastric cancer, intestinal metaplasia has been proposed to be a possible precancerous change. Intestinal metaplasia is rare in the stomach of normal rats, but it is frequently found in rats treated with MNNG or PNNG, and its incidence increases during these treatments [63, 64]. Intestinal metaplasia appeared before or at almost the same time as gastric carcinoma in rats [63, 64]. These results suggest that common factors cause intestinal metaplasia and gastric carcinoma.

Local x-irradiation of the stomach of Wistar rats induced intestinal metaplasia but not gastric tumors [65]. Watanabe and Ito [66] reported that x-irradiation before or after MNNG treatment resulted in a lower incidence of gastric tumors after treatment with MNNG alone, but that the incidence of intestinal metaplasia in groups irradiated with x-rays before or after MNNG treatment was significantly higher than that in a group treated with MNNG alone. A similar inverse correlation between intestinal metaplasia and adenocarcinoma has been reported in rats treated with x-rays and MNU [67].

Tatematsu et al. [68] administered MNNG 50 μg/ml to Wistar rats and examined sequential changes in the incidence of intestinal metaplasia, adenomatous hyperplasia, and well differentiated adenocarcinoma. They classified cells into gastric and intestinal types by paradoxical concanavalin A staining. Intestinal metaplasia first appeared in the pylorus of MNNG-treated rats 16 weeks after the beginning of MNNG treatment and in untreated control rats after 40 weeks. Most parts of the adenomatous hyperplasias and well differentiated adenocarcinomas consisted of gastric-type cells. Similarly, using polyclonal antibody against rat intestinal-type alkaline phosphatase, it was observed that stomach tumors induced by MNNG in rats consisted mainly of gastric-type cells [69]. Thus there is no direct evidence that intestinal metaplasia is a precancerous lesion in rat stomach.

Factors Modulating MNNG-Induced Gastric Carcinogenesis

There is increasing evidence that experimental gastric carcinogenesis is significantly modulated by various host and environmental factors. Most factors that enhance gastric carcinogenesis increase cell proliferation in gastric mucosa [70], and most inhibitory factors have inhibiting effects of cell proliferation.

Dietary Factors

Epidemiological studies have shown that populations with excessive intake of highly salted foods are a high risk group for the development of gastric cancer. Administration of saturated NaCl solution by gastric intubation or 10% NaCl in the diet during MNNG treatment significantly increased the incidence of gastric carcinomas [71, 72]. Treatment with saturated NaCl solution before a single dose of MNNG increased the incidence of carcinomas in the rat glandular stomach [73]. An enhancing effect of NaCl was also observed when it was given to rats after cessation of MNNG treatment [74, 75]. These results indicate that NaCl enhances both the initiation and promotion stages of gastric carcinogenesis induced by MNNG in rats. Rats were given MNNG 100 ppm in their drinking water for 8 weeks and then fed a diet supplemented with NaCl at doses of 10%, 5%, 2.5%, or 0% for the next 82 weeks. The administration of 10% and 5% NaCl significantly enhanced the development of gastric adenocarcinomas and adenomas in a dose-dependent manner [76]. Similar but nonsignificant tendencies to increase were also seen in the group given 2.5% NaCl compared to that in the MNNG-alone group. Thus NaCl exerts dose-dependent tumor-promoting activity on gastric carcinogenesis in rats, even at doses as low as 2.5%, when given after MNNG initiation [76].

Populations with poor diets (i.e. low in protein and high in carbohydrates) have a high risk of gastric cancer. Tatsuta et al. [77] reported that the incidence of gastric adenocarcinomas in Wistar rats given MNNG (50 μg/ml) for 25 weeks followed by a low protein diet (5% casein) was 63%, whereas those given a higher protein diet (10% and 25% casein) were 15% and 18%, respectively. Serum gastrin, the norepinephrine level, and the labeling index in the pyloric mucosa were significantly higher in rats fed a low protein diet. It was suggested that the enhanced sympathetic nervous system resulting from a low protein diet increased cell proliferation and enhanced gastric carcinogenesis [77].

Populations who drink milk have a low risk of gastric cancer [78]. The effect of calcium was tested in rats treated with MNNG (100 ppm) in the drinking water for 8 weeks followed by calcium chloride (0.2%) [79]. The incidence of adenomatous hyperplasia was significantly lower in rats given calcium chloride in a dose-dependent manner. In contrast, rats given a calcium-deficient diet after MNNG treatment had a higher incidence of gastric adenocarcinomas [80].

Epidemiological studies have shown a lower risk of gastric cancer among people who consume a large amount of green tea. It was found that crude tea extracts decrease the mutagenic activity of MNNG in vitro and in the intragastric tract of rats [81]. (−)-Epigalloncatechin gallate (EGCG) is one of the main constituents of green tea, which inhibited tumor promotion by teleocidin in two-stage carcinogenesis in mouse skin. The incidence of gastric carcinomas in rats treated with MNNG plus EGCG was 31%, significantly lower than that in rats treated with MNNG alone [82]. The inhibiting activity of EGCG was suggested to be due to inhibition of cellular kinetics and decrease in the ornithine decarboxylase activity in the gastric mucosa [82].

Gastrectomy and Bile Acid

The incidence of human gastric cancer in the remnant of the stomach after surgery for benign lesions is higher than that in the general population. Gastrectomy of rats before or after MNNG treatment resulted in a higher incidence of gastric adenocarcinomas [83–86]. There was a clear correlation between bile reflux and an increase in the incidence of gastric carcinomas [83–87]. Even without MNNG treatment, adenocarcinomas developed with an incidence of 23% in the remnant of the stomach of Wistar rats [84]. All of these carcinomas were located in the vicinity of the gastrojejunal anastomosis, which is directly exposed to duodenal contents [84]. Among the duodenal contents, bile acids (sodium taurocholate and taurocholic acid) were demonstrated to enhance gastric carcinogenesis induced by MNNG [83, 85]. When gastrectomized rats were fed a high cholesterol (1%) diet, which increases bile acid excretion, a significantly higher incidence of gastric carcinomas developed (61%) in the remnant stomach after MNNG treatment than in gastrectomized rats fed a normal diet (36%) [88]. Histologically, undifferentiated adenocarcinoma was recognized more frequently in the high cholesterol group [88].

Phenolic Compounds

Catechol is a major industrial chemical and a major phenolic component of cigarette smoke. Catechol is not mutagenic to *Salmonella* (mutagenicity assay), but it greatly enhances cell proliferation in the gastric mucosa when given in the diet [70]. Treatment with catechol (0.8% in the diet) after a single intragastric MNNG dose of 150 mg/kg greatly enhanced both forestomach and glandular stomach carcinogenesis [89]. The other derivatives including *p-tert*-butylcatechol and *p*-methylcatechol also significantly enhanced gastric carcinogenesis induced by MNNG. Moreover, catechol and *p*-methylcatechol alone induced adenomatous hyperplasia and adenocarcinomas in the pyloric region [89, 90].

Tanaka et al. [91] analyzed strain differences in catechol carcinogenicity to the stomach. Groups of 30 animals were treated with a powdered diet containing 0.8% catechol for 104 weeks. Induction of glandular stomach adenocarcinomas occurred in 67%, 73%, and 77% of Wistar, Lewis, and SD animals, respectively, but in only 10% of WKY rats [91].

Hirose et al. [92] treated F344 rats with catechol (0.8% in the diet) for 12, 24, 48, 72, or 96 weeks. The incidence of submucosal hyperplasia, adenomas, and adenocarcinomas, the average number of tumors per rat, and the size of the tumors increased time-dependently. After cessation of catechol treatment, although the average number of tumors per rat and labeling indices in both tumorous and nontumorous areas decreased, the size of tumors tended to increase [92].

Helicobacter pylori Infection

Helicobacter pylori was implicated in gastric carcinogenesis through the induction of metaplasia of the gastric mucosa in humans. *H. pylori* has potent urease activity and produces ammonia, a factor causing *H. pylori*-related gastroduodenal muscular lesions. Rats were treated with MNNG (83 μg/ml) for 24 weeks followed by a solution of 0.01% ammonia or tap water for an additional 24 weeks. The administration of ammonia solution significantly increased the incidence and number of gastric carcinomas in the glandular stomach [93]. Increased cell proliferation in the gastric mucosa was observed in rats treated with ammonia solution [93].

Kawaura et al. [94] examined the co-carcinogenic activity of *H. pylori* infection during gastric carcinogenesis induced by MNNG in Wistar WKY male rats. Rats received drinking water containing MNNG (50 μg/ml), and intragastric administration of *H. pylori* for 40 weeks. However, the frequency of glandular stomach tumors did not differ between rats given MNNG alone and those given MNNG and *H. pylori*.

Experimental Gastric Cancer in Transgenic Mice

Several strains of transgenic mice have been reported to develop preneoplastic lesions or adenocarcinomas in the glandular stomach. However, because of the lack of availability of regulatory or promoter sequence for specific expression of transgenes in the glandular stomach mucosa, to date strains of transgenic mice that selectively develop adenocarcinomas with histology similar to that of human gastric cancer have not been established.

Transgenic Mice Carrying Metallothionein-I Promoter/TGF-α Fusion Gene

Transgenic mice overexpressing human TGF-α cDNA under transcriptional regulation with metallothionein-I (MT-I) promoter developed spontaneously adenomatous hyperplasia in the fundic region of the glandular stomach [95] as well as mammary carcinomas and abnormality in the pancreas [96]. MNU was administered to MT-I/TGF-α mice (line MT100). Untreated MT100 mice exhibited a severe age-related gastric fundic hyperplasia. Precancerous lesions, including atypical or adenomatous hyperplasia, were found in the fundic regions of 16 of 22 male and 8 of 22 female MT100 mice but not in 27 male and 24 female nontransgenic mice [96]. There was no significant difference in the incidence of adenocarcinomas induced by MNU in the pyloric region between MT100 mice and nontransgenic mice [97]. Hyperplastic lesions in the gastric fundus induced by TGF-α overexpression appeared to predispose MT100 mice to carcinogenesis by MNU [97].

Transgenic Mice Carrying MMTV-LTR/E1a and E1b Fusion Gene

The adenovirus protein E1a functions to immortalize cells and cooperate with another adenovirus, protein E1b, to effect complete transformation of cells in culture [98]. Transgenic mice carrying both the adenovirus 12 (Ad12) E1a and E1b genes developed gastric tumors but not those carrying only one of the two transgenes. All male transgenic mice died between 3 and 4 months. Most of the mice showed macroscopically visible lesions in the stomach. Interestingly, tumors were restricted at or near the transition from squamous to columnar epithelium. Histologically, they were classified as adenocarcinomas or adenosquamous carcinomas composed of glandular elements with adjacent or overlaying squamous hyperplasia [99, 100].

Transgenic Mice Carrying Bovine Keratin 6 Gene Promoter/Human Papilloma Virus Type 16 Early Region Fusion Gene

Certain human papilloma viruses (HPVs) have been implicated as important contributory factors in the development of cervical carcinoma and other epithelial malignancies. Transgenic mice carrying papilloma virus type 16 early region gene under the bovine keratin 6 promoter showed solitary glands with small dysplastic cells within the gastric mucosa after the age of 100 days. Later this abnormal cell population spread within the glandular stomach mucosa, invaded the submucosa and outer muscular wall of the stomach, and commonly metastasized to local lymph nodes and the liver. These tumors were classified as malignant carcinoids, originating from the neuroendocrine enterochromaffin-like cells. Increased expression of HPV mRNA was evident in the tumors. The mean age at tumor presentation was 246 days in males and 352 days in females [101].

Transgenic Mice Carrying a Murine Amylase 2.2 Promoter/SV40 Large T Antigen Fusion Gene

The mouse pancreatic amylase Amy-2.2 gene was fused to the structural gene for SV40 T antigen, and 51 independent transgenic founder mice carrying the fusion gene were generated. Most of the founders and 100% of their offspring in the derived transgenic lines developed pancreatic acinar cell carcinomas and stomach carcinomas. Northern blot analyses and RNA protection assays showed that Amy-2.2 is expressed in stomach at a rate of approximately 0.05% that in pancreas. Expression of the fusion gene in the stomach therefore appears to represent a previously unrecognized activity of the Amy-2.2 promoter. RNA protection assays demonstrated the properly initiated large T and small t antigen transcripts in pancreas and stomach during tumorigenesis. T antigen protein was also detected in pancreas and stomach by immunohistochemistry [102]. Early

stomach lesions consisted of focal or multifocal areas and tended to localize in the basal to midportion of the gland. Such lesions comprised cells of uncertain deviation that had hyperchromatic nuclei and scant cytoplasm. The distribution of these cells suggests that the lesions may be of chief cell origin. Extensive invasion of the mucosa and submucosa was characteristic of malignant stomach lesions [102].

Transgenic Mice Carrying Rabbit Uteroglobin Promoter/SV40 T Antigen Fusion Gene

All transgenic founders carrying rabbit uteroglobin promoter/SV40 T antigen fusion gene exhibited bronchoalveolar adenocarcinomas, probably due to expression of the transgene in Clara cells. Most founders also developed tumors of the submandibular salivary gland and adenocarcinomas of the stomach [103]. In the stomach, solid, undifferentiated tumors frequently exhibited disturbed muscularis mucosa and infiltrated submucosa. Early stages of morphological alterations in the stomach were characterized by increased numbers of clustered pepsinogen-producing cells [103].

References

1. Sugimura T, Fujimura S (1967) Tumour production in glandular stomach of rat by N-methyl-N'-nitro-N-nitrosoguanidine. Nature 216:943–944
2. Hirota N, Aonuma T, Yamada S, Kawai T, Saito K, Yokoyama T (1987) Selective induction of glandular stomach carcinoma in F344 rats by N-methyl-N-nitrosourea. Jpn J Cancer Res 78:634–638
3. Tatematsu M, Yamamoto M, Iwata H, Fukami H, Yuasa H, Tezuka N, Masui T, Nakanishi H (1993) Induction of glandular stomach cancers in C3H mice treated with N-methyl-N-nitrosourea in the drinking water. Jpn J Cancer Res 84:1258–1264
4. Sugimura T, Fujimura S, Baba T (1970) Tumor production in the glandular stomach and alimentary tract of the rat by N-methyl-N'-nitro-N-nitrosoguanidine. Cancer Res 30:455–465
5. Sugimura T, Kawachi T (1973) Experimental stomach cancer. In: Busch H (ed) Methods in cancer research. Academic, Orlando, pp 245–308
6. Sugimura T, Kawachi T (1978) Experimental stomach carcinogenesis. In: Lipkin M, Good RA (eds) Gastrointestinal tract cancer. Plenum, New York, pp 327–341

7. Ohgaki H, Sugimura T (1988) Experimental stomach cancer. In: Douglass HOJ (ed) Gastric cancer. Churchill Livingstone, New York, pp 27–54

8. Ohgaki H, Kleihues P, Sugimura T (1991) Experimental gastric cancer. Ital J Gastroenterol 23:371–377

9. Martin MS, Martin F, Justrabo E, Michiels R, Bastien H, Knobel S (1974) Susceptibility of inbred rats to gastric and duodenal carcinomas induced by N-methyl-N'-nitro-N-nitrosoguanidine. J Natl Cancer Inst 53:837–840

10. Ohgaki H, Kawachi T, Matsukura N, Morino K, Miyamoto M, Sugimura T (1983) Genetic control of susceptibility of rats to gastric carcinoma. Cancer Res 43:3663–3667

11. Furukawa H, Iwanaga T, Koyama H, Taniguchi H (1982) Effect of sex hormones on carcinogenesis in the stomachs of rats. Cancer Res 42:5181–5182

12. Furukawa H, Iwanaga T, Koyama H, Taniguchi H (1982) Effect of sex hormones on the experimental induction of cancer in rat stomach-a preliminary study. Digestion 23:151–155

13. Kimura M, Fukuda T, Sato K (1979) Effect of aging on the development of gastric cancer in rats induced by N-methyl-N'-nitro-N-nitrosoguanidine. Gann 70:521–525

14. Bralow SP, Gruenstein M, Meranze DR (1973) Host resistance to gastric adenocarcinomatosis in three strains of rats ingesting N-methyl-N'-nitro-N-nitrosoguanidine. Oncology 27:168–180

15. Ohgaki H, Tomihari M, Sato S, Kleihues P, Sugimura T (1988) Differential proliferative response of gastric mucosa during carcinogenesis induced by N-methyl-N'-nitro-N-nitrosoguanidine in susceptible ACI rats, resistant Buffalo rats, and their hybrid F_1 cross. Cancer Res 48:5275–5279

16. Sugimura T, Inoue R, Ohgaki H, Ushijima T, Canzian F, Nagao M (1995) Genetic polymorphisms and susceptibility to cancer development. Pharmacogenetics 5:S161–S165

17. Hirono I, Shibuya C (1972) Induction of stomach cancer by a single dose of N-methyl-N'-nitro-N-nitrosoguanidine through a stomach tube. In: Nakahara W, Takayama S, Sugimura T, Odashima S (eds) Topics in chemical carcinogenesis. University Park Press, Baltimore, pp 121–131

18. Zaidi NH, O'Connor PJ, Butler WH (1993) N-Methyl-N'-nitro-N-nitrosoguanidine-induced carcinogenesis: differential pattern of upper gastrointestinal tract tumours in Wistar rats after single or chronic oral doses. Carcinogenesis 14:1561–1567

19. Maekawa A, Matsuoka C, Onodera H, Tanigawa H, Furuta K, Ogiu T, Mitsumori K, Hayashi Y (1985) Organ-specific carcinogenicity of N-methyl-N-nitrosourea in F344 and ACI/N rats. J Cancer Res Clin Oncol 109:178–182

20. Fujita M, Ishii T, Tsukahara Y, Scimozuma K, Nakano Y, Taguchi T, Hirota N (1989) Establishment of optimum conditions for induction of stomach carcinoma in rats by continuous oral administration of N-methyl-N-nitrosourea. J Toxicol Pathol 2:27–32

21. Kodama M, Kodama T, Fukami H, Ogiu T (1992) Comparative genetics of host response to N-methyl-1-N'-nitro-N-nitrosoguanidine. I. A lack of tumor production in the glandular stomach of Swiss mouse. Anticancer Res 12:441–449

22. Hirose M, Fukushima S, Tanaka H, Asakawa E, Takahashi S, Ito N (1993) Carcinogenicity of catechol in F344 rats and B6C3F1 mice. Carcinogenesis 14:525–529

23. Tatematsu M, Ogawa K, Hoshiya T, Shichino Y, Kato T, Imaida K, Ito N (1992) Induction of adenocarcinomas in the glandular stomach of BALB/c mice treated with N-methyl-N-nitrosourea. Jpn J Cancer Res 83:915–918

24. Tatematsu M, Fukami H, Yamamoto M, Nakanishi H, Masui T, Kusakabe N, Sakakura T (1994) Clonal analysis of glandular stomach carcinogenesis in C3H/HeN↔BALB/c chimeric mice treated with N-methyl-N-nitrosourea. Cancer Lett 83:37–42

25. Sugimura T, Tanaka N, Kawachi T, Kogure K, Fujimura S (1971) Production of stomach cancer in dogs by N-methyl-N'-nitro-N-nitrosoguanidine. Gann 62:67

26. Shimosato Y, Tanaka N, Kogure K, Fujimura S, Kawachi T (1971) Histopathology of tumors of canine alimentary tract produced by N-methyl-N'-nitro-N-nitrosoguanidine, with particular reference to gastric carcinomas. J Natl Cancer Inst 47:1053–1070

27. Koyama Y, Omori K, Hirota T, Sano R, Ishihara K (1976) Leiomyosarcomas of the small intestine induced in dogs by N-methyl-N'-nitro-N-nitrosoguanidine. Gann 67:241–251

28. Kurihara M, Shirakabe H, Murakami T, Yasui A, Izumi T (1974) A new method for producing adenocarcinomas in the stomach of dogs with N-ethyl-N'-nitro-N-nitrosoguanidine. Gann 65:163–177

29. Matsukura N, Morino K, Ohgaki H, Kawachi T (1981) Canine gastric carcinoma as an animal model of human gastric carcinoma. Stomach Intestine 16:715–722

30. Sasajima K, Kawachi T, Sano T, Sugimura T, Shimosato Y (1977) Esophageal and gastric cancers with metastases induced in dogs by N-ethyl-N'-nitro-N-nitrosoguanidine. J Natl Cancer Inst 58:1789–1794

31. Sunagawa M, Takeshita K, Nakajima A, Ochi K, Habu H, Endo M (1985) Duration of ENNG administration and its effect on histological differen-

tiation of experimental gastric cancer. Br J Cancer 52:771–779

32. Kurihara M, Shirakabe H, Izumi T, Miyasaka K, Yamaya F, Maruyama T, Yasui A (1977) Adenocarcinomas of the stomach induced in beagle dogs by oral administration of N-ethyl-N′-nitro-N-nitrosoguanidine. Z Krebsforsch Klin Onkol [Cancer Res Clin Oncol] 90:241–252

33. Kurihara M, Izumi T, Miyakawa K, et al (1979) Radical and endoscopic analyses of growth of experimental dog gastric cancer and morphological alteration of human gastric cancer treated with anticancer agents. Prog Dig Endosc 15:16

34. Fujita M, Taguchi T, Takami M, Usugane M, Takahashi A (1975) Lung metastasis of canine gastric adenocarcinoma induced by N-methyl-N′-nitro-N-nitrosoguanidine. Gann 66:107–108

35. Ohgaki H, Hasegawa H, Kusama K, Morino K, Matsukura N, Sato S, Maruyama K, Sugimura T (1986) Induction of gastric carcinomas in nonhuman primates by N-ethyl-N′-nitro-N-nitrosoguanidine. J Natl Cancer Inst 77:179–186

36. Szentirmay Z, Ohgaki H, Maruyama K, Esumi H, Takayama S, Sugimura T (1990) Early gastric cancer induced by N-ethyl-N′-nitro-N-nitrosoguanidine in a cynomolgus monkey six years after initial diagnosis of the lesion. Jpn J Cancer Res 81:6–9

37. Loktionova NA, Beniashvili DS, Sartania MS, Zabezhinski MA, Kazanova OI, Petrov AS, Likhachev AJ (1993) Individual levels of activity of O^6-alkylguanine-DNA alkyltransferase in monkey gastric mucosa during chronic exposure to a gastrocarcinogen N-ethyl-N′-nitro-N-nitrosoguanidine. Biochimie 75:821–824

38. Rice LE, Stahl SJ, McLeod CG Jr (1992) Pyloric adenocarcinoma in a ferret. J Am Vet Med Assoc 200:1117–1118

39. Fox JG, Wishnok JS, Murphy JC, Tannenbaum SR, Correa P (1993) MNNG-induced gastric carcinoma in ferrets infected with *Helicobacter mustelae*. Carcinogenesis 14:1957–1961

40. Lee A (1995) *Helicobacter* infections in laboratory animals: a model for gastric neoplasias? Ann Med 27:575–582

41. Fox JG (1994) Gastric disease in ferrets: effects of *Helicobacter mustelae*, nitrosamines and reconstructive gastric surgery. Eur J Gastroenterol Hepatol 6(suppl 1):S57–S65

42. Lawley PD, Shah SA (1972) Methylation of ribonucleic acid by the carcinogens dimethyl sulphate, N-methyl-N-nitrosourea and N-methyl-N′-nitro-N-nitrosoguanidine: comparisons of chemical analyses at the nucleoside and base levels. Biochem J 128:117–132

43. Lawley PD, Thatcher CJ (1970) Methylation of deoxyribonucleic acid in cultured mammalian cells by N-methyl-N′-nitro-N-nitrosoguanidine: the influence of cellular thiol concentrations on the extent of methylation and the 6-oxygen atom of guanine as a site of methylation. Biochem J 116:693–707

44. Sugimura T, Fujimura S, Nagao M, Yokoshima T, Hasegawa M (1968) Reaction of N-methyl-N′-nitro-N-nitrosoguanidine with protein. Biochim Biophys Acta 170:427–429

45. Sugimura T, Nagao M, Okada Y (1966) Carcinogenic action of N-methyl-N′-nitro-N-nitrosoguanidine. Nature 210:962–963

46. Schoental R (1966) Carcinogenic activity of N-methyl-N-nitroso-N′-nitroguanidine. Nature 209:726–727

47. Wiestler O, von Deimling A, Kobori O, Kleihues P (1983) Location of N-methyl-N′-nitro-N-nitrosoguanidine-induced gastrointestinal tumors correlates with thiol distribution. Carcinogenesis 4:879–883

48. Kobori O, Schmerold I, Ludeke B, Ohgaki H, Kleihues P (1988) DNA methylation in rat stomach and duodenum following chronic exposure to N-methyl-N′-nitro-N-nitrosoguanidine and the effect of dietary taurocholate. Carcinogenesis 9:2271–2274

49. McKay AF, Wright GF (1947) Preparation and properties of N-methyl-N′-nitro-N-nitrosoguanidine. J Am Chem Soc 69:3028–3030

50. Weisburger JH, Jones RC, Barnes WS, Pegg AE (1988) Mechanisms of differential strain sensitivity in gastric carcinogenesis. Jpn J Cancer Res 79:1304–1310

51. Deschner EE, Tamura K, Bralow SP (1979) Sequential histopathology and cell kinetic changes in rat pyloric mucosa during gastric carcinogenesis induced by N-methyl-N′-nitro-N-nitrosoguanidine. J Natl Cancer Inst 63:171–179

52. Ohgaki H, Kusama K, Hasegawa H, Sato S, Takayama S, Sugimura T (1986) Sequential histologic changes during gastric carcinogenesis induced by N-methyl-N′-nitro-N-nitrosoguanidine in susceptible ACI and resistant BUF rats. J Natl Cancer Inst 77:747–755

53. Yasui W, Sumiyoshi H, Yamamoto T, Oda N, Kameda T, Tanaka T, Tahara E (1987) Expression of Ha-*ras* oncogene product in rat gastrointestinal carcinomas induced by chemical carcinogens. Acta Pathol Jpn 37:1731–1741

54. Livingstone JI, Filipe MI, Wastell C (1994) Expression of transforming growth factor alpha in experimental gastric carcinogenesis. Gut 35:604–607

55. Ohgaki H, Ludeke BI, Meier I, Kleihues P, Lutz WK, Schlatter C (1991) DNA methylation in the digestive tract of F344 rats during chronic expo-

sure to N-methyl-N-nitrosourea. J Cancer Res Clin Oncol 117:13–18

56. Ohgaki H, Vogeley KT, Kleihues P, Wechsler W (1993) *neu* Mutations and loss of normal allele in schwannomas induced by N-ethyl-N-nitrosourea in rats. Cancer Lett 70:45–50

57. Tatematsu M, Saito D, Furihata C, Miyata Y, Nakatsuka T, Ito N, Sugimura T (1980) Initial DNA damage and heritable permanent change in pepsinogen isoenzyme pattern in the pyloric mucosae of rats after short-term administration of N-methyl-N′-nitro-N-nitrosoguanidine. J Natl Cancer Inst 64:775–781

58. Furihata C, Sasajima K, Kazama S, Kogure K, Kawachi T (1975) Changes in pepsinogen isozymes in stomach carcinogenesis induced in rats by N-methyl-N′-nitro-N-nitrosoguanidine. J Natl Cancer Inst 55:925–930

59. Tatematsu M, Furihata C, Hirose M, Shirai T, Ito N (1977) Changes in pepsinogen isozymes in stomach cancers induced in Wistar rats by N-methyl-N′-nitro-N-nitrosoguanidine and in transplantable gastric carcinoma (SG2B). J Natl Cancer Inst 58:1709–1716

60. Tatematsu M, Ichinose M, Tsukada S, Kakei N, Takahashi S, Ogawa K, Hirose M, Furihata C, Miki K, Kurokawa K, Ito N (1993) DNA methylation of the pepsinogen 1 gene during rat glandular stomach carcinogenesis induced by N-methyl-N′-nitro-N-nitrosoguanidine or catechol. Carcinogenesis 14:1415–1419

61. Saito T, Inokuchi K, Takayama S, Sugimura T (1970) Sequential morphological changes in N-methyl-N′-nitro-N-nitrosoguanidine carcinogenesis in the glandular stomach of rats. J Natl Cancer Inst 44:769–783

62. Matsukura N, Itabashi M, Kawachi T, Hirota T, Sugimura T (1980) Sequential studies on the histopathogenesis of gastric carcinoma in rats by a weak gastric carcinogen, N-propyl-N′-nitro-N-nitrosoguanidine. J Cancer Res Clin Oncol 98:153–163

63. Matsukura N, Kawachi T, Sasajima K, Sano T, Sugimura T, Hirota T (1978) Induction of intestinal metaplasia in the stomachs of rats by N-methyl-N′-nitro-N-nitrosoguanidine. J Natl Cancer Inst 61:141–144

64. Sasajima K, Kawachi T, Matsukura N, Sano T, Sugimura T (1979) Intestinal metaplasia and adenocarcinoma induced in the stomach of rats by N-propyl-N′-nitro-N-nitrosoguanidine. J Cancer Res Clin Oncol 94:201–206

65. Watanabe H (1978) Experimentally induced intestinal metaplasia in Wistar rats by x-ray irradiation. Gastroenterology 75:796–799

66. Watanabe H, Ito A (1986) Relationship between gastric tumorigenesis and intestinal metaplasia in rats given x-radiation and/or N-methyl-N′-nitro-N-nitrosoguanidine. J Natl Cancer Inst 76:865–870

67. Watanabe H, Ando Y, Yamada K, Okamoto T, Ito A (1994) Lack of any positive effect of intestinal metaplasia on induction of gastric tumors in Wistar rats treated with N-methyl-N-nitrosourea in their drinking water. Jpn J Cancer Res 85:892–896

68. Tatematsu M, Furihata C, Katsuyama T, Hasegawa R, Nakanowatari J, Saito D, Takahashi M, Matsushima T, Ito N (1983) Independent induction of intestinal metaplasia and gastric cancer in rats treated with N-methyl-N′-nitro-N-nitrosoguanidine. Cancer Res 43:1335–1341

69. Yuasa H, Hirano K, Kodama H, Nakanishi H, Imai T, Tsuda H, Imaida K, Tatematsu M (1994) Immunohistochemical demonstration of intestinal-type alkaline phosphatase in stomach tumors induced by N-methyl-N′-nitro-N-nitrosoguanidine in rats. Jpn J Cancer Res 85:897–903

70. Ohgaki H, Szentirmay Z, Take M, Sugimura T (1989) Effects of 4-week treatment with gastric carcinogens and enhancing agents on proliferation of gastric mucosa cells in rats. Cancer Lett 46:117–122

71. Tatematsu M, Takahashi M, Fukushima S, Hananouchi M, Shirai T (1975) Effects in rats of sodium chloride on experimental gastric cancers induced by N-methyl-N′-nitro-N-nitrosoguanidine or 4-nitroquinoline-1-oxide. J Natl Cancer Inst 55:101–106

72. Takahashi M, Kokubo T, Furukawa F, Kurokawa Y, Tatematsu M, Hayashi Y (1983) Effect of high salt diet on rat gastric carcinogenesis induced by N-methyl-N′-nitro-N-nitrosoguanidine. Gann 74:28–34

73. Shirai T, Imaida K, Fukushima S, Hasegawa R, Tatematsu M, Ito N (1982) Effects of NaCl, Tween 60 and a low dose of N-methyl-N′-nitro-N-nitrosoguanidine on gastric carcinogenesis of rat given a single dose of N-methyl-N′-nitro-N-nitrosoguanidine. Carcinogenesis 3:1419–1422

74. Takahashi M, Kokubo T, Furukawa F, Kurokawa Y, Hayashi Y (1984) Effects of sodium chloride, saccharin, phenobarbital and aspirin on gastric carcinogenesis in rats after initiation with N-methyl-N′-nitro-N-nitrosoguanidine. Gann 75:494–501

75. Ohgaki H, Kato T, Morino K, Matsukura N, Sato S, Takayama S, Sugimura T (1984) Study of the promoting effect of sodium chloride on gastric carcinogenesis by N-methyl-N′-nitro-N-nitrosoguanidine in inbred Wistar rats. Gann 75:1053–1057

76. Takahashi M, Nishikawa A, Furukawa F, Enami T, Hasegawa T, Hayashi Y (1994) Dose-dependent promoting effects of sodium chloride (NaCl) on rat glandular stomach carcinogenesis initiated with N-methyl-N'-nitro-N-nitrosoguanidine. Carcinogenesis 15:1429–1432

77. Tatsuta M, Iishi H, Baba M, Uehara H, Nakaizumi A, Taniguchi H (1991) Enhanced induction of gastric carcinogenesis by N-methyl-N'-nitro-N-nitrosoguanidine in Wistar rats fed a low-protein diet. Cancer Res 51:3493–3496

78. Sugimura T, Wakabayashi K (1990) Gastric carcinogenesis: diet as a causative factor. Med Oncol Tumor Pharmacother 7:87–92

79. Nishikawa A, Furukawa F, Mitsui M, Enami T, Kawanishi T, Hasegawa T, Takahashi M (1992) Inhibitory effect of calcium chloride on gastric carcinogenesis in rats after treatment with N-methyl-N'-nitro-N-nitrosoguanidine and sodium chloride. Carcinogenesis 13:1155–1158

80. Tatsuta M, Iishi H, Baba M, Uehara H, Nakaizumi A, Taniguchi H (1993) Enhancing effects of calcium-deficient diet on gastric carcinogenesis by N-methyl-N'-nitro-N-nitrosoguanidine in Wistar rats. Jpn J Cancer Res 84:945–950

81. Jain AK, Shimoi K, Nakamura Y, Kada T, Hara Y, Tomita I (1989) Crude tea extracts decrease the mutagenic activity of N-methyl-N'-nitro-N-nitrosoguanidine in vitro and in intragastric tract of rats. Mutat Res 210:1–8

82. Yamane T, Takahashi T, Kuwata K, Oya K, Inagake M, Kitao Y, Suganuma M, Fujiki H (1995) Inhibition of N-methyl-N'-nitro-N-nitrosoguanidine-induced carcinogenesis by (−)-epigallocatechin gallate in the rat glandular stomach. Cancer Res 55:2081–2084

83. Kobori O, Shimizu T, Maeda M, Atomi Y, Watanabe J, Shoji M, Morioka Y (1984) Enhancing effect of bile and bile acid on stomach tumorigenesis induced by N-methyl-N'-nitro-N-nitrosoguanidine in Wistar rats. J Natl Cancer Inst 73:853–861

84. Kondo K, Suzuki H, Nagayo T (1984) The influence of gastro-jejunal anastomosis on gastric carcinogenesis in rats. Gann 75:362–369

85. Salmon RJ, Merle S, Zafrani B, DeCosse JJ, Sherlock P, Deschner EE (1985) Gastric carcinogenesis induced by N-methyl-N'-nitro-N-nitrosoguanidine: role of gastrectomy and duodenal reflux. Jpn J Cancer Res 76:167–172

86. Sano C, Kumashiro R, Saito T, Inokuchi K (1984) Promoting effect of partial gastrectomy on carcinogenesis in the remnant stomach of rats after oral administration of N-methyl-N'-nitro-N-nitrosoguanidine. Oncology 41:124–128

87. Langhans P, Heger RA, Stegemann B (1984) The cancer risk in the stomach subjected to nonresecting procedures: an experimental long-term study. Scand J Gastroenterol Suppl 92:138–141

88. Makino M, Kaibara N, Koga S (1989) Enhanced induction by high-cholesterol diet of remnant gastric carcinogenesis by N-methyl-N'-nitro-N-nitrosoguanidine in rats. J Natl Cancer Inst 81:130–135

89. Hirose M, Kurata Y, Tsuda H, Fukushima S, Ito N (1987) Catechol strongly enhances rat stomach carcinogenesis: a possible new environmental stomach carcinogen. Jpn J Cancer Res 8:1144–1149

90. Hirose M, Yamaguchi S, Fukushima S, Hasegawa R, Takahashi S, Ito N (1989) Promotion by dihydroxybenzene derivatives of N-methyl-N'-nitro-N-nitrosoguanidine-induced F344 rat forestomach and glandular stomach carcinogenesis. Cancer Res 49:5143–5147

91. Tanaka H, Hirose M, Hagiwara A, Imaida K, Shirai T, Ito N (1995) Rat strain differences in catechol carcinogenicity to the stomach. Food Chem Toxicol 33:93–98

92. Hirose M, Wada S, Yamaguchi S, Masuda A, Okazaki S, Ito N (1992) Reversibility of catechol-induced rat glandular stomach lesions. Cancer Res 52:787–790

93. Tsujii M, Kawano S, Tsuji S, Takei Y, Tamura K, Fusamoto H, Kamada T (1995) Mechanism for ammonia-induced promotion of gastric carcinogenesis in rats. Carcinogenesis 16:563–566

94. Kawaura A, Yamamoto I, Tanida N, Inouye H, Takahashi A, Tonokatsu Y, Sawada Y, Sawada K, Shimoyama T (1991) Helicobacter pylori is not a co-carcinogen in N-methyl-N'-nitro-N-nitrosoguanidine-induced rat gastric carcinogenesis. Tokushima J Exp Med 38:71–75

95. Takagi H, Jhappan C, Sharp R, Merlino G (1992) Hypertrophic gastropathy resembling Menetrier's disease in transgenic mice overexpressing transforming growth factor alpha in the stomach. J Clin Invest 90:1161–1167

96. Jhappan C, Stahle C, Harkins RN, Fausto N, Smith GH, Merlino GT (1990) TGF alpha overexpression in transgenic mice induces liver neoplasia and abnormal development of the mammary gland and pancreas. Cell 61:1137–1146

97. Tamano S, Jakubczak J, Takagi H, Merlino G, Ward JM (1995) Increased susceptibility to N-nitrosomethylurea gastric carcinogenesis in transforming growth factor alpha transgenic mice with gastric hyperplasia. Jpn J Cancer Res 86:435–443

98. Jones NC (1990) Transformation by the human adenoviruses. Semin Cancer Biol 1:425–435

99. Ullrich SJ, Zeng ZZ, Jay G (1994) Transgenic mouse models of human gastric and hepatic carcinomas. Semin Cancer Biol 5:61–68

100. Koike K, Hinrichs SH, Isselbacher KJ, Jay G (1989) Transgenic mouse model for human gastric carcinoma. Proc Natl Acad Sci USA 86:5615–5619

101. Searle PF, Thomas DP, Faulkner KB, Tinsley JM (1994) Stomach cancer in transgenic mice expressing human papillomavirus type 16 early region genes from a keratin promoter. J Gen Virol 75:1125–1137

102. Ceci JD, Kovatch RM, Swing DA, Jones JM, Snow CM, Rosenberg MP, Jenkins NA, Copeland NG, Meisler MH (1991) Transgenic mice carrying a murine amylase 2.2/SV40 T antigen fusion gene develop pancreatic acinar cell and stomach carcinomas. Oncogene 6:323–332

103. Sandmoller A, Halter R, Gomez La Hoz E, Grone HJ, Suske G, Paul D, Beato M (1994) The uteroglobin promoter targets expression of the SV40 T antigen to a variety of secretory epithelial cells in transgenic mice. Oncogene 9:2805–2815

Multistep Carcinogenesis of Esophageal Carcinoma

Yusuke Nakamura, Takashi Tokino, Minoru Isomura, Johji Inazawa, Takahisa Aoki, Takahiro Mori, Mamoru Shimada, Koh Miura, and Kazufumi Suzuki

Summary. To investigate genetic features of esophageal cancer, we have examined a large number of squamous cell carcinomas of the esophagus (ESCs) for loss of heterozygosity (LOH) using polymorphic DNA markers representing all autosomal chromosomes. Allelic losses at frequencies of at least 30% were observed at loci on chromosomal arms on 3p (33%), 3q (30%), 5q (36%), 9p (57%), 9q (60%), 10p (33%), 13q (43%), 17p (62%), 17q (46%), 18q (38%), 19q (32%), and 21q (37%). By comparing the LOH on each chromosomal arm with the clinicopathologic parameters of patients, we found a significant correlation between LOH on 19q and regional lymph node metastasis. Interestingly, the frequency of LOH on 17q was significantly higher in tumors from female patients (12 of 14 cases) than in those from male patients (20 of 56 cases) ($P = 0.0009$ by Fisher's exact test). Subsequent analysis of allelic losses in DNA extracts isolated from 106 lesions among 32 patients with ESCs revealed that allelic losses on 3p or 17p occurred frequently even in dysplastic lesions, and that allelic losses on these chromosomal arms were observed in cancerous tissues as well. We detected allelic losses of the short and long arms of chromosome 9 at low frequency in lesions with mild dysplasia but often in lesions with severe dysplasia and in intraepithelial cancers. Our results suggested that inactivation of tumor suppressor genes on 3p and 17p occurs at an early stage of esophageal carcinogenesis, and that genes on 9p and 9q are likely to play important roles in malignant changes.

Laboratory of Molecular Medicine, Human Genome Center, Institute of Medical Science, University of Tokyo, 4-6-1 Shirokanedai, Minato-ku, Tokyo 108, Japan

Allelotype Study

Like other cancers, esophageal cancer is thought to result from the accumulation of certain genetic alterations that affect normal control of cell growth and transform a normal cell to a neoplastic cell. Some genetic features associated with esophageal cancer have now been discovered, including amplifications of the c-*myc*, human epithelial growth factor (EGF) receptor, and *cyclin D* genes [1, 2]. Metastasis of tumors seems to be associated with amplification of the *cyclin D* gene [3]. Mutations in genes of the *ras* family have been detected only rarely with esophageal carcinomas [4]. With respect to tumor suppressor genes, loss of heterozygosity (LOH) studies in esophageal cancers have indicated possible involvement of the *TP53*, *RB1*, *APC*, *MCC*, and *DCC* genes [5–8]. Of these candidate genes, additional mutational analyses have been performed only for *TP53*; somatic mutation in this gene is often detected in esophageal cancers [9, 10]. Although one group reported abnormal expression of both *TP53* and *RB1* in esophageal cancers [11], the authors were uncertain whether the *RB1* gene itself was mutated or its expression was down-regulated owing to other genetic changes. In one other study of LOH on chromosomal loci in a small number of esophageal cancers, only the chromosomal arms of 17p frequently showed allelic loss [12].

To investigate localizations of putative tumor suppressor genes involved in the development or progression of esophageal carcinomas, we used 41 restriction fragment length polymorphism (RFLP) markers, including 25 VNTR loci, representing all chromosome arms, to test for LOH. Table 1 indicates the frequency of LOH at each of the 41 loci examined. The most frequent LOH (16 of 21 informative cases, or 76%) was observed at the D9S17 locus on chromosomal band 9q34. The short arm of chromosome 9 also showed frequent LOH at the D9S18 locus (9pter-p13) (17 of 30 informative cases, or 57%). Both arms of chromo-

Table 1. Loss of heterozygosity in esophageal carcinoma

Chromosome location	Probe	Locus	Enzyme	No. patients tested	Allelic loss/ informative cases (%)
1p	MCT58[a]	D1S77	Taq^I	62	4/18 (22)
1q	HHH106	D1S67	Msp^I	65	3/26 (12)
2p	TBAB5.7[a]	D2S47	Pvu^{II}	72	10/41 (24)
2q	YNH24[a]	D2S44	Msp^I	66	10/60 (17)
3p	C^{I}3–515[a]	D3S685	Msp^I	60	15/47 (32)
3p	C^{I}3–373	D3S659	Pvu^{II}	66	10/28 (36)
Total of 3p				75	19/55 (35)
3q	EFD64.2[a]	D3S46	Msp^I	65	13/44 (30)
4p	YNZ32[a]	D4S125	Msp^I	59	7/40 (18)
4q	EFD139.1[a]	D4S163	Msp^I	58	9/35 (26)
5q	APC/cDNA	APC	Msp^I	76	5/21 (24)
5q	L5.71	D5S141	Msp^I	65	13/35 (37)
Total of 5q				78	16/45 (36)
6p	C^{I}6–7[a]	D6S139	Pvu^{II}	73	12/49 (24)
6q	C^{I}6–111[a]	D6S193	Taq^I	63	9/56 (16)
7p	RMU7.4[a]	D7S370	Msp^I	64	2/20 (10)
7q	JCZ67[a]	D7S396	Rsa^I	66	5/44 (11)
8p	C^{I}8–2125[a]		Taq^I	63	9/38 (24)
8q	C^{I}8–134[a]	D8S177	Msp^I	64	4/42 (10)[b]
9p	HHH220	D9S18	Taq^I	73	17/30 (57)
9q	MCT112	D9S15	Msp^I	64	9/22 (41)
9q	EKZ19.3	D9S17	Taq^I	76	16/21 (76)
Total of 9q				77	24/40 (60)
10p	MHZ15	D10S17	Msp^I	65	11/33 (33)
10q	EFD75.1[a]	D10S25	Taq^I	64	6/36 (17)
11p	Ha-RAS1[a]	HRAS	Msp^I	60	4/21 (19)
11q	MCMP1[a]	PYGM	Msp^I	60	5/42 (12)[b]
12p	THH14	D12S16	Taq^I	72	2/7 (29)
12q	YNH15	D12S17	Msp^I	64	3/34 (9)
13q	MHZ47[a]	D13S52	Pvu^{II}	70	23/53 (43)
14q	CMM101[a]	D14S13	Msp^I	65	9/64 (14)
15q	THH55	D15S27	Msp^I	63	2/17 (12)
16p	CMM65[a]	D16S84	Taq^I	60	4/28 (14)
16q	CJ52.209MI	D16S151	Msp^I	64	8/43 (19)
17p	YNZ22[a]	D17S30	Taq^I	74	40/65 (62)
17q	C^{I}17–730[a]	D17S874	Msp^I	90	20/35 (57)
17q	CMM86[a]	D17S74	Taq^I	80	20/54 (37)
Total of 17q				91	32/70 (46)
18p	B74	D18S3	Msp^I	64	2/18 (11)
18q	OS4	D18S5	Taq^I	65	11/29 (38)
19p	JCZ3.1[a]	D19S20	Rsa^I	61	2/25 (8)
19q	EFD4.2[a]	D19S22	Pvu^{II}	73	11/34 (32)
20q	CMM6[a]	D20S19	Taq^I	60	7/59 (12)
21q	MCT15[a]	D21S113	Msp^I	64	11/30 (37)
22q	EFZ31	D22S32	Msp^I	64	1/13 (8)

[a] Variable number of tandem repeat markers.
[b] Amplification of alleles was observed: frequency is described in the text.

some 17 showed frequent LOH: 62% at the locus defined by YNZ22 (D17S5) at 17p13.3 (40/65 informative cases) and 57% at the locus defined by C'17-730 (D17S874) at 17q21.3 (20/35 informative cases).

Figure 1 summarizes the data that revealed LOH on each chromosomal arm. Allelic losses at frequencies of 30% or more were observed on chromosomal arms 3p (35%), 3q (30%), 5q (36%), 9p (57%), 9q (60%), 10p (33%), 13q (43%), 17p (62%), 17q (46%), 18q (38%), 19q (32%), and 21q (37%). LOH on chromosomal arms 5q, 13q, 17p, and 18q, sites of the *APC/MCC*, *RB1*, *TP53*, and *DCC* loci, had been reported previously by others [5–8]. In addition to LOH, we observed increased intensities of bands representing single alleles on chromosomal arms 8q (12%, or 5/42 informative cases), and 11q (32%, or 13/41 informative cases). These alleles involve loci of the c-*myc* (8q), EGF receptor (8q), and *cyclin D* (11q) genes, which are known to be amplified in esophageal carcinoma [1, 2].

We have also examined a correlation of LOH on each chromosomal arm with clinical and pathological features (age, sex, location of tumor, TNM classification, and clinicopathological stage). We found a significant correlation of LOH on chromosome 19q with regional lymph node metastasis ($P = 0.0128$, Fisher's exact test). For the long arm of chromosome 17, the frequency of LOH in tumors from female patients (12/14 informative cases) was significantly higher than those from male patients (20/56 informative cases) ($P = 0.0009$, Fisher's exact text). No other significant correlation between LOH and clinicopathological parameters was detected.

Each of three polymorphic loci on chromosome 9 revealed LOH at high frequency (76% at q34, 41% at q21.1–q13, and 57% at p13-pter). A significant proportion of non-small-cell lung cancers, including squamous cell carcinomas, also have revealed LOH on chromosomal arms 9p [13]. On the long arm of chromosome 9, a gene responsible for multiple self-healing squamous epithelioma, an autosomal dominant disease causing skin tumors that are morphologically indistinguishable from well differentiated squamous cell carcinomas, has been localized to 9q22–31 by linkage analysis [14]. The gene responsible for this hereditary syndrome might be associated with the development of esophageal squamous carcinomas as well. Analysis of squamous cell carcinomas of the lung has revealed

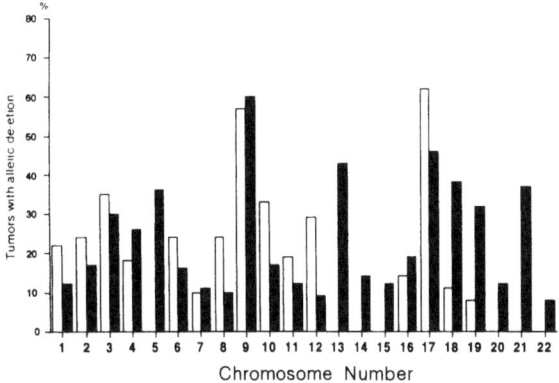

Fig. 1. Frequency of allelic loss at each chromosomal arm. p, *open bars*; q, *closed bars*

frequent LOH on chromosomal arm 9q (67%, or 12/18 informative cases) [15]. These various observations suggest that putative tumor suppressor gene(s) on chromosome 9 may play an important role in squamous cell carcinomas of the lung, skin, and esophagus. Loci on both arms of chromosome 3 also revealed frequent LOH: 35% on 3p and 30% on 3q. Loss of 3p seems to be common among squamous cell carcinomas of the esophagus, lung, nasopharynx, head and neck, and skin [15–18].

The LOH for 5q21, including the *APC/MCC* loci in esophageal cancer, has already been reported; and the authors suggested that inactivation of *MCC* or *APC* might be involved in esophageal carcinogenesis [7]. However, as we detected no alteration by screening one-third of the *APC* genes in 50 esophageal cancers, it is likely that a gene on 5q other than *APC* is related to the genesis of esophageal cancer [18].

Multistep Carcinogenesis

To further investigate genetic alterations that may affect the development or progression of esophageal squamous cell carcinomas (ESCs) we examined LOH on each of the 12 chromosomal arms that showed more than 30% frequency of LOH in early-stage esophageal carcinomas. As shown in Table 2, there was on high frequency of LOH at loci on chromosomes 3p21.3, 9p22, 9q31, and 17p13. LOH frequency on 5q, 13q, 17q, 18q, and 19q was lower in early-stage carcinomas here than appeared in our earlier allelotype study of esophageal carcinomas. These results likely in-

Table 2. LOH on each of nine chromosomal arms at various stages of esophageal carcinogenesis

Chromosomal arm	Allelic losses/informative cases			
	Basal cell hyperplasia	Dysplasia	Early carcinoma	Advanced carcinoma
3p	0/3 (0)	17/30 (57)	15/33 (45)	34/78 (44)
5q		1/8 (13)	1/19 (5)	16/45 (36)
9p	0/4 (0)	9/38 (24)	19/37 (51)	38/54 (70)
9q	0/3 (0)	11/36 (31)	21/33 (64)	36/46 (78)
13q	0/4 (0)	4/28 (14)	7/38 (18)	36/81 (44)
17p	0/4 (0)	15/32 (47)	20/34 (59)	59/90 (66)
17q		1/8 (13)	3/17 (18)	20/35 (57)
18q		1/5 (20)	2/9 (22)	11/29 (38)
19q		0/4 (0)	1/15 (7)	11/34 (32)

Numbers in parentheses are the percent.

dicate that the inactivation of genes on these chromosomal arms is associated with progression of the esophageal carcinoma.

To explore the genetic changes of these four chromosomal arms, we analyzed LOH at microsatellite loci on chromosomal arms 3p, 9p, 9q, and 17p in DNA extracts from lesions at various stages from 32 patients who had developed ESC. No LOH was detected in any of the basal cell hyperplasias examined. LOH was observed frequently on each of the four chromosomal arms in intraepithelial cancerous lesions adjacent to the main cancerous lesions (3p, 32%; 9p, 70%; 9q, 70%; and 17p, 72%). Allelic losses on 3p (9/21, or 43%) and 17p (13 of 24, or 54%) were frequent even in dysplastic lesions.

The results reported here imply that events that inactivate tumor suppressor genes located on chromosomal arms 3p, 9p, 9q, and 17p are likely to play a significant role in an early stage of esophageal carcinogenesis. Our results indicate that accumulation of genetic alterations correlates with the progression of esophageal tumors (Fig. 2). LOH on 3p or 17p was frequent in both mildly dysplastic and severely dysplastic lesions and cancerous tissues. Hence inactivation of tumor suppressor genes on one or both of these chromosomal arms may be important for converting normal stratified squamous epithelial cells to dysplastic cells. Because LOH of 9p or 9q was observed occasionally in mild dysplasias, but frequently in severe dysplasias and in intraepithelial cancerous lesions adjacent to a main tumor, inactivation of tumor suppressor genes on 9p and 9q may be important for transformation to the malignant phenotype.

Detailed Mapping of Putative Tumor Suppressor Gene on Chromosome 9q

Allelic losses on 9q have also been found in many early-stage bladder carcinomas [19, 20], and detailed deletion mapping in those tumors has assigned a candidate locus to chromosomal band 9q34.1–q34.2 [21]. Furthermore, genetic analyses of squamous cell carcinomas of the lung and of the head and neck have disclosed frequent LOH on the long arm of chromosome 9q [15, 22, 23]. These results suggested to us that inactivation of a tumor suppressor gene on 9q is likely to play a significant role in the development of squamous cell carcinoma of the esophagus and other tissues.

To further define a region containing the putative tumor suppressor gene, we examined LOH in 37 ESCs using 14 microsatellite markers mapped to 9q31–q34.1. LOH was observed in 30 of 37 (81%) tumors at one or more of the loci examined, and partial or interstitial deletions at 9q31–q34.1 were detected in 13 of these tumors. On the basis of these results, we constructed a detailed deletion map and defined a commonly deleted region between the D9S262 and D9S154 loci at 9q31–q32. The genetic distance between these two loci is estimated to be approximately 4 cM. We have investigated this region further using six new microsatellite markers isolated from yeast artificial chromosome (YAC) clones covering the deleted region and have narrowly defined the commonly deleted region to a segment between two loci: KM9.1 and D9S177. On the basis of the contig map of cosmid and YAC clones, we esti-

Fig. 2. Model of multistep carcinogenesis of esophageal squamous cell carcinoma

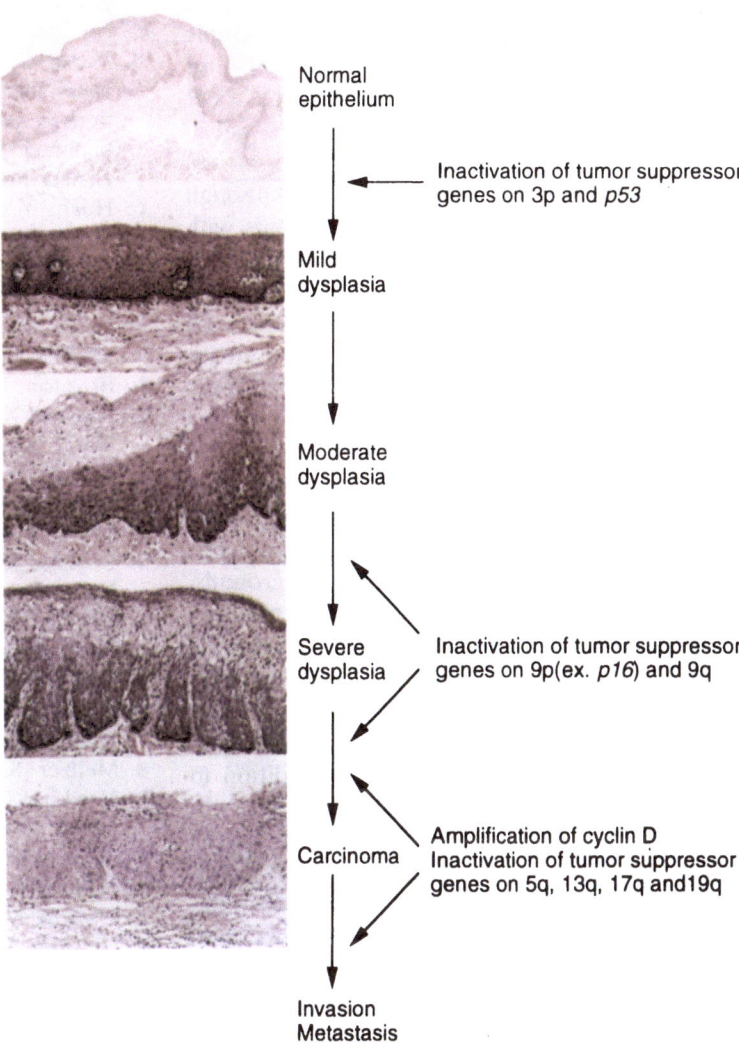

Normal
epithelium

Inactivation of tumor suppressor
genes on 3p and *p53*

Mild
dysplasia

Moderate
dysplasia

Severe
dysplasia

Inactivation of tumor suppressor
genes on 9p(ex. *p16*) and 9q

Carcinoma

Amplification of cyclin D
Inactivation of tumor suppressor
genes on 5q, 13q, 17q and19q

Invasion
Metastasis

mate the physical size of the region of interest to be about 200 kb. Because the distal 9q region also has been implicated as the site of a tumor suppressor gene(s) related to squamous cell carcinomas of other tissues, our map provides useful information for attempts to identify a common gene for carcinomas of this cell type.

We also investigated a possible role of the *PTC* gene on chromosome 9q22.3 (identified as the cause of nevoid basal cell carcinoma syndrome (NBCCS) [24–26]) during carcinogenesis in the esophagus and lung. We examined 20 ESCs and 10 squamous cell carcinomas of the lung for mutations in any coding exon of *PTC* using single-strand conformation polymorphism (SSCP) and direct sequencing. We detected no mutations other than two nondeleterious polymorphisms,

suggesting that inactivation of tumor suppressor gene(s) on 9q other than *PTC* contributes to the development of squamous cell carcinomas in these tissues [27].

Infrequent Replication Error in Esophageal Carcinomas

Genetic defects in the mismatch repair system can be monitored by RER (Replication Error) at microsatellite loci in cancer cells. The RER$^+$ phenotype has been reported in tumors associated with hereditary nonpolyposis colorectal cancer (HNPCC) or Muir-Tore syndrome, which develop multiple primary cancers [28–30]. Moreover, it has been reported that genetic instability may play an important role in the development of multiple primary cancers not associated with HNPCC or Muir-Torre syndrome [31]. However, the RER phenotype has not been investigated in detail in patients with squamous cell carcinoma of the esophagus or of the head and neck. Although esophageal cancer is infrequent in patients with HNPCC or Muir-Torre syndrome, it is well known that patients with ESC have a high statistical risk of developing a second primary cancer in the head or neck [32]. The increased risk has been attributed to life style, such as heavy smoking and excessive consumption of alcohol [33]. It is also possible that genetic background including an abnormality in the mismatch repair pathway may increase the risk for developing multiple primary tumors in various tissues including the esophagus. To investigate whether any genetic backgrounds, such as defects in the DNA-mismatch repair system, influence the development of these multiple primary tumors, we examined replication errors (RER) at six microsatellite loci in DNA extracts of 46 tumors from 33 patients who had developed primary cancers in various tissues in addition to the esophagus. The RER$^+$ phenotype was observed in only three tumors from 2 of the 33 patients examined. Our results suggest that development of multiple primary tumors in these patients would not be affected by an abnormality in the DNA repair system(s) detected as the RER phenotype. However, it is notable that a single patient who developed multiple cancers revealed the RER$^+$ phenotype at multiple microsatellite loci in both tumors, indicating that a defect in the DNA repair gene(s) may have played an important role in the development of tumors in this patient.

References

1. Lu S-H, Hsieh L-L, Luo F-C, Weinstein IB (1988) Amplification of the EGF receptor and c-*myc* genes in human esophageal cancers. Int J Cancer 42:502–505

2. Jiang W, Kahn SM, Tomita N, Zhang Y-J, Lu S-H, Weinstein IB (1992) Amplification and expression of the human *cyclin D* gene in esophageal cancer. Cancer Res 52:2980–2983

3. Mori M, Tokino T, Yanagisawa A, Kanamori M, Kato Y, Nakamura Y (1992) Association between chromosome 11q13 amplification and prognosis of patients with oesophageal carcinomas. Eur J Cancer 28A:755–757

4. Victor T, Toit RD, Jordaan AM, Bester AJ, vanHelden PD (1990) No evidence for point mutations in codons 12, 13, and 61 of the *ras* gene in a high-incidence area for esophageal gastric cancers. Cancer Res 50:4911–4914

5. Huang Y, Boynton RF, Blount PL, Silverstein RJ, Yin J, Tong Y, McDaniel TK, Newkirk C, Resau JH, Sridhara R, Reid B, Meltzer SJ (1992) Loss of heterozygosity involves multiple tumor suppressor genes in human esophageal cancers. Cancer Res 52:6525–6530

6. Boynton RF, Huang Y, Blount PL, Reid BJ, Raskind WH, Haggitt RC, Newkirk C, Reseau JH, Yin J, McDaniel TK, Meltzer SJ (1991) Frequent loss of heterozygosity at the retinoblastoma locus in human esophageal cancers. Cancer Res 51:5766–5769

7. Boynton RF, Blount PL, Yin J, Brown VL, Huang Y, Tong Y, McDaniel T, Newkirk C, Resau JH, Raskind WH, Haggitt RC, Reid BJ, Meltzer SJ (1992) Loss of heterozygosity involving the *APC* and *MCC* genetic loci occurs in the majority of human esophageal cancers. Proc Natl Acad Sci USA 89:3385–3388

8. Meltzer SJ, Yin J, Huang Y, McDaniel TK, Newkirk C, Iseri O, Vogelstein B, Resau JH (1991) Reduction to homozygosity involving *p53* in esophageal cancers demonstrated by the polymerase chain reaction. Proc Natl Acad Sci USA 88:4976–4980

9. Hollstein MC, Metcalf RA, Welsh JA, Montesano R, Harris CC (1990) Frequent mutation of the *p53* gene in human esophageal cancer. Proc Natl Acad Sci USA 87:9958–9961

10. Bennett WP, Hollstein MC, He A, Zhu SM, Resau JH, Trump BF, Metcalf RA, Welsh JA, Midgley C, Lane DP, Harris CC (1991) Archival analysis of *p53* gene and protein alterations in Chinese esophageal cancer. Oncogene 6:1779–1784

11. Huang Y, Boynton RF, Blount PL, Silverstein RJ, Yin J, Tong Y, McDaniel TK, Newkirk C, Resau JH, Sridhara R, Reid B, Meltzer SJ (1992) Loss of heterozygosity involves multiple tumor suppressor genes in human esophageal cancers. Cancer Res 52:6525–6530

12. Wagata T, Ishizaki K, Imamura M, Shimada Y, Ikenaga M, Tobe T (1991) Deletion of 17p and amplification of the int-2 gene in esophageal carcinomas. Cancer Res 51:2113–2117

13. Huang Y, Meltzer SJ, Yin J, Tong Y, Chang EH, Srivastava S, McDaniel TK, Boynton RF, Zou Z-Q (1993) Altered messenger RNA and unique mutational profiles of *p53* and *Rb* in human esophageal carcinomas. Cancer Res 53:1889–1894

14. Goudie DR, Yuille MAR, Affara NA, Ferguson-Smith MA (1993) Mapping of the gene for multiple self-healing squamous epithelioma by haplotype analysis in families with common ancestry. Cytogenet Cell Genet 64:114

15. Tsuchiya E, Nakamura Y, Weng S-Y, Nakagawa K, Tsuchiya S, Sugano H, Kitagawa T (1992) Allelotype of non-small cell lung carcinoma: comparison between loss of heterozygosity in squamous cell carcinoma and adenocarcinoma. Cancer Res 52:2478–2481

16. Huang DP, Lo K-W, Choi PHK, Ng AYT, Tsao S-Y, Yiu GKC, Lee JCK (1991) Loss of heterozygosity on the short arm of chromosome 3 in nasopharyngeal carcinoma. Cancer Genet Cytogenet 54:91–99

17. Yokoyama S, Yamakawa K, Tsuchiya E, Murata M, Sakiyama S, Nakamura Y (1992) Deletion mapping on the short arm of chromosome 3 in squamous cell carcinoma and adenocarcinoma of the lung. Cancer Res 52:873–877

18. Mori T, Yanagisawa A, Kato Y, Miura K, Nishihira T, Mori S, Nakamura Y (1994) Accumulation of genetic alterations during esophageal carcinogenesis. Hum Mol Genet 3:1969–1971

19. Cairns P, Shaw ME, Knowles MA (1993) Initiation of bladder cancer may involve deletion of a tumor-suppressor gene on chromosome 9. Oncogene 8:1083–1085

20. Habuchi T, Ogawa O, Kakehi Y, Ogura K, Koshiba M, Hamazaki S, Takahashi R, Sugiyama T, Yoshida O (1993) Accumulated allelic losses in the development of invasive urothelial cancer. Int J Cancer 53:579–584

21. Orlow I, Lianes P, Lacombe L, Dalbagni G, Reuter VE, Cardo CC (1994) Chromosome 9 allelic losses and microsatellite alterations in human bladder tumors. Cancer Res 54:2848–2851

22. Merlo A, Gabrielson E, Askin F, Sidransky D (1994) Frequent loss of chromosome 9 in human primary non-small cell lung cancer. Cancer Res 54:640–642

23. Sato S, Nakamura Y, Tsuchiya E (1994) Difference of allelotype between squamous cell carcinoma and adenocarcinoma of the lung. Cancer Res 54:5652–5655

24. Wicking C, Berkman J, Wainwright B, Chenevix-Trench G (1994) Fine genetic mapping of the gene for nevoid basal cell carcinoma. Genomics 22:505–511

25. Goldstein A, Stewart C, Bale SJ, Dean M (1994) Localization of the gene for the nevoid basal cell carcinoma syndrome (NBCCS). Am J Hum Genet 54:765–773

26. Hahn H, Christiansen J, Wicking C, Zaphiropoulos PG, Chidambaram A, Gerrard B, Vorechovsky I, Bale AE, Toftgard R, Dean M, Wainwright B (1996) A mammalian patched homolog is expressed in target tissues of sonic hedgehog and maps to a region associated with developmental abnormalities. J Biol Chem 271:12125–12128

27. Suzuki K, Daigo Y, Fukuda S, Tokino T, Isomura M, Isono K, Wainwright B, Nakamura Y (1997) No evidence of mutation in the human *PTC* gene, responsible for NBCC syndrome, in human primary squamous cell carcinomas of the esophagus and lung. Jpn J Cancer Res (in press)

28. Aaltonen LA, Peltomaki P, Leach FS, Sistonen P, Rylkkanen L, Mecklin J-P, Jarvinen H, Powell SM, Jen J, Hamilton SR, Petersen GM, Kinzler KW, Vogelstein B, de la Chapelle A (1993) Clues to the pathogenesis of familial colorectal cancer. Science 260:812–816

29. Peltomaki P, Lothe RA, Aaltonen LA, Pylkkanen L, Nystrom-Lahti M, Seruca R, David L, Holm R, Ryberg D, Haugen A, Brogger A, Borresen A-L, de la Chapelle (1993) A microsatellite instability is associated with tumors that characterize the hereditary non-polyposis colorectal carcinoma syndrome. Cancer Res 53:5853–5855

30. Honchel R, Halling KC, Schaid DJ, Pittelkow M, Thibodeau SN (1994) Microsatellite instability in Muir-Torre syndrome. Cancer Res 54:1159–1163

31. Horii A, Han H-J, Shimada M, Yanagisawa A, Kato Y, Ohta H, Yasui W, Tahara E, Nakamura Y (1994) Frequent replication errors at microsatellite loci in tumors of patients with multiple primary cancer. Cancer Res 54:3373–3375

32. Kuwano H, Morita M, Tsutsui S, Kido Y, Mori M, Sugimachi K (1991) Comparison of characteristics of esophageal squamous cell carcinoma associated with head and neck cancer and those with gastric cancer. J Surg Oncol 46:107–109

33. Franceschi S, Talamini R, Barra S, Baron AE, Negri E, Bidoli E, Serraino D, Vecchia CL (1990) Smoking and drinking in relation to cancers of the oral cavity, pharynx, larynx, and esophagus in northern Itlay. Cancer Res 50:6502–6507

Oxidative Damage During the Gastric Precancerous Process

Pelayo Correa[1], Mark Miller[2], and Elizabeth E. Mannick[2]

Summary. Reactive oxygen species (ROS) and reactive nitrogen species (RNS) may play a role in human carcinogenesis. Epidemiologic studies have indicated that infection with *Helicobacter pylori* increases the risk of gastric cancer. This chapter explores the possibility that such an association is the result of long-standing inflammation and the release of ROS and RNS by white blood cells.

Introduction

Research on cancer causation historically has focused on epidemiologic studies of the association between external agents and neoplastic events in affected individuals. Such studies have provided strong evidence for the carcinogenicity of some external chemical mixtures, most prominently tobacco smoke. Unlike this major cause of cancers of the lung and other organs, no such equivalent cause has been found for most other frequent human cancers. No external carcinogen has been identified as a major cause of cancers of the breast, colon, prostate, or most other major causes of death from neoplasia. This lack has inspired investigators to focus on the possibility that the carcinogen(s) responsible may be formed "in situ." The long incubation period of such tumors suggests that the locally synthesized carcinogens are delivered to the target cells in minute amounts over a long period, usually decades.

In the case of the stomach, it has been shown that in the presence of chronic gastritis high levels of nitrite are usually present in the gastric lumen. Nitrites are mostly formed by bacterial reductases acting on nitrate derived from food. Nitrites can nitrosate food-derived species, such as chloroindoles, to produce highly mutagenic compounds. Chloroindoles are abundant in some foods eaten frequently by populations at high risk of cancer (e.g. fava beans in Colombia and Chinese cabbage in China) [1]. Nitrosation of Japanese fish has been used in experimental carcinogenesis in rodents [2]. As yet, no definitive proof has been provided that products of food nitrosation are carcinogenic in humans.

Chronic infectious diseases are suspected to play a carcinogenic role in humans. Several major human cancers have been linked to infectious agents, but the mechanisms for this association are unclear. The role of hepatitis virus in primary liver carcinoma is well documented epidemiologically [3]. Similarly, papilloma viruses are causally related to human cervical cancer, and again the mechanism of carcinogenesis is unclear [4]. The most recent infectious agent linked to a major human cancer is *Helicobacter pylori*. The World Health Organization has classified the bacterium as a human carcinogen [5]. This chapter discusses hypotheses related to possible mechanisms of action of *H. pylori* in human carcinogenesis, especially the role of reactive oxygen species (ROS) and reactive nitrogen species (RNS). We describe the process in terms of histopathology, chemistry, cellular defense mechanisms, and immunochemistry.

Histopathology

The gastric precancerous process for the most frequent tumor (intestinal type) has been described in terms of sequential steps identified by their morphologic characteristics: chronic gastritis, at-

[1]Department of Pathology, Louisiana State University Medical Center, 1901 Perdido Street, New Orleans, LA 70112, USA
[2]Department of Pediatrics, Louisiana State University Medical Center, 1901 Perdido Street, New Orleans, LA 70112, USA

rophy, intestinal metaplasia, dysplasia [6]. There is epidemiologic evidence supporting the involvement of *H. pylori* in all of the steps [7].

Helicobacter pylori produces a potent urease that splits urea into carbon dioxide and ammonia. The latter compound damages the mucous layer (together with bacterial lipases) and stimulates excessive proliferation of epithelial cells [8]. The bacteria remain outside the tissue of the gastric mucosa, in the gastric lumen, close to the surface epithelium. Bacterial chemotaxis attracts monocytes and polymorphonuclear neutrophils, which migrate from the capillaries in the lamina propia. These migrating white blood cells contain toxins capable of destroying the bacteria, but most inflammatory cells do not reach the bacteria present in the lumen. They degenerate and die in the stroma itself or while traversing the layer of epithelial cells that line the foveola, around the gland necks, or in the gastric lumen. The toxins intended to kill the bacteria are instead released in "oxidative bursts" and are capable of damaging the DNA and the proteins of the host cells. This process has been called "frustrated phagocytosis" and may be of critical importance in carcinogenesis.

cascade of effects, including mitochondrial dysfunction, lipid peroxidation, modification of protein structure and function, and genotoxicity. The latter effect is of great concern in terms of promoting the precancerous process because if mutations initiated by these agents are not repaired before cellular replication they may remain part of the transformed genomic burden. The types of alterations caused by reactive oxygen and nitrogen species are primarily point mutations, particularly $G:C \rightarrow A:T$ mutations (Table 1), which are a common type of transformation in cancer. The 12 potential sites for alkylation of DNA include the ring nitrogen positions in adenine, guanine, cytosine, and thymine; the oxygen atoms of guanine, thymine, and cytosine; and the phosphate groups. Experimental data confirm that the O^6 alkylation of guanine represents the most important reaction. Mutations at this site are strongly linked to carcinogenicity.

Oxygen free radicals and NO-derived products promote deamination of DNA. Nitric oxide promotes *N*-nitrosation of aromatic amines ($Ar-NH_2$) to form the nitrosamine ($Ar-NH-NO$) intermediate, which then decomposes and rearranges to

Reactive Oxygen and Nitrogen Species and DNA Damage

Reactive species are produced as part of the cellular defense mechanisms stimulated by *H. pylori* infection (Fig. 1). These species may initiate a

Table 1. Alterations and mutations that may arise from the deamination of DNA bases by NO_x

Conversion	Type of mutation
Cytosine + $NO_x \rightarrow$ uracil	$G:C \rightarrow A:T$
mCytosine + $NO_x \rightarrow$ thymine	$G:C \rightarrow A:T$
Guanine + $NO_x \rightarrow$ xanthine	$G:C \rightarrow A:T$
Adenine + $NO_x \rightarrow$ hypoxanthine	$A:T \rightarrow G:C$

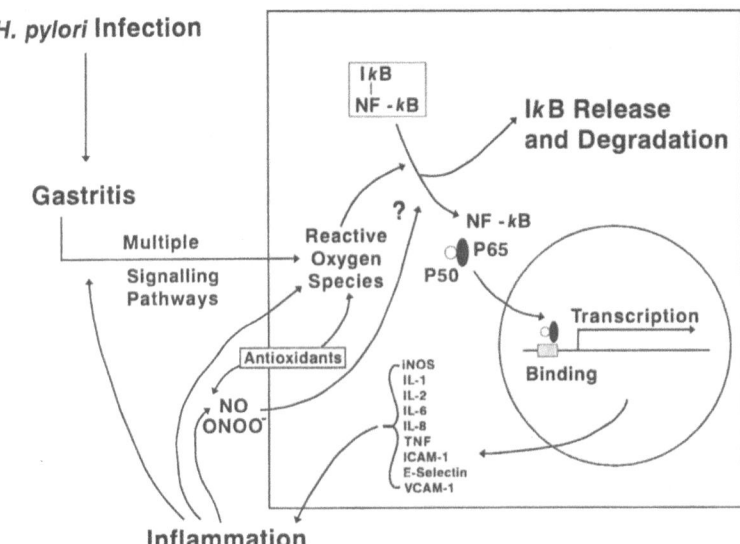

Fig. 1. Events related to ROS and RNS brought about by infection of the gastric mucosa with *H. pylori*

produce the diazonium ion $(Ar-N_2^+)$, which in turn decomposes to the hydroxyl derivative of the aromatic amine (Ar-OH). These reactions have been proposed for the oxidative deamination of cytosine, methylcytosine, guanine, or adenine (Table 1) and the observed increased formation of oxidative DNA adducts following exposure to oxidative or nitrosative species. It has been described that nitro-guanine adducts can be detected in response to peroxynitrite exposure [9, 10], the chemical processes and potential endogenous mediators for mutations. Nitric oxide has also been shown to compromise the ability of natural repair processes, for example, poly(ADP-ribose) or Fpg to repair DNA damage [11, 12]. Thus in addition to causing DNA damage, these endogenous compounds may limit the mechanisms to prevent these mutations from being permanently incorporated into the genome [13].

An interesting aspect of research in the field of reactive nitrogen species and inflammation is the formation of nitroso (NO) and nitro (NO_2) adducts from endogenous sources [14–17]. A wide range of exogenous nitrosated compounds have been linked to the development of gastrointestinal cancer [18, 19], and it appears that they may operate through mechanisms that are similar, if not identical, to the effects of endogenous compounds. For example, exogenous nitrosamines resemble intermediate products formed during nitrosative reactions produced endogenously. Thus the ability of compounds to promote gastrointestinal cancer may not be some spurious toxicological phenomenon but, rather, a means of duplicating the reactions elicited in the natural precancerous process.

Cellular Defenses Against Reactive Oxygen or Nitrogen Species

Cellular defenses against both species are similar; sulfhydryl groups in the form of glutathione quench these reactive species [20, 21]. Enzymatic degradation of superoxide and hydrogen peroxide is mediated by superoxide dismutase and catalase, respectively. To date, a comparable enzymatic pathway has not been discovered for the nitric oxide cascade. The two pathways can also interact. Nitric oxide and superoxide react at almost diffusion-limited kinetics to form peroxynitrite, ONOO− [22, 23]. Whereas these substrates possess unpaired electrons, thereby defining them

as free radicals, these electrons pair up in peroxynitrite. Peroxynitrite is therefore not a free radical but an oxidant that is considerably more reactive than either of its parent molecules, with a biological half-life of approximately 1 s. It reacts with numerous proteins, enzymes, lipids, and DNA to cause cell injury and toxicity. Because of its potency and ephemeral existence, it is difficult to quantify. In addition to being an oxidant, it also is an excellent nitrating agent, particularly in the presence of metals; and it avidly nitrates tyrosine residues in proteins to form the stable product nitrotyrosine. Nitrotyrosine formation in vivo can be evaluated by immunohistochemical staining, Western blotting, or high-performance liquid chromatography techniques [14, 17, 24]. Nitrotyrosine levels are particularly low in noninflamed states but increase markedly during inflammation or immune activation and co-localize with inducible nitric oxide synthase expression [14, 25, 26]. Bicarbonate and ascorbic acid [22, 27] rapidly degrade peroxynitrite, and ascorbic acid has been demonstrated to prevent peroxynitrite-induced cell death in cultured epithelial cells [28]. This finding may have great relevance for gastritis because those at the greatest risk for the development of gastric cancer have the lowest luminal levels of ascorbic acid [29].

A cellular defense mechanism against marked DNA damage is the process of apoptosis, or programmed cell death [30, 31]. We have noted that marked apoptosis accompanies gastritis and co-localizes with sites of inducible nitric oxide synthase expression and nitrotyrosine formation [26]. Both nitric oxide and peroxynitrite promote apoptosis [28]. Importantly, treatment of patients with antibiotics to clear the *H. pylori* or use of the supplemental antioxidants β-carotene and ascorbic acid lowers the frequency of such lesions [26]. Thus cell toxicity and death can be manipulated by clearing the source of immune activation or modifying the host response.

Antioxidants also have the potential to diminish the entire immune cascade, including the release of cytokines, by compromising activation of the nuclear transcription factor NF-KappaB [32]. *H. pylori* infection has been associated with NF-KappaB activation, a result confirmed in our laboratories. Antioxidants may therefore not only reduce the bioactivity of free radicals but also dampen the release of cytokines and expression of adhesion molecules that contribute to the host response. To a large extent the activation of NF-

KappaB involves a proteosome that is activated by reactive oxygen species, which places greater importance on the potential utility of antioxidants for terminating the cascade of events in the precancerous process.

Immunochemical Studies

Evidence of nitric oxide is assessed by staining the enzyme-inducible nitric oxide synthase (iNOS), which is involved in the synthesis of nitric oxide by inflammatory cells and represents abnormal synthesis of the product, in contrast to the constitutive synthase involved in physiologic functions, (Figs. 2–4). As seen in the microphotographs in Figs. 2–4, polymorphonuclear leukocyte cells stained positive for iNOS in the stroma, epithelium, and lumen, indicating migration into the gastric cavity. Positively stained cells are also seen around epithelial cells in the glandular necks. These changes indicate potential for damage to the normal gastric mucosal cells, specifically the epithelial cells, by oxidative bursts of the polynuclear cells. Figure 5 shows positive staining for nitrotyrosine, indicating damage to proteins associated with *H. pylori* infection.

iNOS is a marker of activated host defense mechanisms and, with the exception of pregnancy,

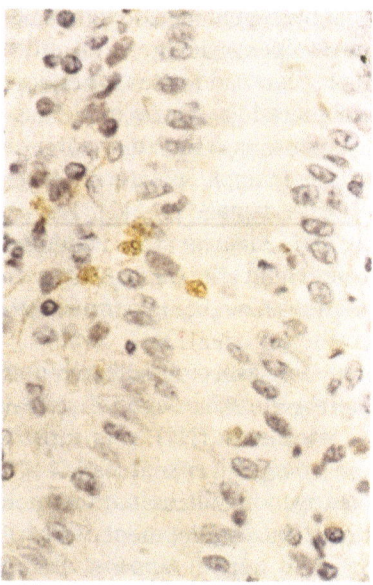

Fig. 3. Microphotograph of gastric foveola of a patient with *H. pylori*-associated active gastritis. Immunostaining for inducible nitric oxide synthase (iNOS) was used. Positively stained polymorphonuclear leukocytes are seen migrating from the stroma, through the epithelium, to the lumen

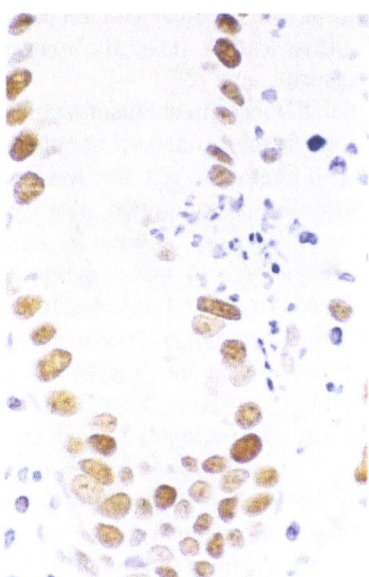

Fig. 2. Microphotograph of a gastric foveola of a patient with *H. pylori*-associated active gastritis. Immunostaining for proliferating cell nuclear antigen (PCNA) indicates active DNA synthesis. Polymophonuclear neutrophils (PMNs) are seen migrating from the stroma to the gastric lumen, where *H. pylori* was identified with silver stain. The migrating PMNs break through the epithelium and come into intimate contact with dividing epithelial cells. (This topographic setup allows oxidative bursts to contact dividing cells)

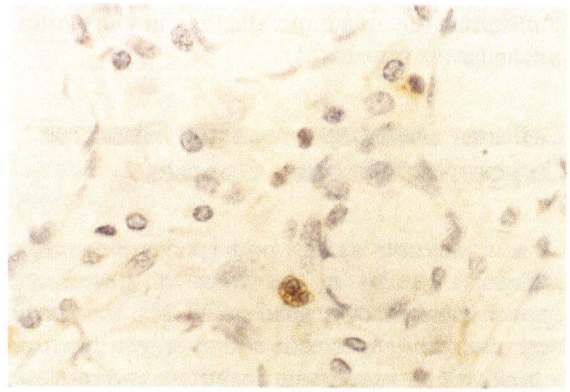

Fig. 4. Microphotograph of the glandular neck region of a patient with *H. pylori*-associated active gastritis. Immunostaining for inducible nitric oxide synthase (iNOS) was used. Positively stained polymorphonuclear leukocytes are seen in the immediate vicinity of the gland necks, where DNA synthesis normally takes place

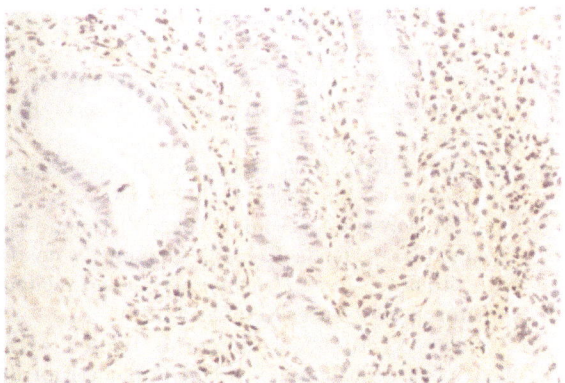

Fig. 5. Microphotograph of the foveolar region of a patient with *H. pylori*-associated active gastritis. Immunostaining for nitrotyrosine. Positive staining of cells and stroma indicates damages to proteins, presumably from peroxynitrite

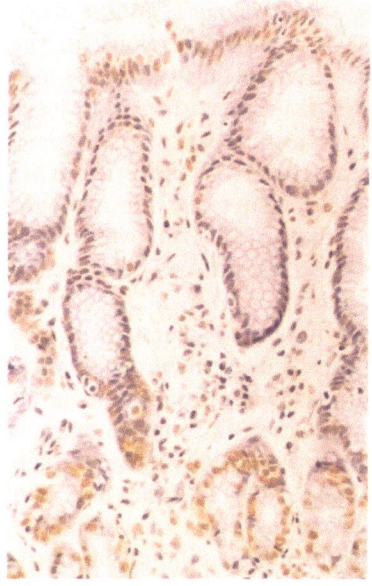

Fig. 6. Microphotograph of the neck and foveolar regions of a patient with *H. pylori*-associated active gastritis. Immunostaining for apoptosis (TUNEL stain) was used. Positively stained cells are seen at the surface (normal location) but also prominently in the neck region, probably related to the adjacent inflammatory infiltrate

is associated with cell toxicity [33]. Cellular damage, including genotoxicity, may result in different outcomes. Severe damage to cells usually compromises not only the DNA but also the cellular membranes, resulting in complete destruction of the integrity of the cell, namely necrosis. Less damage may induce DNA fragmentation, which may be beyond cellular repair mechanisms. Under these circumstances, a cellular defense may be the initiation of programmed cell death, (apoptosis), which prevents the survival of transformed cells. Apoptosis can be assessed in situ with the TUNEL assay as shown in (Fig. 6). The normal site of apoptosis is at the surface epithelium in cells predetermined to desquamate. In gastric mucosa with *H. pylori*-associated chronic gastritis, apoptosis is abnormally observed at the level of the glandular necks, where cell replication normally takes place. It has been suggested that this abnormally located apoptosis results from disruption of the normal adhesion of epithelial cells to their basement membrane (anchorage) by the cytokines released by the inflammatory cells in the lamina propia. This phenomenon has been labeled "anoikis" (homelessness) [34]. As seen in Figs. 2–6, apoptosis is prominent in the *H. pylori*-associated gastritis, indicating a degree of damage that is insufficient to induce necrosis but sufficient to induce programmed cell death. This phenomenon may explain why *H. pylori* has been causally linked to atrophy (gland loss), a precancerous change, in epidemiologic studies. Reactive oxygen and nitrogen species can initiate apoptosis in low

concentrations, and higher burdens may evoke necrosis. Thus the co-localization of enzymes that produce large amounts of nitric oxide with apoptosis is suggestive of a causal link. This link has been confirmed in cell culture and is further suggested by chemotherapeutic approaches wherein both iNOS and apoptosis staining are reduced. It does not prove causality, as other inflammatory mediators and cytokines released during gastritis also promote apoptosis [35].

Apoptotic cells are destined not to replicate and obviously do not generate neoplastic clones. These clones could be generated by levels of DNA damage that are insufficient to induce apoptosis but sufficient to induce mutations. They are detected by techniques of molecular biology dealt with in other chapters.

Conclusions

Whether cell damage by carcinogens synthesized "in situ" by inflammatory cells is of relevance to human carcinogenesis is conjectural at the present time. The process appears to be highly complex, and further research is justified.

Strong epidemiologic evidence links *H. pylori* infection with gastric neoplasia in humans. At least three hypothetical pathways are suggested by the human experience. *H. pylori* plays an important role in gastric lymphoma, suggesting that carcinogenic influences brought about by the bacterium may target the mucosa-associated lymphoid tissue (MALT), which colonizes the gastric mucosa after its infection and apparently induces trisomy 3 [36] and 1; 14 translocations [37]. *H. pylori* is also associated with the intestinal type of gastric adenocarcinoma in which molecular alterations of cell proliferation and differentiation similar to those of colon carcinoma have been described, including involvement of *p53*, *APC*, and *DCC* genes [37–39]. It has been reported that the diffuse type of gastric carcinoma is associated with *H. pylori* infection [40]. The nuclear alterations indicative of DNA damage are less well characterized in such tumors; there seems to be selective damage directed to the synthesis and preservation of cellular membranes and basal membrane proteins: adhesion molecules, laminin, and type IV collagen. Hypothetically, all three types of alteration linked to *H. pylori* may be induced by oxygen- and nitrogen-reactive species. Nitric oxide resulting from *H. pylori* infection may be the common link of the three gastric neoplastic pathways proposed, as an active agent or a marker of the so far poorly understood processes. Hopefully, future research will elucidate the role of oxygen- and nitrogen-reactive species, their interaction with antioxidants, and other defense mechanisms for determining the outcome of *H. pylori* infection.

References

1. Yang D, Tannenbaum SR, Buchi G, Lee G (1984) 4-Chloro-6-methoxy-indole is the precursor of a potent mutagen that forms during nitrosation of the fava bean (Vicia faba). Carcinogenesis 5:1219–1224
2. Weisburger JH, Marquardt H, Hirota N, Mori H, William SM (1980) Induction of cancer of the glandular stomach in rats by an extract of nitrite treated fish. J Nate Cancer Inst 64:163
3. IARC (1994) Hepatitis virus. In: IARC monographs on the evolution of carcinogenic risk to humans, vol 59. IARC, Lyon, France
4. De Villiers E (1992) Epidemiology of cervical cancer and human papilloma viruses. Oxford University Press, Oxford
5. IARC (1994) Schistosomes, liver flukes and *Helicobacter pylori*. In: IARC monographs on the evaluation of carcinogenic risk to humans, vol 61. IARC, Lyon, France
6. Correa P (1992) Human gastric carcinogenesis: a multistep and multifactorial process. Cancer Res 52:6735–6740
7. Correa P (1995) *Helicobacter pylori* and gastric carcinogenesis. Am J Surg Pathol 19:S37–S43
8. Tsujii M, Kawano S, Tsujii S, Takei Y, Tamura K, Fusamoto H, Kamada T (1992) Ammonia, a possible promotor in *Helicobacter pylori*-related carcinogenesis. Cancer Lett 65:15–18
9. Yermilov V, Rubio J, Becci M, Friesen MD, Pignatelli B, Ohshima H (1995) Formation of 8-nitroguanine by the reaction of guanine with peroxynitrite in vitro. Carcinogenesis 16:2045–2050
10. Yermilov V, Rubio J, Ohshima H (1995) Formation of 8-nitroguanine in DNA treated with peroxynitrite in vitro and its rapid removal from DNA by depurination. FEBS Lett 376:207–210
11. Messmer UC, Reimer DM, Brune B (1996) Nitric oxide induced poly(ADP-ribose) polymerase leavage in RAW 264.7 macrophage apoptosis is blocked by Bcl-2. FEBS Lett 384:162–166
12. Wink DA, Laval J (1995) The Fpg protein, a DNA repair enzyme, is inhibited by the biomediator nitric oxide in vitro and in vivo. Carcinogenesis 15:2125–2129
13. Ohshima H, Bartsch H (1994) Chronic infections and inflammatory processes cancer risk factors: possible role of nitric oxide in carcinogenesis. Mutat Res 305:253–254
14. Miller MJS, Thompson JH, Zhang X-J, Sadowska-Krowicka H, Kakkis JL, Munshi UK, Sandoval M, Rossi JL, Eloby-Childress S, Beckman JS, Ye YZ, Rodi CP, Manning PT, Currie MG, Clark DA (1995) Role of inducible nitric oxide synthase expression and peroxynitrite formation in guinea pig ileitis. Gastroenterology 109:1475–1483
15. Grisham MB, Ware K, Gilleland HE Jr, Gilleland LB, Abell CL, Yamada T (1992) Neutrophil-mediated nitrosame formation: role of nitric oxide in rats. Gastroenterology 103:1260–1266
16. Ohshima H, Bandaletora TY, Brouet I, Bartsch H, Kirby G, Ogunbiyi F, Vatansapt V, Pipitgool V (1995) Increased nitrosamine and nitrate biosynthesis mediated by nitric oxide synthase induced in hamsters infected with liver fluke (*Opisthorchis viverrini*). Carcinogenesis 15:271–275
17. Ischiropoulos NW, Royall JA, Ye YZ, Kelly DR, Beckman JS (1995) Evidence for in vivo peroxynitrite production in human acute lung injury. Am J Respir Crit Care Med 151:1250–1254
18. Sugimura T, Fugimura S (1967) Tumour production in glandular stomach of rat by N-methyl-N'-N-nitrosoguanidine. Nature 216:943–944
19. Saito T, Sasaki O, Tamada R, Iwamatsu M, Inokuchi K (1978) Sequential studies of develop-

ment of gastric carcinoma in dogs induced by N-methyl-N'-nitro-N-nitrosoguanidine. Cancer 42(3): 1246–1254

20. McKenzie SJ, Baker MS, Buffinton GD, Doe WF (1996) Evidence of oxidant-induced injury to epithelial cells during inflammatory bowel disease. J Clin Invest 98:136–141

21. Radi R, Beckman JS, Bush KM, Freeman BA (1991) Peroxynitrite oxidation of sulfhydryls. J Biol Chem 266:4244–4250

22. Pryor WA, Squadrito GL (1995) The chemistry of peroxynitrite: a product from the reaction of nitric oxide with superoxide. Am J Physiol 268:L699–L722

23. Radi R, Beckman JS, Bush KM, Freeman BA (1991) Peroxynitrite-induced membrane lipid peroxidation: the cytotoxic potential of superoxide and nitric oxide. Arch Biochem Biophys 288:481–487

24. Kaur H, Halliwell B (1994) Evidence of nitric oxide-mediated oxidative damage in chronic inflammation: nitrotyrosine in serum and synovial fluid from rheumatoid patients. FEBS Lett 350:9–12

25. Seago ND, Thompson JH, Zhang X-J, Clark DA, Miller MJS (1995) Inducible nitric oxide synthase and guinea-pig ileitis induced by adjuvant. Mediat Inflamm 4:19–24

26. Mannick EE, Bravo LE, Zarama G, Realpse JL, Zhang X-J, Ruiz B, Fontham ETH, Mera R, Miller MJS, Correa P (1996) Inducible nitric oxide synthase, nitrotyrosine, and apoptosis in *Helicobacter pylori* gastritis: effect of antibiotics and antioxidants. Cancer Res 56:3238–3243

27. Uppu RM, Squadrito GL, Pryor WA (1996) Accelation of peroxynitrite oxidations by carbon dioxide. Arch Biochem Biophys 327:335–343

28. Sandoval M, Zhang X-J, Liu X, Mannick EE, Clark DA, Miller MJS (1997) Peroxynitrite-induced apoptosis in T84 and RAW 264.7 cells: attenuation by L-ascorbic acid. Free Radical Biol Med 22:489–495

29. Ruiz B, Rood JC, Fontham ETH, Malcom GT, Hunter FM, Sobhan M, Johnson WD, Correa P (1994) Vitamin C concentration in gastric juice before and after anti-*Helicobacter pylori* treatment. Am J Gastroenterol 89:533–539

30. Cui S, Reichner JS, Mateo RB, Albina JE (1994) Activated murine macrophages induce apoptosis in tumor cells through nitric oxide dependent or independent mechanisms. Cancer Res 54:2462–2467

31. Sandoval M, Liu X, Oliver PD, Zhang X-J, Clark DA, Miller MJS (1995) Nitric oxide induces apoptosis in a human colonic epithelial cell line, T84. Mediat Inflamm 4:248–250

32. Shin WS, Hong YH, Peng HB, DeCaterina R, Libby P, Liao JK (1996) Nitric oxide attenuates vascular smooth muscle cell activation by interferon-gamma: the role of constitutive NF-kappa B activity. J Biol Chem 271:11317–11324

33. Miller MJS, Voelker CA, Olister SA, Thompson JH, Zhang X-J, Rivera D, Eloby-Childress S, Liu X, Clark DA, Pierce MR (1996) Fetal growth retardation in rats may result from apoptosis: role of peroxynitrite. Free Radical Biol Med 21:619–629

34. Strater J, Ulrich W, Barth TFE, Koretz K, Elsing C, Moller P (1996) Rapid onset of apoptosis in vitro follows disruption of B1 integrin/matrix interactions in human colonic crypt cells. Gastroenterology 110:1776–1784

35. Shin WS, Hong YH, Peng HB, DeCaterina R, Libby P, Liao JK (1996) Nitric oxide attenuates vascular smooth muscle cell activation by interferon-gamma: the role of constitutive NF-kappa B activity. J Biol Chem 271:11317–11324

36. Wotherspoon AC, Finn TM, Isaacson PG (1995) Trisomy 3 in low grade B cell lymphomas of mucosa associated lymphoid tissue (MALT). Blood 85:2000–2004

37. Spencer J, Diss TC, Isaacson PG (1989) Primary B cell gastric lymphoma: a genotypic analysis. Am J Pathol 135:557–564

38. Tahara E (1993) Molecular mechanisms of gastric carcinogenesis. J Cancer Res Clin Oncol 119:265–272

39. Correa P, Shiao YH Phenotypic and genotypic events in gastric carcinogenesis. Cancer Res 54:1941s–1943s

40. Solcia E, Fiocca R, Luinetti O, Villani L, Padovan L, Calistri D, Ranzani GN, Chiaravalli A, Capella C (1996) Intestinal and diffuse gastric cancers arise in different background of *Helicobacter pylori* gastritis through different gene involvement. Am J Surg Pathol 20:S8–S22

Multiple Genetic Alterations and Abnormal Growth Factor Network in Human Esophageal Carcinomas

Kazuhiro Yoshida[1], Wataru Yasui[2], Yoshihiro Kagawa[1], and Eiichi Tahara[2]

Summary. Esophageal carcinoma is the most malignant gastrointestinal neoplasm. Multiple genetic alterations of oncogenes and tumor suppressor genes take place in esophageal squamous cell carcinomas. Co-amplification of cyclin D1, hst-1, and int-2 gene is found in 40% of the primary tumors and almost all metastatic tumors. The prognosis of the patient with gene amplification is evidently poorer than those without amplification. Multiple alterations of tumor suppressor genes and negative cell cycle regulators, including p53 gene, Rb gene, BRCA1 gene, p16 (MTS1), p15 (MTS2), and p21 (WAF1/CIP1), play an important role in the development and progression of esophageal carcinomas. Furthermore, multiple growth factor–receptor loops exist and participate in the autocrine growth of the esophageal cancer. They include epidermal growth factor (EGF), transforming growth factors (TGF) α and β, and platelet-derived growth factor (PDGF). Overexpression of EGF, TGF-α, and EGFR is closely correlated with the malignant behavior of tumor cells and patient prognosis. These growth factors stimulate production of the interstitial degradation enzymes and down-regulation of E-cadherin function, which may lead to cell invasion and metastasis.

Introduction

Esophageal carcinoma, one of the most malignant gastrointestinal cancers, occurs at a high frequency in Japan and certain areas of China. The incidence of esophageal carcinoma in men is higher than in women; and the prognosis for men is worse than for women, suggesting that esophageal carcinoma is closely related to diet and sex hormones. The development of human esophageal squamous cell carcinoma is a multistep, progressive process [1, 2]. An early indicator of this process is an increased proliferation of esophageal epithelial cells morphologically including basal cell hyperplasia, dysplasia, and carcinoma in situ, which are regarded as precancerous lesions. In this process, multiple genetic alterations and overexpression of growth factor–receptor systems are involved [3], including amplification and overexpression of epidermal growth factor receptor (EGFR), amplification of cyclin D1/hst-1/int-2 gene [4–6], loss of heterozygosity (LOH) at multiple chromosomal loci (e.g., 3p, 5q, 9p, 9q, 13q, 17p, 17q) [7, 8], mutation of the p53 gene, total deletion or mutation of the MTS1 gene [9, 10], and overexpression of growth factors. In the present review, the roles of multiple genetic alterations and growth factor–receptor systems that contribute to the development and progression of esophageal carcinomas are described.

Genetic Alterations in Esophageal Carcinomas

The process of tumorigenesis at the cellular level is related to disorders of the control of cell proliferation and differentiation. Most of the cancer

[1] Department of Surgical Oncology, Research Institute for Radiation Biology and Medicine, Hiroshima University School of Medicine, 1-2-3 Kasumi, Minami-ku, Hiroshima 734, Japan
[2] First Department of Pathology, Hiroshima University School of Medicine, 1-2-3 Kasumi, Minami-ku, Hiroshima 734, Japan

cells contain genetic alterations that relate to the control of this process, including growth factors and their receptors, signal transduction, and transcription factors [11]. Two basic types of genetic damage are encountered frequently in cancer cells: dominant (with targets known as proto-oncogenes) and recessive (with targets known as tumor suppressor genes). The genetic events affecting proto-oncogenes often result in increased stimulatory function, whereas those affecting tumor suppressor genes may cause loss of inhibitory function. The interaction of signaling molecules with their receptors induces receptor activation and initiation of a signal transduction cascade mediated by multiple second messengers and receptor-activated protein kinases. In cells with activated oncogenes many of these pathways become disturbed, often constitutively activated, resulting in autonomous proliferation and other phenotypic changes. There are several major biochemical mechanisms of action for oncogenes [11]: (1) abnormal signaling by a structurally abnormal cytokine/growth factor including amplification, deletion, rearrangement, and point mutation of the gene; (2) aberrant phosphorylation of proteins at either serine, threonine, or tyrosine residues by altered receptors and other signal transducing kinases; and (3) disturbed regulation of gene transcription by abnormal transcription factors. Tumor suppressor genes can be defined as genes whose repression, inactivation, dysfunction,

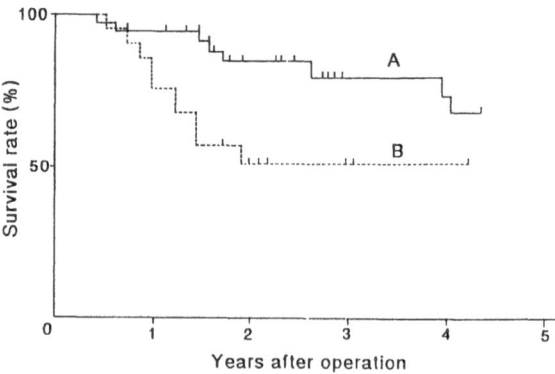

Fig. 1. Survival curve of an esophageal carcinoma patient after esophagectomy without *cyclin* D gene amplification (*A*) and with gene amplification (*B*)

or loss results in cell transformation [12]. They were initially described in hereditary cancers, such as retinoblastoma (*Rb* gene) [13], Wilms' tumors (*WT* gene) [14], and familial adenomatous polyposis coli (*APC* gene) [15]. It has been shown through unbridled cellular proliferation that cell cycle regulators are candidate oncogenes or tumor suppressor genes. The genetic abnormalities of oncogenes and tumor suppressor genes involved in the development of esophageal carcinomas are shown in Table 1.

Activation of Oncogenes

Regarding oncogenes in esophageal carcinomas, amplification of *hst*-1/*int*-2 genes, EGFR gene, and c-*myc* gene has been reported [4–6, 16]. We analyzed the co-amplification of *hst*-1/*int*-2 genes by slot blot analysis using DNAs from formalin-fixed paraffin-embedded tissues of 18 dysplastic lesions, 100 primary esophageal carcinomas after surgical resection, and 18 metastatic esophageal carcinomas obtained at autopsy. No amplification was detected in dysplasia, whereas it was detected in 41 cases (41%) of primary tumors and 100% of metastatic carcinomas. The amplification of these genes correlated with tumor staging and depth of tumor invasion. Moreover, the prognosis for patients with gene amplification was poorer than for those without gene amplification [4, 5] (Fig. 1). Although the co-amplification of *hst*-1 and *int*-2 genes was frequently associated with esophageal carcinoma, mRNA expression has not been found so far.

Table 1. Genes altered in esophageal cancer

Gene alterations	Incidence (%)
hst-1/*int*-2/*cyclin* D (amplification)	40–50
EGFR (amplification)	10–15
c-*myc* (amplification)	14
p53 (17q13) (LOH, mutation)	30–50
APC (5q21) (LOH)	66
Rb (13q14) (LOH)	36–54
MTS1/CDK4 (9q21) (loss, mutation)	50
BRCA (17q) (LOH)	62
LOH of 3p	35
9p	57
9q	60
13q	43
17p	62
17q	46
LOH of 5q, 10p, 18q, 19q, 21p	>30

LOH, loss of heterozygosity.

Much attention has been paid to this hot locus for the candidate gene related to the carcinogenesis of esophageal cancer. Motokura et al. [17] isolated a potential oncogene, *prad* 1, from a rearranged chromosome 11q13 found in parathyroid tumors. Interestingly, the cDNA sequence of the gene was identical to that of *cyclin* D1 gene [18]. The *cyclin* D1 gene encodes a cell cycle regulatory protein that governs G1 progression, S phase entry, or both. Three types of *cyclin* D genes have been discovered and form complexes with *cyclin*-dependent kinases (CDKs) 2, 4, and 5.

What is interesting in the study is that the incidence of distant metastasis and local recurrence is higher in patients with gene amplification. Amplification of *cyclin* D1 gene was detected in one epithelial tumor and two submucosal tumors. The patient with the epithelial tumor suffered from breast cancer 2 years 4 months after esophagectomy. Liver and skin metastases were observed in one case of submucosal tumor, and the patient died 2 years after esophagectomy. Tumor cells with amplified and overexpressed *cyclin* D1 gene might have predominant growth in the local lesion, with deep invasion into the esophageal wall and a proliferative course leading to metastasis. At the time of operation when deciding on the therapeutic plan for the patient, it would be valuable to know if the tumor has amplified *cyclin* D1 gene. Jiang et al. [19] demonstrated amplification and expression of *cyclin* D1 gene in human esophageal carcinoma cells. Amplification and overexpression of *cyclin* D1 gene might lead to uncontrollable cell growth and proliferation. We have also confirmed overexpression of *cyclin* D1 gene with gene amplification in esophageal carcinomas. The expression of *cyclin* D1 gene was increased after treatment with exogenous EGF and transforming growth factor α (TGF-α). In addition, the *cyclin* D2 and *cyclin* E genes were found to be amplified in colorectal carcinomas [20]. Although overexpression of the *cyclin* gene-provoked cellular transformation is not yet proved, amplification or overexpression of the *cyclin* gene family plays an important role in the carcinogenesis of human esophageal cancer and is a good biologic marker of malignancy for human esophageal carcinomas.

Although the amplification of EGFR gene and c-*myc* gene has been reported in esophageal carcinomas, the incidence of amplification is not high compared to that of the *hst*-1 and *int*-2 genes.

The significance of this phenomenon is not yet known. Point mutations of the *ras* gene family are rare events in esophageal carcinoma tissue [21].

Abnormality in Cell Cycle Regulator Genes

Carcinomas are characterized by uncontrolled cell growth. Cellular proliferation follows an orderly progression through the cell cycle, which is governed by protein complexes composed of cyclins and cyclin-dependent kinases [22]. These complexes exert their regulatory functions by phosphorylation of key proteins involved in cell cycle transitions, such as the product encoded by the retinoblastoma gene (pRb). Cyclin D1, functionally forming a complex with CDK4/CDK6, is involved in G1–S transition and may play an important role in carcinogenesis. Mutations and overexpression of cyclins and cyclin-dependent kinases, mainly cyclin D1 and CDK4, have been reported [22]. The expression of cyclin D family members is mediated by many growth factors including EGF and TGF-α, whereas the expression of cyclin E and cyclins A and B is cell cycle-dependent. We have already described the frequent amplification of *cyclin* D1 gene in esophageal carcinomas and its significance for tumor progression.

Several candidates for CDK-inhibitory molecules have been identified. Because of their recessive nature in cell cycle control and the fact that some of them are mutated in human tumors, it has been suggested that they may also function as tumor suppressor genes. These genes include *p21 (SDI1/WAF1/CIP1)* [23–25], *p27 (KIP1)* [26], *p16 (MTS1)* [27], and *p15 (MTS2)* [28]. The *p16* mutations have been reported in a variety of human tumors, including esophageal carcinomas, breast tumors, and brain tumors [27]. The P16 protein binds to CDK4 and inhibits the cyclin D1–CDK complex, which phosphorylates pRb. The gene encoding P15 (*MTS2*) also binds to CDK4 and CDK6. Most esophageal cancer cell lines contain homozygous deletions of the *p16* and *p15* genes associated with overexpression of cyclin D1, CDK4, p27^{KIP1}, and phosphorylated Rb protein, suggesting loss of the *p16* gene; subsequent overexpression of cyclin D1 and CDK4 could confer autonomous growth of esophageal cancer cells [29].

Tumor Suppressor Genes

The loss of genes at specific chromosomal loci has been demonstrated to be involved in the development of a number of human cancers, including hereditary and nonhereditary lesions. It is now believed that gene loss on specific chromosomes is associated with carcinogenesis, as tumor suppressor genes may be located on or near those loci. As suggested in Knudson's two-hit models [30], allelic loss or LOH and mutations of the other allele is required to inactivate the tumor suppressor genes. In esophageal carcinomas, allelic losses at frequencies of at least 30% were observed at loci on chromosomal arms 3p, 3q, 5q, 9p, 9q, 10p, 13q, 17p, 17q, 18q, 19q, and 21q [7, 8] (Table 1).

The most common type of mutation or LOH in human tumors seems to be that affecting the *p53* gene, which is located on chromosome 17p13. As mentioned above, alterations in the gene occur at an early stage of esophageal carcinogenesis (e.g., dysplasia and carcinoma in situ) [31]. Point mutation of the *p53* gene is detected in about 40% of esophageal carcinomas, most of which are missense mutations. Considering the base substitution spectrum, G:C to T:A transversion is common in esophageal carcinomas, which is similar to that in carcinomas of the lung and liver and different from that observed in colorectal carcinomas, which share transition of CpG to TpG [32, 33]. Point mutations of the *p53* gene result in altered conformation and increased stability of the product, leading to the accumulation of P53 protein. This protein accumulation and gene mutation were reported to occur at the early stages of esophageal carcinogenesis. In addition, the prognosis of the patient with mutated P53 protein-positive tumors is poorer than those without mutated P53 protein [34].

The gene encodes a 53-kDa nuclear phosphoprotein, which is a negative regulator of the G1–S phase transition in the cell cycle. A current model of P53 function is that it is activated when DNA damage occurs and serves to block DNA replication; hence it allows time for repair of DNA. Wild-type *p53* functions as a transcription factor for several genes, such as *p21* (*SDI1/WAF1/CIP1*), *GADD45*, and *bax* [23–25, 35]. The promoters of these genes have a P53-binding site, and transcription is activated by wild-type *p53* but not by the mutated one. The *p21* gene is a negative regulator of the cell cycle; it does so by inhibiting enzyme activity of various cyclin–cyclin-dependent kinase (CDK) complexes. GADD45 binds to PCNA, a normal component of CDK complexes, and is involved in DNA replication and repair synthesis. BAX, complexing with BCL-2, induces apoptosis. Therefore P53 inactivation may confer esophageal tumorigenesis through abnormal cell growth, DNA repair, and cell survival.

As mentioned in a previous section, the negative cell cycle regulators are also considered to be tumor suppressor genes because the loss of cell cycle inhibitors would lead to unbridled cell proliferation. The loss of *p15* and *p16* genes, each of which is located on chromosome 9p21, may contribute to uncontrolled growth of esophageal cancer [9, 10, 27]. Moreover, the loss of P21 protein contributes to the highly malignant nature of esophageal carcinoma (unpublished observation). Although mutations of the *APC* gene are rare [36], LOH of the *Rb* gene on chromosome 13q [37] and *BRCA1* on chromosome 17q [38] is frequently observed in human esophageal carcinomas. Another candidate tumor suppressor gene, the *FHIT* gene on chromosome 3p14.2, has been isolated [39]. As frequent abnormalities of this gene are reported in head and neck cancer cells [40], it is interesting to examine the alteration of the gene in human esophageal carcinomas.

Genetic instability is also an important phenomenon in human cancers. For example, mutations of *MSH2* and *MLH1*, which are mismatch repair genes, are responsible for hereditary nonpolyposis coli cancer (HNPCC) [41, 42]. Mutations of these genes may cause defects in the DNA-mismatch repair system. Replication

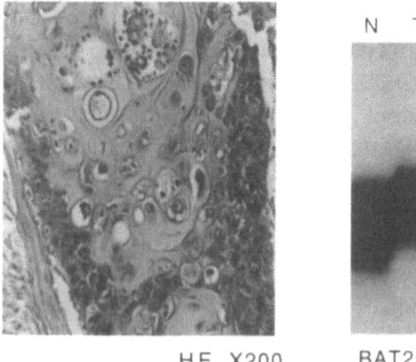

Fig. 2. Microsatellite instability assay showing an RER-positive result in tumor tissue. *N*, normal tissue; *T*, tumor tissue

errors (RER) can be detected by examining microsatellite loci in DNA from tumor tissues and their normal counterparts (Fig. 2). Whether a defect in DNA repair gene plays an important role in carcinogenesis of human esophageal carcinoma is not yet known [43, 44]. Further studies are being conducted to elucidate the pathogenesis of human esophageal carcinomas.

Abnormal Growth Factor Network in Esophageal Carcinomas

The functions of growth factors are mediated through autocrine or paracrine pathways [45]. Most of the cancer cells produce autocrine growth factors, which act through receptors on their cell membrane. Paracrine growth factors, which are produced by cancer cells or interstitial cells, act on cells adjacent to the cells that produce them. The first event of signal transduction through growth factor receptors is dimerization of the receptors, which leads to phosphorylation of tyrosine kinase on the receptors [46]. The interaction between receptors and their intracellular component is mediated through *src* homology domains, which are commonly identified structures in intracellular substrate that include phospholipase C-γ, Ras GTPase-activating protein, phosphatidylinositol-3′-kinase, and members of the *src* family of tyrosine kinases [47–49]. The signals through receptors such as EGFR and PDGFR are mediated through Ras and then through the phosphorylation cascade of *raf*-1 and MAP kinase, which is transported to the nucleus of the cells for proliferation and differentiation [50].

Epidermal Growth Factor and Receptor Family

Epidermal growth factor and TGF-α act through the EGFR (Table 2) and share many biological activities. The expression of either TGF-α or EGFR alone is not sufficient to induce the transformed phenotype in NIH 3T3 cells; both TGF-α and EGFR overexpression is essential to transform the cells. In many cancer cells both EGF and TGF-α act as autocrine growth factors through EGFR [51]. On the other hand, membrane-bound TGF-α binds to EGFR on the surface of contiguous cells and induces receptor

autophosphorylation, leading to signal transduction, which is regarded as juxtacrine growth stimulation [52].

The EGFR is encoded by the proto-oncogene c-*erb*B1 [53]. Amplification and overexpression of the EGFR gene are detected not only in esophageal carcinomas but in a variety of other tumors as well, such as brain tumors, breast carcinomas, and gastric carcinomas [54–57]. Ozawa et al. [58] reported that EGFR was expressed in high numbers in squamous cell carcinomas of the esophagus. We have demonstrated that EGF binding capacity ranges from 4.0×10^5 to 9.0×10^5 sites/cell with a dissociation constant (K_d) of 10^{-9} M [51]. An elevated EGFR level is now regarded as a significant prognostic indicator for esophageal carcinoma [59]. Moreover, esophageal carcinoma cells express EGF and TGF-α mRNA and proteins [60]. The expression of EGF mRNA was detected in 8 (29.6%) of 27 tumors including the cell lines, whereas the TGF-α and EGFR genes were expressed in 21 (77.8%) and 24 (88.9%) of the 27 tumors, respectively [61] (Fig. 3). The EGF content of TE-1 cells is 210 pg/10^6 cells measured by an enzyme-linked immunosorbent assay (ELISA). The number of EGFR sites and EGF content are about 10 times higher than those in gastric carcinoma cells, which might be one of the reasons for the rapid growth of esophageal carcinomas compared to that of other carcinomas. Anti-EGF monoclonal antibody or anti-TGF-α monoclonal antibody inhibited the growth of TE-1 esophageal carcinoma cells. These results suggest that EGF or TGF-α, the ligand of hyperproduced EGFR in esophageal carcinomas, may act as autocrine growth factors.

Table 2. Growth factors and receptors in esophageal carcinomas

Growth factor	Receptor
EGF family	
EGF	EGFR
TGF-α	EGFR
Amphregulin	ERBB3
	ERBB2
PDGF family:	PDGF α- and β-receptor
PDGF A- and B-chains	
Sex hormone	ER
TGF-β family	TGF-β type I, II, III receptor

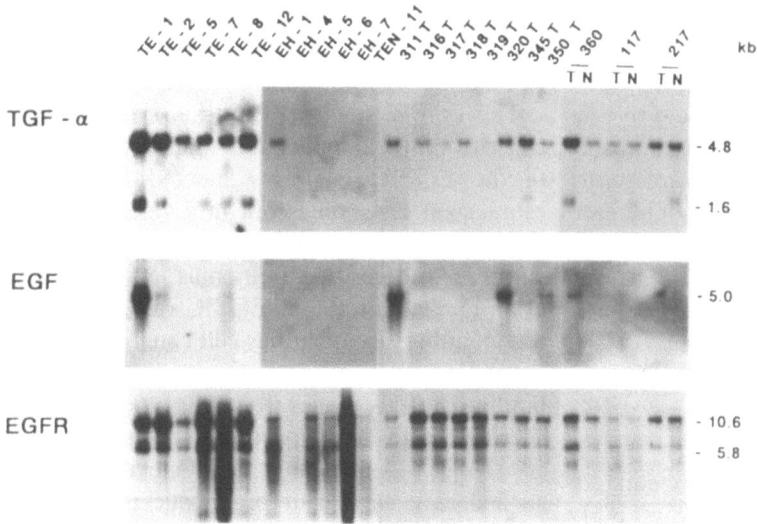

Fig. 3. Expression of mRNA for transforming growth factor-α (*TGF-α*), epidermal growth factor (*EGF*), and EGF receptor (*EGFR*) in human esophageal carcinoma cell lines and tissues. *T*, tumor tissue; *N*, adjacent normal mucosa

The effect of EGF and TGF-α on the expression of mRNA for EGF, EGFR, and *ERBB2* gene was different; that is, TGF-α increased EGF, EGFR, and ERBB2 mRNA expression, whereas EGF decreased the expression [61]. The mechanism of these effects remains to be elucidated.

Two new members of the EGF family, Cripto and Amphiregulin, have been identified [62, 63]. Cripto, a protein of 188 amino acids, has a central portion of the molecule that shares structural homology with EGF and TGF-α. Expression of this molecule is widely detected in a variety of tumor tissues. The expression is correlated with tumor invasion and patient prognosis in gastric and colorectal carcinomas [64, 65].

Amphiregulin is a heparin-binding growth factor whose C-terminal region has homology to EGF. Amphiregulin induces tyrosine autophosphorylation of the EGFR and indirectly ERBB3 [66]. EGF or TGF-α induces mRNA of amphiregulin by gastric carcinoma cells, indicating involvement of the molecule in the autocrine growth stimulatory loop induced by EGF or TGF-α.

Platelet-Derived Growth Factor/Receptor and Estrogen Receptor

Platelet-derived growth factor (PDGF) is made up of two related A- and B-chains, which form homodimers (AA, BB) and heterodimers (AB). Two distinct types of PDGF receptor, α- and β-receptors, have been identified (Table 2). The α-receptor binds all three isoforms of PDGF with equally high affinity, whereas the β-receptor binds only PDGF BB with high affinity [67]. The PDGF B-chain precursor bears a close similarity to the protein of the transforming gene, v-*sis*, of the simian sarcoma virus [68, 69].

Esophageal carcinomas express PDGF A- and B-chains and PDGF B-receptor, suggesting the existence of a multiautocrine loop in the growth and progression of tumor cells. We have detected the expression of PDGF A-chain in all the primary esophageal carcinomas tested [27]. PDGF B-chain and PDGF B-receptor mRNA expression are detected in 66.7% and 74.1%, respectively, of esophageal carcinomas. PDGF B-type receptor was detected in 53% of gastric carcinoma tissues, and its expression was closely related to fibrous stroma. Esophageal carcinomas examined here had no relation to fibrous stroma [70].

What is interesting is that EGF or TGF-α induces the expression of EGF, TGF-α, and EGFR genes, suggesting an autostimulation mechanism. Moreover, the expression of PDGF A- and B-chains is also increased after EGF or TGF-α treatment by TE-1 cells [61]. Pandiell and Massague [71] showed that membrane-bound pro-TGF-α is cleaved by an elastase-like enzyme, which suggests the existence of mechanisms that control the switch of TGF-α from a juxtacrine to a paracrine growth factor. This cleavage is activated by protein kinase C (PKC)-dependent and PKC-independent mechanisms. EGFR and PDGF receptor might activate phospholipase C, resulting in activation of PKC. These findings suggest that

EGF and TGF-α regulate the expression of PDGF, and that PDGF also controls the switch of TGF α-mediated cell growth.

The initial alteration in the regulation of EGF or TGF-α might lead to enhanced expression of the EGF, TGF-α, or EGFR gene. The advantage conferred by EGFR overexpression may be subsequently enhanced and stabilized by gene amplification. EGFR mRNA overexpression can precede gene amplification, which implies that EGFR overexpression takes place in the absence of EGFR gene amplification in human cancers. These clones may exhibit predominant growth and then have a proliferative advantage to metastasis [72]. Above all, EGF and TGF-α not only act as autocrine growth regulators but also function as multigrowth factor modulators leading to uncontrolled growth and progression in human esophageal carcinomas.

Estrogen receptor (ER) has been found to be present in a variety of human tumors, including breast, uterine, gastric, hepatocellular, pancreatic, rectal, and lung carcinomas. Sex hormone receptors (Table 2), including the ER and androgen receptor, have been detected also in human esophageal carcinoma [71]. Interestingly, Matsuoka et al. [73] reported that growth of the esophageal carcinoma cell line with ERs and testosterone receptors was inhibited by administration of estrogen and enhanced by testosterone, which may be one reason for the high incidence of esophageal carcinomas in men and the good prognosis in women.

Transforming Growth Factor β

Transforming growth factor β (TGF-β) exhibits characteristics different from those of other growth factors. Although TGF-β was originally isolated as a fibroblast-transforming factor, it acts as a growth suppressor for benign and malignant epithelial cells. TGF-β is a heterodimer peptide of 25 kDa and consists of five family members (TGF-β1–5). The biological activity of the molecule is regulated by its latent TGF-β-binding protein and proteolytic enzymes [74]. Three distinct receptors for TGF-β (types I, II, and III) have been identified (Table 2) [75]. Type I and II receptors are responsible for its biological functions [76, 77]. The structure of type II receptor includes a cysteine-rich extracellular domain and a cytoplasmic serine/threonine kinase domain. The type II

receptor requires both kinase activity and association with type I receptor to signal growth inhibition. The growth inhibitory mechanism of TGF-β is that it inhibits phosphorylation of CDK2 and subsequently inhibits phosphorylation of *Rb* gene product, which stops the cell cycle to G_1 phase [26]. The expression of TGF-β mRNA is commonly detected in esophageal carcinoma cells and tissues [71]. The biological significance of the molecule in the esophagus is not yet known.

Molecular Mechanism of Invasion and Metastasis of Esophageal Carcinomas

Cancer invasion and metastasis involve a complicated process that includes enzymatic proteolysis, cell motility, and cell adhesion through cancer–stroma interaction [78, 79]. Extracellular degenerative enzymes are assumed to play an important role in tumor invasion and metastasis [80]. Kerr et al. [81] demonstrated that transin RNA is induced by EGF, PDGF, and the tumor promoter 12-O-tetradecanoylphorbol-13-acetate in NIH 3T3 fibroblasts; other authors have reported an opposite regulatory action of TGF-β on extracellular proteolytic activities by carcinoma cells and fibroblasts. It is intriguing that EGF and TGF-α induce the expression of mRNA for interstitial collagenase, stromelysin, and type IV collagenase genes, which might lead to invasive growth of the tumor cells [61, 82]. The increased Fos protein with transcription factor JUN/AP-1 binds to the promoter region of collagenase and stromelysin genes, which increases the transcription of these genes. A TGF-β inhibitory element was found to be present in the promoter region of these genes, suggesting complicated regulation of their expression [81]. Further studies are needed on the transcriptional regulation of these genes in esophageal carcinomas.

E-Cadherin is one of the important components of cell adhesion molecules and may be a crucial determinant of tumor metastasis [83]. The expression of E-cadherin is reduced in 45% of cancers of various organs, including the esophagus, stomach, and breast [84]. The frequency of reduced E-cadherin expression is higher in tumors with infiltrative growth than those with expansive growth. For esophageal cancer the frequency of downregulation of E-cadherin expression in tumors with extensive lymph node metastasis was significantly higher compared to that of their counterparts [85].

E-cadherin is now regarded as a product of suppression or impairment of transcripts of the E-cadherin structural gene and protease cleavage of E-cadherin peptides. Moreover, linkage between transmembranous cadherins and actin filament of the cytoskeleton is necessary to form strong cell–cell adhesion, including the catenins vinculin and actin [86]. Catenins are a series of cadherin-associated cytophasmic proteins composed of α-, β-, and γ-catenins. α-Catenin directly binds to the cytoplasmic domain of cadherin, a connection that is the first step in the complicated linkage between cadherin and actin filament. After this connection, α-catenin binds to vinculin, which can cross-link actin filaments. The cadherin–catenin complex is indispensable for cadherin function and cell–cell adhesion. The reduction of α-catenin expression, as well as that of E-cadherin, is significantly associated with tumor dedifferentiation, infiltrative growth, and lymph node metastasis [87]. In esophageal carcinomas, reduced α-catenin expression is more significantly correlated with the invasive phenotype with lymph node metastasis than is E-cadherin expression [86]. E-cadherin function is down-regulated through the tyrosine phosphorylation of β-catenin induced by hepatocyte growth factor (HGF) and EGF. β-Catenin may be a key molecule for cadherin-mediated cell adhesion activity during the process that effects cell movement and cell migration and eventually cell infiltration and metastasis. Interestingly, EGF induces tyrosine phosphorylation of β-catenin and E-cadherin and may modulate cadherin–catenin adhesion through tyrosine kinase receptors. The down-regulation of E-cadherin by EGF may be a significant factor that facilitates cell invasion [29]. Moreover, the *APC* gene product associated with α- and β-catenin may be important to malignant cell transformation [88, 89].

Above all, esophageal carcinomas exhibit multiple autocrine growth factor–receptor loops that may participate not only in cell growth but also in tumor invasion and metastasis. Understanding the biology of esophageal cancer is indispensable to precise diagnosis and proper cancer treatment.

References

1. Tahara E (1995) Genetic alterations in human gastrointestinal cancers. Cancer 75:1410–1417

2. Qui SL, Yang GR (1988) Precursor lesion of esophageal cancer in high-risk populations in Henan province, China. Cancer 62:551–557

3. Tahara E (1996) Molecular diagnosis of gastrointestinal cancers: the application to clinical practice. Int J Clin Oncol 1:63–68

4. Yoshida K, Kawami H, Kuniyasu H, Nishiyama M, Yasui W, Hirai T, Toge T, Tahara E (1994) Coamplification of *cyclin* D, *hst*-1 and *int*-2 genes is a good biological marker of high malignancy for human esophageal carcinomas. Oncol Rep 1:493–496

5. Kitagawa Y, Ueda M, Ando N, Shinozawa Y, Shimizu N, Abe O (1991) Significance of *int*-2/*hst*-1 coamplification as a prognostic factor in patients with esophageal carcinoma. Cancer Res 51:1504–1508

6. Tsuda T, Tahara E, Kajiyama G, Sakamoto H, Terada M, Sugimura T (1989) High incidence of coamplification of *hst*-1 and *int*-2 genes in human esophageal carcinomas. Cancer Res 49:5505–5508

7. Aoki T, Du X, Nishihira T, Matsubara T, Nakamura Y (1994) Allelotype of esophageal carcinoma. Genes Chromosom Cancer 10:177–182

8. Shibagaki I, Shimada Y, Wagata T, Ikenaga M, Imamura M, Ishizaki K (1994) Allelotype analysis of esophageal squamous cell carcinoma. Cancer Res 54:2996–3000

9. Igaki H, Sasaki H, Kishi T, Sakamoto H, Tachimori Y, Kato H, Watanabe H, Sugimura T, Terada M (1994) Highly frequent homozygous deletion of the *p16* gene in esophageal cancer cell lines. Biochem Biophys Res Commun 203:1090–1095

10. Zhou X, Tarmin L, Yin J, Jiang HY, Suzuki H, Rhyu MG, Abraham JM, Meltzer SJ (1994) The *MTS1* gene is frequently mutated in primary human esophageal tumours. Oncogene 9:3737–3741

11. Piris MA, Sanchez-Beato M, Villuendas R, Martinez JC (1996) Oncogenes and tumour-suppressor genes. In: Cell proliferation in cancer. Oxford Press, Oxford, pp 45–81

12. Weinberg RA (1991) Tumour suppressor genes. Science 254:1138–1146

13. Brookstein R, Shew JY, Chen PL, Scully P, Lee WH (1990) Suppression of tumourigenicity of human prostate carcinoma cells by replacing a mutated *Rb* gene. Science 247:712–715

14. Haber DA, Buckler AJ, Glaser T, Call KM, Pelletier J, Sohn RL, Douglass EC, Housman DE (1990) An internal deletion within an 11p13 zinc finger gene contributes to the development of Wilm's tumour. Cell 61:1257–1269

15. Kinzler KW, Nilbert MC, Su L-K, Vogelstein B, Bryan TM, Lery DB, Smith KJ, Pressinger AC, Hedge P, Mckechnie D, Finniear R, Markham A, Groffen J, Boguski MS, Altschul SF, Horii A, Ando

H, Miyoshi Y, Miki Y, Nishisho I, Nakamura Y (1991) Identification of *FAP* locus genes from chromosome 5q21. Science 253:661–665

16. Kanda Y, Nishiyama Y, Shimada Y, Imamura M, Nomura H, Hiai H, Hukumoto M (1994) Analysis of gene amplification and overexpression in human esophageal carcinoma cell lines. Int J Cancer 58: 291–297

17. Motokura T, Bloom T, Kim HG, Juppner H, Ruderman JV, Kronenberg HM, Arnold A (1991) A novel cyclin encoded by a *bcl*-II linked candidate oncogene. Nature 350:512–515

18. Lew DJ, Vjekoslav D, Reed SI (1991) Isolation of three novel human cyclins by rescue of C1 *cyclin* (Cln) function in yeast. Cell 66:1197–1206

19. Jiang W, Kahn SM, Tomita N, Zhang Y-J, Lu S-H, Weinstein B (1992) Amplification and expression of the human *cyclin* D gene in esophageal cancer. Cancer Res 52:2980–2983

20. Leach FS, Elledge SJ, Sherr CJ, Willson JKV, Markowitz S, Kinzler KW, Vogelstein B (1993) Amplification of cyclin genes in colorectal carcinomas. Cancer Res 52:1986–1989

21. Galiana C, Fusco A, Martel N, Nishihira T, Hirohashi S, Yamasaki H (1993) Possible role of activated *ras* genes in human esophageal carcinogenesis. Int J Cancer 54:978–982

22. Cordon-Cardo C (1995) Mutaion of cell cycle regulators: biological and clinical implications for human neoplasia. Am J Pathol 147:545–560

23. Noda A, Ning Y, Venable SF, Percira-Smith OM, Smith JR (1994) Cloning of senescent cell derived inhibitors of DNA synthesis using an expression screen. Exp Cell Res 11:90–98

24. Harper JW, Adami GR, Wei N, Keyomarsi K, Elledge SJ (1993) The *p21 cdk*-interacting protein Cip is a potent inhibitor of G1 *cyclin*-dependent kinase. Cell 75:805–816

25. El-Deiry WS, Tokino T, Velculescu VE, Levy DB, Parsons R, Trent JM, Lin D, Mercer E, Kinzler KW, Vogelstein B (1993) WAF-1, a potential mediator of *p53* tumour suppression. Cell 75:817–825

26. Toyoshima H, Hunter T (1994) P27, a novel inhibitor of G1 cyclin-cdk protein kinase activity, is related to P21. Cell 78:67–74

27. Serrano M, Hannon GJ, Beach D (1993) A new regulatory motif in cell-cycle control causing specific inhibition of cyclin D/CDK4. Nature 366:704–707

28. Hammon GJ, Beach D (1994) p15INK4B is a potential effector of TGF-β induced cell cycle arrest. Nature 371:257–261

29. Tahara E, Semba S, Tahara H (1996) Molecular biological observations in gastric cancer. Semin Oncol 23:307–315

30. Knudson AG (1989) Mutation and cancer: statistical study of retinoblastoma. Proc Natl Acad Sci USA 68:820–823

31. Wang Li D, Zhou Q, Hong JY, Qui SL, Yang CS (1996) P53 protein accumulation and gene mutations in multifocal esophageal precancerous lesions from symptom free subjects in a high incidence area for esophageal carcinoma in Henan, China. Cancer 77:1244–1249

32. Hollstein MC, Metcalf RA, Welsh JA, Montesano R, Harris CC (1990) Frequent mutation of the *p53* gene in human esophageal cancer. Proc Natl Acad Sci USA 87:9958–9961

33. Hollstein M, Sidransky D, Vogelstein B, Harris CC (1991) *p53* mutations in human cancers. Science 253:49–53

34. Shimaya K, Shiozaki H, Inoue M, Tahara H, Monden T, Shimano T, Mori T (1993) Significance of P53 expression as a prognostic factor in esophageal squamous cell carcinoma. Virchows Arch [A] 422:271–276

35. Miyahita T, Reed JC (1995) Tumor suppressor *p53* is a direct transcriptional activator of the human *bax* gene. Cell 80:293–299

36. Powell SM, Papadopous N, Kinzler KW, Smolinski KN, Meltzer SJ (1994) *APC* gene mutation cluster regions are rare in esophageal cancers. Gastroenterology 107:1759–1763

37. Boynton RF, Huang Y, Blount PL, Reid BJ, Raskind WH, Haggitt RC, Newkirk C, Resau JH, Yin J, McDaniel T (1991) Frequent loss of heterozygosity at the retinoblastoma locus in human esophageal cancers. Cancer Res 51:5766–5769

38. Mori T, Aoki T, Matsubara T, Iida F, Du X, Nishihira T, Mori S, Nakamura Y (1994) Frequent loss of heterozygosity in the region including *BRCA1* on chromosome 17q in squamous cell carcinoma of the esophagus. Cancer Res 54:1638–1640

39. Ohta M, Onoue H, Cotticelli MG, Kastury K, Baffa R, Palazzo J, Siprashvili Z, Mori M, McCue P, Druck T, Croce CM, Huebner K (1996) The *FHIT* gene, spanning the chromosome 3p14.2 fragile site and renal carcinoma-associated t(3;8) breakpoint, is abnormal in digestive tract cancers. Cell 84:587–597

40. Mao L, Fan YH, Lotan L, Hong WK (1996) Frequent abnormalities of *FHIT*, a candidate tumour suppressor gene, in head and neck cell lines. Cancer Res 56:5128–5131

41. Fishel R, Lescoe MK, Rao MRS, Copeland NG, Jenkins NA, Garber J, Kane M, Kolodner R (1993) The human mutator gene homolog *MSH2* and its association with hereditary nonpolyposis colon cancer. Cell 75:1027–1038

42. Papadopoulos N, Nicolaides NC, Wei YF, Ruben SM, Carter KC, Rosen CA, Haseltine WA, Fleischmann RD, Fraser CM, Adams MD (1994) Mutation of a mutL homolog in hereditary colon cancer. Science 263:1625–1629

43. Nakashima H, Mori M, Mimori K, Inoue H, Shibuta K, Baba K, Mafune K, Akiyoshi T (1995) Microsatellite instability in Japanese esophageal carcinoma. Int J Cancer 64:286–289

44. Ogasawara S, Maesawa C, Tamura G, Satodate R (1995) Frequent microsatellite alterations on chromosome 3p in esophageal squamous cell carcinoma. Cancer Res 55:891–894

45. Sporn MB, Roberts AB (1985) Autocrine growth factors and cancer. Nature 313:745–747

46. Ullrich A, Schlessinger J (1990) Signal transduction by receptors with tyrosine kinase activity. Cell 61:203–212

47. Pawson T, Gish GD (1992) SH2 and SH3 domains; from structure to function. Cell 71:359–362

48. Koch CA, Anderson D, Moran MF, Ellis C, Pawson T (1991) SH2 and SH3 domains; elements that control interactions of cytoplasmic signaling proteins. Science 252:668–674

49. Tahara E, Yasui W, Yokozaki H (1996) Abnormal growth factor networks in neoplasia. In: Cell proliferation in cancer. Oxford Press, Oxford, pp 133–153

50. Heidecker G, Kelch W, Morrison DK, Rapp UR (1992) The role of Raf-1-phosphorylation in signal transduction. Adv Cancer Res 58:53–73

51. Yoshida K, Yasui W, Ito H, Tahara E (1990) Growth factors in progression of human esophageal and gastric carcinomas. Exp Pathol 40:291–300

52. Wong ST, Winchell LF, McCune BK, Earp HS, Teixido J, Massague J, Herman BM, Lee DC (1989) The TGF-α precursor on the cell surface binds to the EGF receptor on adjacent cells, leading to signal transduction. Cell 56:495–506

53. Downward J, Yarden Y, Mayes E, Scrace G, Totty N, Stockwell P, Ullrich A, Schlessinger J, Waterfield WD (1984) Close similarity of epidermal growth factor receptor and v-erb-B oncogene protein sequences. Nature 307:521–527

54. Hunts J, Ueda M, Ozawa S, Abe O, Patan I, Shimizu N (1985) Hyperproduction and gene amplification of the epidermal growth factor receptor in squamous cell carcinoma. Jpn J Cancer Res 76:663–666

55. Wong AJ, Binger SH, Binger DD, Kinzler KW, Hamilton SR, Vogelstein B (1987) Increased expression of epidermal growth factor receptor gene in malignant gliomas is invariably associated with gene amplification. Proc Natl Acad Sci USA 84:6899–6903

56. Sainsbury JRC, Farndon JR, Needham GK, Malcolm AJ, Harris AL (1987) Epidermal growth factor receptor status as predictor of early recurrence or of death from breast cancer. Lancet 1:1398–1401

57. Yoshida K, Tsuda T, Mtsumura T, Tsujino T, Hattori T, Ito H, Tahara E (1989) Amplification of epidermal growth factor receptor (EGFR) gene and oncogenes in human gastric carcinomas. Virchows Arch [B] 57:285–290

58. Ozawa S, Ueda M, Ando N, Abe O, Shimizu N (1988) Epidermal growth factor receptors in cancer tissue of esophagus, lung, pancreas, colorectum, breast and stomach. Jpn J Cancer Res 79:1201–1207

59. Mukaida H, Toi M, Hirai T, Yamashita Y, Toge T (1991) Clinical significance of the expression of epidermal growth factor and its receptor in esophageal cancer. Cancer 68:142–148

60. Yoshida K, Tsuda T, Tsujino T, Ito M, Niimoto M, Tahara E (1990) EGF and TGFα, the ligand of hyperproduced EGFR in human esophageal carcinoma cells, act as autocrine growth factors. Int J Cancer 45:131–135

61. Yoshida K, Kuniyasu H, Yasui W, Kitadai Y, Toge T, Tahara E (1993) Expression of growth factors and their receptors in human esophageal carcinomas; regulation of expression by epidermal growth factor and transforming growth factor-α. J Cancer Res Clin Oncol 119:401–407

62. Ciccordicola A, Dono R, Obici S, Simeone A, Zollo M, Persico MG (1989) Molecular characterization of a gene of the EGF family expressed in undifferentiated human NTERA2 teratocarcinoma cell. EMBO J 8:1987–1991

63. Shoyab M, Plowman GD, McDonald VL, Bradley JG, Todaro GJ (1989) Structure and function of human amphiregulin: a member of the epidermal growth factor family. Science 243:1074–1076

64. Ciardiello F, Dono R, Kim N, Persico MG, Slamon DS (1991) Expression of cripto, a novel gene of the epidermal growth factor gene family, leads to the in vitro transformation of a normal mouse mammary epithelial cell line. Cancer Res 51:1051–1054

65. Kuniyasu H, Yoshida K, Yokozaki H, Yasui W, Ito H, Toge T, Ciardiello F, Persico G, Saeki T, Salmon DS, Tahara E (1991) Expression of cripto, a novel gene of the epidermal growth factor family, in human gastrointestinal carcinomas. Jpn J Cancer Res 82:969–973

66. Johnson GR, Kannan B, Shoyab M, Stromberg K (1993) Amphiregulin induces tyrosine phosphorylation of the epidermal growth factor receptor and p185 erbB2. J Biol Chem 268:2924–2931

67. Matsui T, Heidaran M, Miki T, Toru M, Popescu N, La Rochelle W, Kraus M, Pierce J, Aaronson SA (1989) Isolation of a novel receptor cDNA establishes the existence of two PDGF receptor genes. Science 243:800–803

68. Waterfield MD, Scrace GT, Whittle N, Stroobant P, Johnsson A, Wasteson A, Westmark B, Heldin CH, Huang JS, Deuel TF (1983) Platelet-derived growth factor is structurally related to the putative transforming protein P28sis of simian sarcoma virus. Nature 304:35–39

69. Bejcek BE, Li DY, Deuel TF (1989) Transformation by v-*sis* occurs by an internal autoactivation mechanism. Science 245:1496–1499

70. Tsuda T, Yoshida K, Tsujino T, Nakayama H, Kajiyama G, Tahara E (1989) Coexpression of platelet-derived growth factor (PDGF) A chain and PDGF receptor genes in human gastric carcinomas. Jpn J Cancer Res 80:813–817

71. Pandiell A, Massague J (1991) Cleavage of the membrane precursor for transforming growth factor α is a regulated process. Proc Natl Acad Sci USA 88:1726–1730

72. Enoki Y, Niwa O, Yokoro K, Toge T (1990) Analysis of clonal evolution in tumour consisting of pSV2 neo-transfected mouse fibrosarcoma clones. Jpn J Cancer Res 81:141–147

73. Matsuoka H, Sugimach K, Ueo H, Kuwano H, Nakao S, Nakayama M (1987) Sex hormone response of a newly established squamous cell line derived from clinical esophageal carcinoma. Cancer Res 47:4134–4140

74. Taipale J, Miyazono K, Heldin CH, Keski-Oja J (1994) Latent transforming growth factor-beta 1 associates to fibroblast extracellular matrix via latent TGF-beta binding protein. J Cell Biol 124:171–181

75. Massague J (1992) Receptors for the TGF-β family. Cell 69:1067–1070

76. Tahara E, Kuniyasu H, Yasui W, Yokozaki H (1994) Abnormal expression of growth factors and their receptors in stomach cancer. Gann Monogr Cancer Res 42:163–173

77. Ito M, Yasui W, Kyo E, Yokozaki H, Nakayama H, Ito H, Tahara E (1992) Growth inhibition of transforming growth factor β on human gastric carcinoma cells: receptor and postreceptor signaling. Cancer Res 52:295–300

78. Tarin D (1996) Metastasis: secondary proliferation in distant organs. In: Cell proliferation in cancer. Oxford Press, Oxford, pp 316–336

79. Folkman J, Klagsbrun M (1987) Angiogenic factors. Science 235:442–447

80. Liotta LA, Tyggvason K, Garbisa S, Hart I, Foltz CM, Shafie S (1980) Metastatic potential correlates with enzymatic degradation of basement membrane collagen. Nature 284:67–68

81. Kerr LD, Holt JT, Matrisian LM (1988) Growth factors regulate transin gene expression by c-*fos*-dependent and c-*fos*-independent pathways. Science 242:1424–1427

82. Yoshida K, Tsujino T, Yasui W, Kameda T, Sano T, Nakayama H, Toge T, Tahara E (1990) Induction of growth factor receptor and metalloproteinase genes by epidermal growth factor and/or transforming growth factor alpha in human gastric carcinoma cell line MKN-28. Jpn J Cancer Res 81:793–798

83. Frixen UH, Behrrens J, Sachs M, Eberle G, Voss B, Warda A (1991) E-Cadherin-mediated cell–cell adhesion prevents invasiveness of human carcinoma cells. J Cell Biol 113:173–185

84. Shiozaki H, Tahara H, Oka H, Miyata M, Kobayashi K, Tamura S (1991) Expression of immuno-reactive E-cadherin adhesion molecules in human cancers. Am J Pathol 139:17–23

85. Kadowaki T, Shiozaki H, Inoue M, Tamura S, Oka H, Doki Y (1994) E-Cadherin and α-catenin expression in human esophageal cancer. Cancer Res 54:196–201

86. Shiozaki H, Oka H, Inoue M, Tamura S, Monden M (1996) E-Cadherin mediated adhesion system in cancer cells. Cancer 77:1605–1613

87. Yasui W, Kuniyasu H, Akama Y, Kitahara K, Nagafuchi A, Ishihara S, Tsukita S, Tahara E (1995) Expression of E-cadherin, α-catenins in human gastric carcinomas: correlation with histology and tumor progression. Oncol Rep 2:111–117

88. Rubinfeld B, Souza B, Albert B, Muller I, Chamberlain O, Masiarz SC (1993) Association of the *APC* gene product with beta-catenin. Science 262:1731–1734

89. Su LK, Vogelstein B, Kinzler KW (1993) Association of the *APC* tumour suppressor protein with catenins. Science 262:1734–1737

Genetic Alterations in the Precursors of Gastric Cancer

Atsushi Ochiai and Setsuo Hirohashi

Summary. The presence of multiple genetic alterations has been established in human cancers. The evolution of sequential histological changes from normal cells through invasive cancer provides the opportunity to elucidate the molecular basis of this progression. The paradigm for such studies involves the identification of molecular genetic events that occur during the evolution of various human carcinomas, including gastric cancer. Several studies have demonstrated that multiple genetic alterations, comprising oncogene and tumor-suppressor gene mutations and loss of heterozygosity, play roles in cancer development and progression. Two histological forms of gastric carcinoma (intestinal and diffuse) and their different histogenetic and etiological backgrounds suggest that different spectra of genetic changes are involved in different tumor types. That same genetic alterations, including oncogenes and tumor-suppressor genes, have been detected in the precursors of both intestinal- and diffuse-type gastric cancers, but no specific genetic alterations have been detected in the latter. The genetic alterations in precursor lesions of gastric cancer and chronic atrophic gastritis, a precancerous condition, are summarized here. Also presented are the results of investigations into *p53* tumor-suppressor gene mutations in nonneoplastic gastric mucosa exhibiting chronic atrophic gastritis with intestinal metaplasia, an early genetic change.

Introduction

Gastric cancers have been classified by Lauren into two subtypes—intestinal and diffuse [1]—which correspond to Nakamura et al.'s classification of gastric adenocarcinomas: differentiated and undifferentiated, respectively [2]. Intestinal-type (differentiated) gastric cancer, which is more prevalent in males and older individuals than females and the young, is composed of cells resembling intestinal columnar epithelial cells and is associated with widespread intestinal metaplasia in the vicinity of the tumor [1, 3, 4]. Diffuse-type (undifferentiated) gastric cancer is characterized by poorly cohesive tumor cells that show wide, diffuse infiltration of the gastric wall. With respect to the histogenesis of these two gastric cancer subtypes, the results of morphological and epidemiological studies support the hypothesis that there is a link between intestinal metaplasia and intestinal-type gastric cancer. Results obtained in histopathological studies on the surrounding mucosa of minute adenocarcinomas (tumor diameters less than 5 mm) showed that intestinal-type adenocarcinomas arise in metaplastic mucosa, and diffuse type lesions occur in nonmetaplastic gastric mucosa [5, 6].

Chronic infection with *Helicobacter pylori* [7] and excess salt and nitrosamine compound intake [8] are suspected to be important causal factors in gastric cancer. Correa hypothesized that carcinogenesis of the stomach is a multistage process [9], and the progression from normal epithelial cells to tumor cells involves at least six stages: superficial gastritis, chronic atrophic gastritis, intestinal metaplasia of the complete (small intestinal) type followed by the incomplete (colonic) type, gastric adenoma, dysplasia, and carcinoma. It is not clear which steps of the gastric carcinogenetic process such carcinogenic agents affect. Furthermore, no direct correlations between these carcinogenic agents and intestinal metaplasia as a precancerous condition have been established. Identification of the precancerous lesions in nonneoplastic gastric mucosa comprising chronic atrophic gastritis and intestinal metaplasia should provide important information on gastric carcinogenetic pathways.

Molecular genetic studies have established that most human tumors display multiple genetic al-

Pathology Division, National Cancer Center Research Institute, 5-1-1 Tsukiji, Chuo-ku, Tokyo 104, Japan

terations [10, 11]. The molecular biology of gastric carcinomas is expected to reflect the heterogeneity of their causes and histological subtypes, and clonal divergence within tumors is likely to add heterogeneous gene products to those associated with different cancer types. Such alterations are also considered to underlie the multistage processes of carcinogenesis and tumor progression, although in most cases the precise sequence of genetic events is unclear. It has become clear that gastric carcinomas also display multiple genetic alterations [12–14], including alterations of oncogenes, tumor-suppressor genes, and chromosomal loss of heterozygosity (LOH). The genetic alterations detected in gastric cancers to date are summarized in Table 1. An accumulation of genetic alterations was found in both intestinal- and diffuse-type gastric cancers. Two *ras* gene family members (Ki-*ras* and Ha-*ras*), c-*erb*B-2 gene, and *APC* and *p53* tumor-suppressor genes were found mainly in intestinal-type gastric cancers, whereas k-*sam* and c-*met* genes were detected in diffuse-type gastric cancers. Detection of these genetic alterations in precancerous conditions, such as chronic atrophic gastritis, should provide information useful for identifying precancerous lesions of gastric carcinomas. However, in general, the frequencies of genetic alterations detected in gastric cancers are too low to enable the causal genetic changes that occur at the early stages of gastric carcinogenesis to be determined.

Among the genetic changes observed in gastric cancers, *p53* tumor-suppressor gene mutations have been detected most frequently. We and other investigators have detected *p53* gene mutations in human gastric cancers, even in the early stages [15, 16]; and about 40% of intestinal-type gastric cancers had *p53* gene mutations in both the early and advanced stages. We examined the regional differences related to heterogeneous differentiation and invasiveness of *p53* mutations in advanced gastric carcinomas and found that most of the advanced gastric cancers showed the same *p53* mutations, despite their different histological morphologies and invasion sites [17]. The finding that the *p53* gene mutation frequecy in both early and advanced gastric adenocarcinomas is the same suggests that *p53* mutations occur at an early gastric carcinogenetic step.

As well as accumulating information about genetic alterations in gastric carcinomas, genetic changes in precursor lesions of, and precancerous conditions associated with, gastric cancer have been reported. The genetic alterations in precursor lesions of gastric cancer and chronic atrophic gastritis, a precancerous condition, are summarized here; and the findings of investigations into *p53* tumor-suppresor gene mutations in chronic atrophic gastritis with intestinal metaplasia are presented.

Genetic Alterations in Precancerous Lesions and Precancerous Conditions

Precancerous Conditions and Precancerous Lesions

It has been suggested that precursors of gastric cancer are divided into two categories: precancerous conditions and precancerous lesions [18]. Precancerous conditions are clinical entities associated with an increased incidence of gastric cancer development, whereas precancerous lesions are pathological lesions from which gastric carcinomas have been reported to develop. A summary of precancerous lesions of gastric cancer and precancerous conditions associated with it is presented in Table 2.

The precancerous lesion of many gastric cancers is adenoma of the stomach. Hirota et al. reported that about 21% of gastric adenomas were accompanied by cancer [19], whereas the incidence of cancer developing in chronic ulcers lasting more than 5 years is around 0.5% to 2.0%, and

Table 1. Genetic alterations in gastric cancers

Genetic alterations	Frequency		Reference
	Intestinal	Diffuse	
Gene mutation			
Ki-*ras*	3/17	0/18	30
p53	40/100	0/18	16
APC	9/36	3/21	34
Gene amplification			
c-*erb*B-2	5/13	0/17	49
k-*sam*	0/35	10/48	50
c-*met*		15/64	51
Loss of heterozygosity			
5		3/13	52
13q		14/36	53
17		17/23	54
18		8/19	55

Table 2. Precursors of gastric cancer

Gastric adenoma
Gastric dysplasia
Chronic atrophic gastritis
   With intestinal metaplasia
   Gastritis Verruciform
Hyperplastic polyp
Chronic peptic ulcer
Postresection gastric stump
Menetrier's disease

the incidence of cancer in stomachs resected for clinically benign ulcers is about 2% [20]. The malignant transformation rate of chronic peptic ulcer is lower than expected previously, but hyperplastic polyps and gastritis verruciform, which were thought to be reactive changes, have been proved to develop into gastric cancers. Daibo et al. reported that 10 of 477 hyperplastic polyps (2.1%) were associated with a focal carcinoma [21].

Intestinal Metaplasia and Gastric Cancer

The term "metaplasia" means the replacement of one adult tissue by another. Intestinal metaplasia of the stomach is defined as the replacement of antral or fundic gastric mucosa by glands composed of epithelium resembling that of the small intestine. Intestinal metaplasia has been classified into complete (small intestinal) and incomplete (colonic) types based on the findings of light microscopy and histochemical studies [22]. The incomplete type was subdivided into two subtypes, according to the histochemical characteristics: one with *O*-acetylated sialomucin and the other with sulfomucin [23]. Matsukura et al. classified intestinal metaplasia into complete and incomplete types according to their enzymological features [24]. The former exhibited sucrase, trehalase, leucine aminopeptidase, and alkaline phosphatase activities, whereas the latter had sucrase and leucine aminopeptidase, but no trehalase or alkaline phosphatase, activities. The classification criteria used in studies are not always the same. For example, incomplete metaplasia has been defined as that without Paneth cells, lacking certain enzymes, or with the presence of mucous cells in place of absorptive cells; moreover, the types of mucin used for distinguishing small intestinal and colonic types of

metaplasia differ. There is a definite need for a unified concept for classification.

Histological investigations on small gastric cancers (tumors with diameters <5mm) have indicated a high degree of association between intestinal-type gastric cancer and incomplete-type metaplasia in the surrounding mucosa. Hirota et al. reported that the frequency of metaplasia surrounding the gastric mucosa decreased, in the following order: gastric carcinoma (87.3%), benign gastric ulcer (84.1%), gastric polyps (65.0%), duodenal ulcers (38.4%). The association of nonmetaplastic gastritis with carcinoma is less frequent (12.7%) [25]. These data indicate that there is a close relation between gastric carcinoma and chronic gastritis with intestinal metaplasia.

Sipponen et al. reported a correlation between the occurrence of sulfomucin-positive intestinal metaplasia and gastric cancer detected in an endoscopic survey of a large Finnish population [26]. Thirty-one percent of the patients with gastric cancer showed sulfomucin-positive intestinal metaplasia, whereas this lesion occurred in only 6% of the benign cases. Sulfomucin-positive intestinal metaplasia was present frequently in the immediate vicinity of intestinal-type carcinomas; and the mucin profiles of sulfomucin-positive intestinal metaplasia and intestinal-type carcinomas were similar, indicating there is a close relation between intestinal metaplasia and intestinal-type sulfomucin-producing carcinomas.

Genetic Alterations in Precancerous Lesions

Most investigations into genetic changes in precancerous lesions have been carried out on adenomas. The genetic alterations in precancerous lesions of gastric cancer are summarized in Table 3. Ki-*ras*, *p53*, and *APC* tumor-suppressor gene mutations have been reported in gastric adenomas.

Ki-ras Gene

Three members of the *ras* oncogene family (H-, Ki-, and N-*ras*) were first detected in human cancers as transforming genes in the transfection assay using NIH/3T3 cells [27, 28]. These genes, which encode closely related 21 kDa proteins, are highly conserved among species. The Ras proteins bind guanine nucleotides with high affinity and serve as transducer molecules for signals regulating cell proliferation and differentiation. Muta-

Table 3. Genetic alterations in gastric adenomas

Gene	Reference
Oncogene	
Ki-*ras*	30
Tumor-suppressor genes	
APC	35
p53	40

tions at the codon 12, 13, and 61 amino acid positions confer transforming activity; and point mutation of the c-Ki-*ras* oncogene has been detected frequently in adenocarcinomas of the colon, pancreas, and bile duct [29]. Fewer than 10% of gastric carcinomas have been reported to show Ki-*ras* mutations, which were found in one of seven gastric adenomas [30]. Studies on *ras* expression have shown increased Ras p21 protein levels not only in carcinomas but also in noncancerous epithelia such as dysplasia, intestinal metaplasia, and regenerating epithelium adjacent to peptic ulceration [31].

APC *Tumor-Suppressor Gene*

The *APC* gene, which was isolated as a tumor-suppressor gene for familial adenomatous polyposis (FAP), is located at chromosome 5q21 [32, 33], and *APC* gene mutations have been detected in colorectal carcinomas occurring in FAP patients and sporadically. Most mutations lead to truncation of the *APC* gene product. Among gastric carcinomas, *APC* gene mutations were detected in both intestinal (differentiated) and diffuse (undifferentiated) types, especially in very well differentiated adenocarcinomas [34]. Some signet-ring cell carcinomas were also found to possess *APC* gene mutations, and *APC* gene mutations were present in 6 of 30 gastric adenomas (20%) [35].

p53 *Tumor-Suppressor Gene*

The p53 protein, originally identified as a protein that forms a stable complex with the SV40 large T antigen, was thought to be an oncogene but is now defined as a tumor-suppressor gene. It is located on chromosome 17p13, the inactivation of which has been suggested to be involved in carcinogenesis of various organs. Mutations of the *p53* gene are clustered at four hot spots in highly conserved regions; and the locations of the muta-

tions and types of base change they show have been demonstrated to differ among cancers of different organs [36, 37]. In gastric cancers, approximately 40% of intestinal-type adenocarcinomas showed *p53* gene mutations [38, 39], and Tohdo et al. reported that 4 of 10 gastric adenomas possessed such mutations [40].

Shiao et al. reported that dysplastic epithelium of the stomach also possessed *p53* gene mutations. Most mutation patterns in gastric adenomas were G:C to A:T, which is also the main mutation pattern of gastric adenocarcinomas [41].

Genetic Alterations in Chronic Atrophic Gastritis

Detection of genetic alterations in mucosa showing chronic atrophic gastritis is considered difficult because chronic atrophic gastritis is so common it can be difficult to obtain a sample of the precancerous lesion present in the mucosa. The genetic alterations detected in gastric mucosa obtained from patients with chronic atrophic gastritis are summarized in Table 4. The genetic alterations in chronic atrophic gastritis were also found in several genes, including *ras*, *tpr-met*, *cripto*, and *p53* tumor-suppressor genes, and telomere reduction in chronic atrophic gastritis has been reported.

ras *Gene*

The mutation of the *ras* gene in chronic atrophic gastritis has also been reported. Tahara et al. observed the point mutation of the Ki-*ras* gene in 1 of 10 endoscopic biopsy specimens of metaplastic mucosa obtained from 10 patients [42].

tpr-met *Gene*

The *tpr-met* oncogenic rearrangement was first observed in MNNG-transformed cells of an osteosarcoma cell line (HOS). The rearrangement involved fusion of the translocated promoter region (*tpr*) locus present on chromosome 1 to the 5′

Table 4. Genetic alterations in chronic atrophic gastritis

Genetic alteration	Positive cases (no.)
Ki-*ras* mutation	1/10
tpr-met expression	9/13
cripto overexpression	10/12

regions of *met* gene sequences located on chromosome 7 [43]. Soman et al. reported that expression of *tpr-met* protein was also detected in gastric cancer, and they observed *tpr-met* expression in 9 of 13 patients with nonneoplastic mucosa associated with chronic gastritis [44].

cripto *Gene*

The *cripto* gene, which encodes 188 amino acids and is a member of the family of transforming genes of the epidermal growth factor (EGF), was cloned from an undifferentiated human teratocarcinoma cell line, NTERA2 clone D1 (NT2D1) [45]. The cDNA of this gene encodes 188 amino acids, the central portion of which is structurally homologous with human EGF, human transforming growth factor-α (TGF-α), and human amphiregulin. Overexpression of the *cripto* gene has been detected in gastric and colonic carcinomas; nonneoplastic mucosa with intestinal metaplasia has also been found to overexpress it [46].

Telomere Reduction

Telomere shortening has been proposed to be the major mitotic clock mechanism whereby cells know how many times to divide. Telomere DNA length decreases with in vitro and in vivo division of human somatic cells [47, 48]. In immortalized cells in vitro, telomere length is stabilized by the activation of telomerase, which elongates telomeres de novo. Tahara et al. reported telomere reduction in gastric mucosa with intestinal metaplasia [42].

p53 Alteration in Chronic Atrophic Gastritis

Detection of *p53* Protein Nuclear Accumulation in the Mucosa of Chronic Atrophic Gastritis

To investigate the earliest genetic alterations that occur in the mucosa with chronic atrophic gastritis, we carried out systematic investigations of *p53* gene mutations in noncancerous gastric mucosa. Sixteen patients who underwent resection for gastric cancer at the National Cancer Center Hospital in Tokyo from 1992 to 1993 were selected for a retrospective study to detect *p53* alterations in nonneoplastic gastric mucosa. Of these 16 patients, 7 had single early gastric cancer, one had

advanced cancer, and 8 had double or multiple gastric cancers. All the gastric cancers examined were intestinal-type adenocarcinomas and comprised papillary adenocarcinomas (pap, 1 lesion) and well differentiated (tub1, 22 lesions) and moderately differentiated (tub2, 6 lesion) tubular adenocarcinomas, according to the histological classification of the general rules for gastric cancer study in surgery and pathology of the Japanese Research Society for Gastric Cancer [49]. All the resected stomachs were fixed with formalin, and step-cut sections of virtually the entire stomach were examined histologically. To examine the nonneoplastic gastric mucosa, 756 serial sections 3 μm thick were cut from blocks of nonneoplastic gastric mucosa from the 16 gastric cancer patients and stained with hematoxylin and eosin (H&E). Intestinal metaplasia was detected in 477 of these 756 sections; complete-type intestinal metaplasia with absorptive epithelial cells, goblet cells, and Paneth cells was detected in 125 of the 477, and incomplete-type intestinal metaplasia lacking absorptive cells and Paneth cells was observed in 352.

The methods used for immunohistochemical staining of formalin-fixed paraffin-embedded sections with the antibody RSP-53 are described in detail elsewhere [16, 17]. RSP-53 (Nichirei, Tokyo, Japan) is a polyclonal antibody against p53 protein raised in rabbits immunized against amino acids 54–69 of synthetic p53 peptide; it reacts with both wild and mutant forms of p53 protein. The p53-positive foci detected comprised 5 single lesions in 5 patients with a single gastric cancer and 14 lesions in 6 patients with multiple gastric cancers. A total of 19 foci of p53-positive glands were detected by immunohistochemical staining among the 756 sections of nonneoplastic gastric mucosa examined. As shown in Table 5, 17 of the 19 (89.5%) p53-positive lesions were detected in tissues showing intestinal metaplasia with or without atypia, and 2 (10.5%) were in pseudoploric glands of the regenerative gastric mucosa. Of the 17 (23.5%) p53-positive intestinal mataplastic lesions, 4 showed mild atypia, which consisted of round or oval nuclei, structural atypia, or both.

Figure 1 shows representative features of p53-positive intestinal metaplasia with slight to mild atypia (case 8) in comparison with the surrounding intestinal metaplastic glands. However, it was not easy to distinguish p53-positive from surrounding p53-negative metaplastic glands exhibit-

Table 5. p53 Alterations detected by immunohistochemistry and PCR-SSCP and mucin histochemistry in nonneoplastic gastric mucosa

Case no.	Histology of cancer	Histology of p53-positive glands	Sulfomucin production	p53 Alteration delected by PCR-SSCP
1	tub2	IM, incomplete	−	ND
2	tub1, tub1	IM, incomplete	−	−
3	tub1	IM, incomplete	+	−
4	tub1, tub2	IM, incomplete	+	ND
5		Regenerative mucosa	−	ND
6		Regenerative mucosa	−	ND
7		IM, incomplete	−	ND
8	tub2	IM, incomplete	−	exon 5
9	tub1, multiple	IM, incomplete	−	exon 7
10		IM, incomplete	−	−
11		IM, incomplete	−	exon 5
12		IM, incomplete	−	IS
13		IM, incomplete	−	IS
14		IM, incomplete	−	IS
15	tub2	IM, incomplete	+	exon 5
16	pap, tub1	IM, incomplete	−	−
17	tub2, tub2	IM, incomplete	−	IS
18	tub1, multiple	IM, incomplete	−	−
19	tub1	IM, incomplete	−	−

IM, intestinal metaplasia; PG, pyloric gland; tub1, well-differentiated tubular adenocarcinoma; tub2, moderately differentiated tubular adenocarcinoma; ND, not detected for complete PCR-SSCP analysis of exons 5 to 8; IS, insufficient specimen.

ing various levels of regenerative atypia. All the p53-positive intestinal metaplastic lesions were of the histologically incomplete type and possessed neither Paneth cells nor brush borders at the base of the glands. Nuclear accumulation of p53 protein was not observed in whole metaplastic glands but was present in their lower halves, which are thought to be proliferative zones. Slightly fewer goblet cells were observed in areas showing p53-positive intestinal metaplasia than in those that did not. A few scattered foveolar epithelial nuclei were p53-positive.

p53 Gene Mutations in Chronic Atrophic Gastritis

To confirm the presence of *p53* gene mutations in the nonneoplastic intestinal metaplasia associated with chronic atrophic gastritis, at least two sheets of 10μm thick sections from each lesion were stained with RSP53, and the p53-positive glands were excised selectively with microscissors under a light microscope. The method used to extract the DNA from formalin-fixed, paraffin-embedded sections is described elsewhere [15]. Briefly, the excised tissues containing p53-positive glands were treated with proteinase K (Sigma) for 24 hours at 37°C followed by phenol/chloroform extraction; the DNAs extracted were examined by polymerase chain reaction single-strand conformation polymorphism (PCR-SSCP) analysis of exons 5 to 8 of the *p53* gene, as described previously [15]. To avoid tissue and DNA contamination from other dysplastic or carcinomatous tissues, at least two independent experiments were performed. Oligonucleotide primers with sequences corresponding mainly to those of the exons used to amplify exons 5 to 8 were designed on the basis of the published sequence of the *p53* gene and synthesized using a DNA synthesizer (model 391; Applied Biosystems Japan, Tokyo, Japan) followed by purification with an oligonucleotide purification column. The primers used for p53 analysis (exons 5 to 8) in the present study are described elsewhere [15, 16]. They were labeled with $[\gamma^{32}P]dATP$, and a PCR assay comprising 34 cycles, each consisting of amplification for 3 minutes at 94°C, 1 minute at 55°C, and 2 minutes at 72°C, was carried out. The PCR products were diluted serially and applied to 1% (w/v) (exons 5,

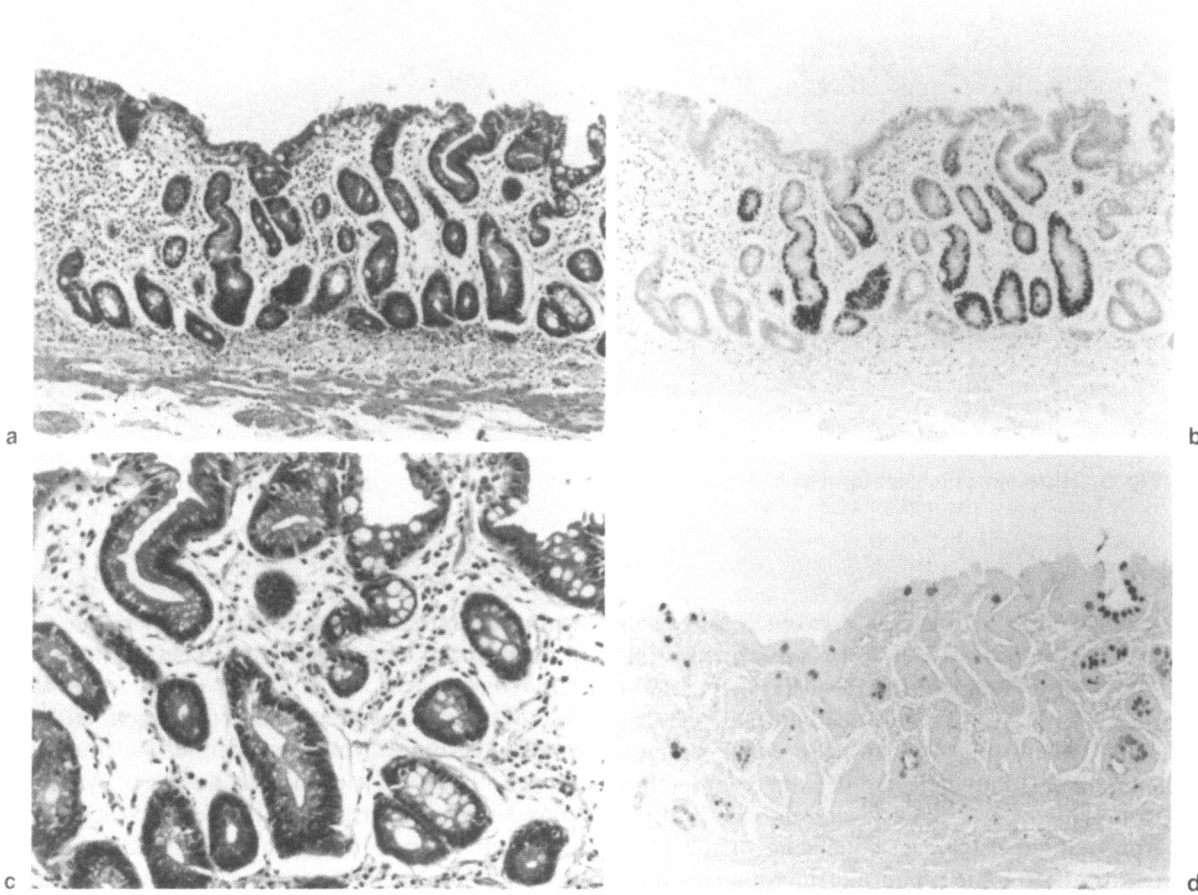

Fig. 1a–d. Histology of p53-positive intestinal metaplasia. **a,c** H&E staining. **b** p53 Immunohistochemistry. **d** HID-alcianblue staining for sulfomucin

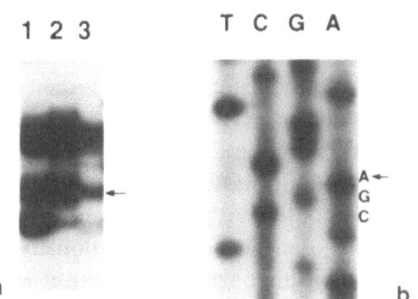

Fig. 2a,b. PCR-SSCP analysis **a** and direct sequencing **b** of DNA from a lesion in patient 9 on exon 7

6, and 7) and 2% (w/v) (exon 8) polyacrylamide gels without glycerol and to 4% (w/v) (exon 5) and 1% (w/v) (exons 6, 7, and 8) polyacrylamide gels containing 5% (v/v) glycerol. After electrophoresis, the gels were dried on filter paper and autoradiographed overnight using x-ray film (Kodak XRP-1) at −80°C. The abnormally migrating bands detected by PCR-SSCP analysis were eluted from the gels and amplified using phosphated and nonphosphated oligonucleotide primers, as described previously [15]. Each amplified DNA was annealed with the appropriate [γ^{32}P]dATP-labeled primer, and the sequence reaction was performed using a Sequenase version 2.0 kit (United States Biochemicals, Cleveland, OH, USA). These samples were electrophoresed on 5% to 8% (w/v) acrylamide sequence gel containing 7.5 M urea, which was then dried on filter paper and subjected to autoradiography. The sequencing primers used for each of the exons were the same as those used for the PCR-SSCP analysis.

Not enough DNA could be obtained from the p53-positive glands in all the samples, and com-

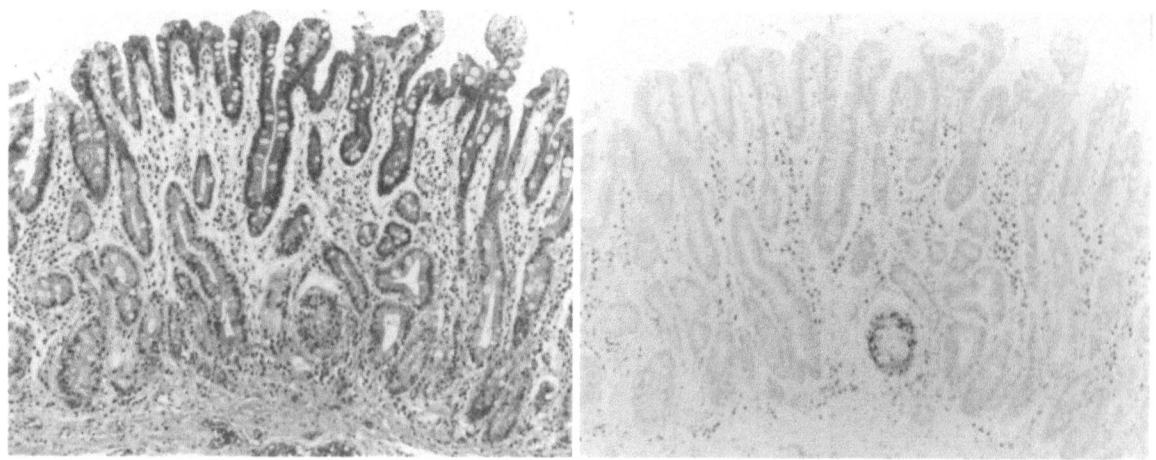

Fig. 3. Histology of mutant form of p53 in the mucosa of chronic atrophic gastritis **a** using PAB240 antibody **b**

plete PCR-SSCP analysis of exons 5 to 8 of the DNAs from only 10 of 19 lesions was possible. The DNAs obtained from 4 of these 10 patients (nos. 8, 9, 11, and 15) showed abnormal migration bands when subjected to PCR-SSCP analysis. These bands were detected in exon 5 of the DNA from patients 8, 11, and 15 and in exon 7 of that from patient 9. Direct sequencing of the DNA extracted from each abnormal migrating band was performed by PCR-SSCP analysis, the results of which, together with those of direct sequencing of the p53-positive intestinal metaplastic tissues, are shown in Table 5 and Fig. 2. Three mutations were found in exon 5 (patients 8, 11, and 15) and one in exon 7 (patient 9). Direct sequencing analysis of these abnormal migrating bands showed a CCC to CGC mutation at codon 117 in exon 5, TGC to AGC at codon 182 in exon 5, and GGC to AGC at codon 245 in exon 7. These findings are summarized in Table 5.

Table 6. p53-Positive cells and glands in 50 cases of nonneoplastic gastric mucosa

p53-Positive cells	Cases (no.)
By antibody to mutant and wild-type p53 (RSP 53)	
A few cells	13
Several cells	18
More than 10 cells	3
By antibody to mutant form of p53 (PAB 240)	
A few cells	4
Glands (more than 10 cells)	1

Immunohistochemical Detection of *p53* Mutations in Chronic Atrophic Gastritis

To investigate the frequency of *p53*-mutated lesions in chronic atrophic gastritis, 454 sections of nonneoplastic gastric mucosa obtained from 50 consecutive patients who underwent gastric resection were stained immunohistochemically with a *p53*-mutation-specific antibody. The resected gastric tumors comprised 27 intestinal-type and 22 diffuse-type gastric cancers and one malignant lymphoma of the stomach.

Mutant form p53 protein in chronic atrophic gastritis was detected immunohistochemically by applying a monoclonal antibody, PAb 240 (Novocastra), which is specific for mutant p53 protein, to AMeX-fixed tissues. A total of 454 sections of nonneoplastic gastric mucosa obtained from surgically resected stomachs were fixed with AMeX and embedded in paraffin. The specificity of the PAb 240 antibody for mutant forms of p53 protein was confirmed by performing both Western blotting analysis and immunohistochemical staining of cell lines with and without *p53* mutations. This antibody did not react with wild-type p53 in human bronchial epithelial cells transfected with SV40 large T antigen, but it did react with an HCC cell line. Table 6 shows the immunohistochemical staining results. Examination of the 454 sections revealed that the Pab 240 antibody reacted with only one gland from one patient and one or two cells from four patients (Fig. 3). The frequency of p53-positive glands is estimated to be about 0.0087 positive foci/cm of the H&E

section. These results indicate that *p53* gene mutations had occurred in the nonneoplastic mucosa of chronic atrophic gastritis, especially incomplete-type intestinal metaplasia.

Conclusions

Evidence obtained from molecular genetic analyses of precancerous conditions, lesions, and gastric carcinomas suggests that gastric cancers develop from nonneoplastic gastric mucosa with chronic atrophic gastritis through multiple steps, thereby accumulating multiple genetic alterations. First, some genetic changes occur in gastric mucosa with chronic atrophic gastritis or intestinal metaplasia, a precancerous condition. Epithelial cells with genetic alterations, if they acquire growth advantages or genetic instability, expand clonally and accumulate additional mutations, leading to precancerous lesions (adenoma and dysplasia), early carcinoma, a locally aggressive tumor, and finally an advanced tumor with metastatic capability.

The data accumulated on genetic alterations during the various steps in gastric cancer progression also indicate that the multiple gastric carcinogenetic steps in the two histological subtypes of gastric cancer, intestinal and diffuse, differ. The former, which is associated with intestinal metaplasia in the vicinity of the tumor, may have a similar carcinogenic pathway to colorectal cancer, as these two cancers both show *ras*, *p53*, and *APC* gene mutations. On the other hand, the genetic changes in the early stage of diffuse-type gastric cancer have not yet been elucidated, and K-*sam* and c-*met* gene amplification has been detected only in the late stages of this type of gastric cancer. Although *tpr-met* rearrangement in chronic atrophic gastritis has been reported, all precancerous lesions have been proved to possess this type of gene rearrangement. The precursor lesion of diffuse-type gastric cancer remains to be elucidated. To clarity this lesion, further developments in molecular biological and genetic techniques are needed.

The genetic alterations discussed here undoubtedly play important roles in the multistage progression of gastric carcinomas. Studies are needed to clarify the genetic alterations that occur during the early gastric carcinogenetic stages in order to discover the risk factors for and mechanisms of genetic susceptibility to gastric cancer. Elucidation of these multiple genetic alterations in gastric carcinogenesis should clarify the differences between the natural histories of intestinal- and diffuse-type gastric cancers and hopefully provide important information that will help prevent gastric cancer.

References

1. Lauren P (1965) The two histological main types of gastric carcinoma: diffuse and so-called intestinal-type carcinoma; an attempt at a histoclinical classification. Acta Pathol Microbiol Scand 64:31–49
2. Nakamura K, Sugano H, Takagi K, Kumakura K (1967) Histogenesis of carcinoma of the stomach with special reference to 50 primary microcarcinomas: light- and electron-microscopic and statistical studies. Jpn J Cancer Clin 15:627–647
3. Morson BC (1955) Carcinoma arising from areas of intestinal metaplasia in the gastric mucosa. Br J Cancer 9:377–385
4. Jass JR (1980) Role of intestinal metaplasia in the histogenesis of gastric carcinoma. J Clin Oncol 33:801–810
5. Nakamura K, Sugano H, Takagi K (1967) Histopathological study on early carcinoma of the stomach: some considerations on the ulcer cancer by analysis of 144 foci of the superficial spreading carcinomas. Gann 58:377–387
6. Nakamura K, Sugano H, Takagi K (1968) Carcinoma of the stomach in incipient phase: its histogenesis and histological appearances. Gann 59:251–258
7. Blaser MJ (1987) Gastric *Campylobacter*-like organisms, gastritis and peptic ulcer disease. Gastroenterology 93:37–383
8. Sugimura T, Wakabayashi K (1990) Gastric carcinogenesis: diet as a causative factor. Med Oncol Tumor Pharamacother 7:87–92
9. Correa P (1970) Carcinoma and intestinal metaplasia of the stomach in Colombian migrants. J Natl Cancer Inst 44:297–306
10. Marx J (1989) Many gene changes found in cancer. Science 246:1386–1388
11. Fearon ER, Vogelstein B (1990) A genetic model for colorectal tumorigenesis. Cell 61:759–767
12. Hirohashi S, Sugimura T (1991) Genetic alterations in human gastric cancer. Cancer Cells 3:49–52
13. Tahara E (1993) Molecular mechanism of stomach carcinogenesis. J Cancer Res Clin Oncol 119:455–465
14. Stemmermann G, Heffelfinger SC, Noffsinger A, Hui UZ, Miller MA, Fenoglio-Preiser CM (1994) The molecular biology of esophageal and gastric cancer and their precursors: oncogenes, tumor suppressor genes, and growth factors. Hum Pathol 25:968–981

15. Yokozaki H, Kuniyasu K, Kitadai Y, Nishimura K, Todoh H, Auhan A, Tahara E (1992) *p53* point mutations in primary human gastric carcinomas. Cancer Res Clin Oncol 119:67–70

16. Uchino S, Noguchi M, Ochiai A, Saito T, Kobayashi M, Hirohashi S (1993) *p53* mutation in gastric cancer: a genetic model for carcinogenesis is common to gastric and colorectal cancer. Int J Cancer 54:759–764

17. Cho JH, Noguchi M, Ochiai A, Uchino S, Hirohashi S (1994) Analysis of regional differences of *p53* mutation in advanced gastric carcinoma: relation to heterogeneous differentiation and invasiveness. Mod Pathol 7:205–211

18. Morson BC, Sobin LH, Grundmann E, Johansen A, Negayo T, Serckkhanssen A (1980) Precancerous conditions and epithelial dysplasia in the stomach. J Clin Pathol 33:711–721

19. Hirota T, Okada T, Itabashi M, Kitaoka H (1984) Histogenesis of human gastric cancer—with special reference to the significance of adenoma as a precancerous lesion. In: Ming SC (ed) Precursors of gastric cancer. Praeger, New York, pp 233–252

20. Bajtai A, Juhaz J (1984) Possible correlation between stomach ulcer and cancer. In: Ming SC (ed) Precursors of gastric cancer. Praeger, New York, pp 273–284

21. Daibo M, Itabashi M, Hirota T (1987) Malignant transformation of gastric hyperplastic polyps. Am J Gastroenterol 82:1016–1025

22. Teglbjaerg P, Nielsen HO (1978) "Small intestinal type" and "colonic type" intestinal metaplasia of the human stomach, and their relationship to the histogenetic types of gastric adenocarcinoma. Acta Pathol Micobiol Scand [A] 86:351–355

23. Iida F, Murata F, Nagata T (1978) Histochemical studies of mucosubstances in metaplastic epithelium of the stomach with special reference to the development of intestinal metaplasia. Histochem J 56:229–237

24. Matsukura N, Suzuki K, Kawachi T, Aoyagi M, Sugimura T, Kitaoka H, Numajiri H, Shirota A, Itabashi M, Hirota T (1980) Distribution of marker enzymes and mucin in intestinal metaplasia in human stomachs and relation of complete and incomplete types of metaplasia to minute gastric carcinomas. J Natl Cancer Inst 65:231–240

25. Hirota T, Okada T, Itabashi M, Yoshida H, Matsukura H, Kitaoka H, Hirayama T (1984) Significance of intestinal metaplasia as a precancerous condition of the stomach. In: Ming SC (ed) Precursors of gastric cancer. Praeger, New York, pp 179–193

26. Sipponen P, Seppala K, Varis K, Hjelt L, Ihamaki T, Kekki M, Siurala M (1980) Intestinal metaplasia with colonic-type sulphomucins in the gastric mucosa; its association with gastric carcinoma. Acta Pathol Microbiol Scand [A] 88:217–224

27. Land H, Parada LF, Weinberg RA (1983) Cellular oncogenes and multistep carcinogenesis. Science 222:771–778

28. Barbacid M (1987) *ras* genes. Annu Rev Biochem 56:779–827

29. Sukumar S (1990) An experimental analysis of cancer: role of *ras* oncogenes in multistep carcinogenesis. Cancer Cells 2:199–244

30. Kihana T, Tsuda H, Hirota T, Shimosato Y, Sakamoto H, Terada M, Hirohashi S (1991) Point mutation of c-Ki-*ras* oncogene in gastric adenoma and adenocarcinoma with tubular differentiation. Jpn J Cancer Res 82:308–314

31. Czerniak B, Herz F, Gorczyca W, Koss LG (1989) Expression of *ras* oncogene p21 protein in early gastric carcinoma and adjacent gastric epithelia. Cancer 64:1467–1473

32. Joslyn G, Carlson M, Thliverris A, Albertsen H, Gelbert L, Samowits W, Groden J, Stevens F, Spirio L, Robertson M, Sargeant L, Kraocho K, Wolff E, Burt R, Hughes JP, Warrington J, McPherson J, Wasmuth J, Lepaslier D, Abderrahim H, Cohen D, Leppert M, White R (1991) Identification of deletion mutations and three new genes at the familial polyposis locus. Cell 66:601–613

33. Kinzler KW, Nilbert MC, Su L-K, Vogelstein B, Bryan TM, Levy DB, Smith KJ, Preisinger AC, Hedge P, McKechnie D, Finniear R, Markham A, Groffen J, Boguski MS, Altschul SF, Horii A, Ando H, Miyoshi Y, Nakamura Y (1991) Identification of FAP locus genes from chromosome 5q21. Science 253:661–665

34. Nakatsuru S, Yanagisawa A, Ichii S, Tahara E, Kato Y, Nakamura Y, Horii A (1992) Somatic mutations of the *APC* gene in gastric cancer: frequent mutations in very well differentiated adenocarcinoma and signet-ring cell carcinoma. Hum Mol Genet 1:559–563

35. Tamura G, Maesawa C, Suzuki Y, Tamada H, Satoh M, Ogasawara S, Kashiwaba M, Satodate R (1994) Mutations of the *APC* gene occur during early stages of gastric adenoma development. Cancer Res 54:1149–1151

36. Nigro JM, Baker SJ, Preisinger AC, Jessup JM, Hostetter R, Cleary K, Bigner SH, Davidson N, Baylin S, Devilee P, Glover T, Collins FS, Weston A, Modali R, Harris CC, Vogelstein B (1989) Mutations in the *p53* gene occur in diverse human tumor types. Nature 342:705–708

37. Hollstein M, Sidransky D, Vogelstein, Harris CC (1991) *p53* mutations in human cancers. Science 253:49–53

38. Yokozaki H, Kuniyasu K, Kitadai Y, Nishimura K, Todo H, Ayhan A, Tahara E (1992) *p53* point mu-

tations in primary human gastric carcinomas. Cancer Res Clin Oncol 119:67–70

39. Uchino S, Noguchi M, Ochiai A, Saito T, Kobayashi M, Hirohashi S (1993) *p53* mutation in gastric cancer: a genetic model for carcinogenesis is common to gastric and colorectal cancer. Int J Cancer 54:759–764

40. Tohdo H, Yokozaki H, Haruma K, Kajiyama G, Tahara E (1993) *p53* gene mutations in gastric adenomas. Virchow Arch B Cell Pathol 63:191–195

41. Shiao YH, Rugge M, Correa P, Lehmann PH, Scheer DW (1994) *p53* alteration in gastric precancerous lesions. Am J Pathol 144:511–517

42. Tahara E, Kuniyasu H, Yashi W, Yokozaki H (1994) Gene alterations in intestinal metaplasia and gastric cancer. Eur J Gastroenterol Hepatol 6(suppl 1):pS97–102

43. Park M, Dean M, Cooper CS, Schmidt M, O'Brien SJ, Blair DG, Vande Woude GF (1986) Mechanism of met oncogene activation. Cell 45:895–904

44. Soman NR, Correa P, Ruiz B, Wogan GN (1991) The TPR-MET oncogenic rearrangement is present and expressed in human gastric carcinoma and precursor lesions. Proc Natl Acad Sci USA 88:4892–4896

45. Ciccodicloa A, Dono R, Obici S, Simeone A, Zollo M, Persico MG (1989) Molecular characterization of a gene of the EGF family expressed in undifferentiated human NTERA2 teratocarcinoma cells. EMBO J 8:1987–1991

46. Kuniyasu H, Yoshida K, Yokozaki H, Yasui W, Ito H, Toge T, Ciardiello F, Persico MG, Saeki T, Salomon DS, Tahara E (1991) Expression of *cripto*, a novel gene of the epidermal growth factor family, in human gastrointestinal carcinomas. Jpn J Cancer Res 82:969–973

47. Harley CB, Futcher AB, Greider CW (1990) Telomere shortening during aging of human fibroblasts. Nature 345:458–560

48. Counter CM, Avilion AA, LeFeuver CE, Stewart NG, Greider CW, Harley CB, Bacchetti S (1992) Telomere shortening associated with chromosome instability is arrested in immortal cells which express telomerase activity. EMBO J 11:1921–1929

49. Japanese Research Society for Gastric Cancer (1981) The general rules for the gastric cancer study in surgery and pathology. Jpn J Surg 11:127–139

Molecular Bases of Human Stomach Carcinogenesis

Hiroshi Yokozaki, Hiroki Kuniyasu, Shuho Semba,
Wataru Yasui, and Eiichi Tahara

Summary. Multiple genetic alterations, including inactivation of tumor-suppressor genes, activation of oncogenes, and reactivation of telomerase, are implicated in human stomach carcinogenesis. Among them, replication errors (RERs) at microsatellite loci, reactivation of telomerase, activation of c-*met*, inactivation of *p53*, and deranged *CD44* transcription are common events of both well-differentiated and poorly differentiated gastric carcinomas. In addition to these common events, K-*ras* mutation, *APC* inactivation, loss of *DCC*, and amplification of c-*erb*B2 are preferentially found in well-differentiated gastric carcinomas, whereas gene mutations, loss of the cadherin/catenin system, and amplification of K-*sam* are frequently observed in poorly differentiated cancers. In addition, a paracrine loop formed between cancer cells and stromal cells through the hepatocyte growth factor/c-*met* system plays an important role in morphogenesis and invasion of gastric carcinoma with different status of adhesion molecules and signal transduction systems in vivo. Reduction or loss of *p27* protein, associated with overexpression of *cyclin E*, may confer the progression and metastasis. In regard to precancerous lesions of the stomach, some of the intestinal metaplasias and adenomas exhibited the same genetic alterations (e.g. mutations of *APC* and *p53*, RERs, and reactivation of telomerase) and telomere shortening as those found in well-differentiated carcinomas. Moreover, human telomerase RNA overexpression, which correlates well with the number of *Helicobacter pylori* present, may precede telomerase reactivation in human stomach carcinogenesis. These observations suggest overall that there are two distinct genetic pathways in human stomach carcinogenesis, and some well-differentiated cancers share the same multistep genetic alterations as those established for colorectal cancers.

First Department of Pathology, Hiroshima University School of Medicine, 1-2-3 Kasumi, Minami-ku, Hiroshima 734, Japan

Introduction

The most fascinating hypothesis that links the findings of molecular biology and human carcinogenesis is the one by Fearon and Vogelstein concerning multistep human colorectal carcinogenesis [1]. The stepwise alterations in several tumor-suppressor genes, such as adenomatous polyposis coli (*APC*) gene, *p53* gene, and deleted in colorectal cancer (*DCC*) genes, as well as activation of oncogenes such as K-*ras* gene point mutation, were contrasted chronologically and morphologically in the so-called adenoma–carcinoma sequence of the colorectum. The multiple alterations of genes susceptible for carcinogenesis are also found in stomach cancer [2] (Table 1). In this chapter, we offer a detailed overview of the multistep genetic alterations in stomach carcinogenesis.

Genetic Instability in Human Stomach Carcinogenesis

One of the exciting concepts in human carcinogenesis is the possible participation of genetic or genomic instabilities, which can establish a background of multiple gene abnormalities. The polymerase chain reaction (PCR)-based assay for the altered length of cytosine-adenine (CA) repeat microsatellites, which are scattered all over the human genome, can assess part of the genetic instabilities in human cancers.

Although the frequency of microsatellite instability in human gastric cancer differs depending on the number and nature of microsatellites examined, it is estimated to be around 30% of primary cancers [3–7]. Han et al. detected microsatellite instability in 64% of poorly differentiated and 17% of well-differentiated gastric cancers [3]. Rhyu et al. found microsatellite instability in 31% of gastric cancers [4]. Seruca et al. found that most gastric cancers with microsatellite instability dis-

Table 1. Alterations in tumor suppressor genes, cyclins, oncogenes, and telomerase activity in gastric cancer

Alterations	Well differentiated[a] (%)	Poorly differentiated[a] (%)
Tumor-suppressor genes		
p53 LOH, mutation	60	75
APC LOH, mutation	40–60	0
DCC LOH	50	0
LOH of 1p	30	38
LOH of 1q	44	0
LOH of 7q	53	33
Cyclin and CDK inhibitors		
Cyclin E gene amplification	33	7
Cyclin E overexpression	57	63
p21 overexpression	77	76
p16 loss	12	31
p27 loss	46	69
Oncogenes		
K-*ras* mutation	10	0
c-*met* amplification	19	39
K-*sam* amplification	0	33
c-*erb*B-2 amplification	20	0
Receptor and protein		
EGFR overexpression	50	25
EGF overexpression	40	20
TGFα overexpression	60	55
Osteopontin	86	65
IL-8	75	86
Adhesion molecules		
E-Cadherin, mutation and loss	0	50
CD44 aberrant transcript including intron 9	100	100
Replication error	20–40	20–70
Telomere reduction[b]	62	53
Telomarase activity	100	90

[a] In young patients (under 35 years old).
[b] Under 10 Kb.

played abundant T lymphocyte infiltration and exhibited a relatively good prognosis [8]. We detected CA repeat instability in 33% of well differentiated tumors and in 18% of the poorly differentiated type by analyzing 25 cases of gastric carcinomas [7]. Moreover, we found microsatellite instability in 42% of gastric adenomas and 33% of intestinal metaplasias of the stomach, both of which are considered precancerous lesions of well-differentiated gastric carcinomas [7]. Our results overall indicated that microsatellite instability may occur as an early event of stomach carcinogenesis, contributing to malignant progression, as reported by Strickler et al. [5].

Another important finding on microsatellite instability in human cancer is that multiple primary cancers, including stomach, colon, and gallbladder carcinomas arising in a single case, frequently display replication errors at multiple microsatellites [9]. This finding indicates the possibility of the existence of background abnormalities in some of the DNA mismatch repair genes in these patients. Moreover, detection of microsatellite instability in a cancer may serve as a good molecular marker for the assessment of a second cancer risk in the same patient.

In addition to microsatellite instabilities, telomere length reduction may bring about chromosomal instability, additional genetic alterations, reactivation of telomerase (which is the ribonucleoprotein enzyme that synthesizes telomeric DNA in germline tissues and in immortal tumor cells), and ultimately cancer development [10]. It is known that in normal somatic cells the length of telomeres progressively shorten in the absence of telomerase activity with each cell division and aging, and this shortening of telomeres may function as a mitotic clock by which cells count their division, leading to replicative cellular senescence [11]. Intestinal metaplasias and carcinomas of the stomach display shorter telomere length than that of the normal gastric mucosa [12]. Interestingly, telomere reduction in primary tumors is closely related with increase in tumor staging. However, long telomeres (over 15 kb) are sometimes seen in poorly differentiated gastric cancer (see chapter by H. Tahara et al., this volume).

Most tumor tissues, all metastatic tumors, and all cultured tumor cell lines of gastric cancer express telomerase activity, which is necessary for the immortality of the cell [13, 14]. However, the corresponding normal gastric mucosa is negative for telomerase activity. Therefore the reactivation of telomerase and ensuing telomere stabilization may occur concomitantly with the acquistion of immortality by tumor cells. More interestingly, more than 50% of intestinal metaplasias share short telomeres (under 8 kb). Twenty-three percent of intestinal metaplasias and 50% of stomach adenomas exhibit detectable telomerase activity, indicating that reactivation of telomerase may occur at an early stage of stomach carcinogenesis [13]. Considering the strong correlation between telomerase activity and malignant transformation,

selection for cell immortality may be a critical step in the development of gastric cancers, as is reported in other organs. Measurement of telomerase activity may thus serve as a powerful additional tool for cancer diagnosis.

The RNA component of telomerase (TR) has been cloned [15] and the expression of TR has been assessed in several cancer tissues as well as in cell lines [16]. Blasco et al. [17] reported that TR expression increased in preneoplastic and early stage tumors, whereas telomerase activity was evident only in late-stage tumors in two mouse models. We also found that most primary gastric carcinomas expressed higher levels of TR than that of the corresponding gastric mucosa [18]. Moreover, the expression of human TR, which correlated well with *Helicobacter pylori* infection, may precede telomerase reactivation during human stomach carcinogenesis [18].

Alterations of Tumor-Suppressor Genes in Human Stomach Carcinogenesis

Stomach cancer shows frequent loss or inactivation of multiple tumor-suppressor genes, including *p53*, *APC*, and *DCC*. Loss of heterozygosity (LOH) on chromosome 17p (*p53* locus) and mutation of the *p53* gene are observed in more than 60% of gastric carcinomas [19–21], regardless of histological type. Gastric cancer cell lines also dis-

Table 2. Alterations of tumor-suppressor genes and oncogenes in human gastric cancer cell lines

Cell line	*p53* mutation	*APC* mutation	Gene amplification
KATO-III	Deletion	Partial deletion (exon 7)	K-*sam*, c-*met*
HSC-39	Missense mutation codon 245 GGC-AGC	No mutation	c-*myc*, c-*met*
TMK-1	Missense mutation codon 173 GTG-ATG	No mutation	
MKN-1	Missense mutation codon 143 GTG-GCC	No mutation	
MKN-7	Missense mutation codon 278 CCT-TCT	Silent mutation codon 1179 TAT-TAC	c-*erb*B2 *cyclin E*
MKN-28	Missense mutation codon 257 ATC-CTC	Nonsense mutation codon 1470 CGA-TGA	
MKN-45	No mutation	No mutation	c-*met*
MKN-74	No mutation	No mutation	

play frequent *p53* gene mutations [22] (Table 2). Moreover, these alterations take place even in the mucosal cancers. Mutation of the *p53* gene was also found in 33% of gastric adenomas [23]. Among the adenomas studied, most of those with severe atypia had missense or frameshift mutations of the gene, whereas the ones with mild to moderate atypia had only silent mutations [23]. Sakurai et al. [24] studied long-term, followed-up cases of gastric adenomas and reported that *p53* missense mutation was the key indicator for malignant transformation of the lesion. Ochiai et al. [25] investigated nonneoplastic gastric mucosa in 756 sections from 16 resected stomachs containing gastric adenocarcinomas and identified *p53* mutations in 4 of 19 foci with nuclear accumulation of p53 protein. We also found LOH of the *TP53* polymorphic locus in 14% of intestinal metaplasias and 22% of gastric adenomas [7]. Although some investigators insist on the absence of the adenoma–carcinoma sequence in stomach carcinogenesis [26], these accumulating findings overall suggest that some of the adenomas and intestinal metaplasias of the stomach have irreversible genetic alterations and possess definite characteristics of precancerous lesions.

Because *p53* gene mutation is a relatively general event in human carcinogenesis, the mutation spectrum of this gene can serve as an indicator for the effect of putative carcinogens in a certain organ [27]. The mutation spectrum of *p53* in gastric carcinomas displays an intermediate pattern between carcinoma of the colon and that of the esophagus [20, 28, 29]. *p53* mutations at A:T group is frequent in well differentiated gastric carcinomas, whereas G:C to A:T transitions are predominant in poorly differentiated cancers. It is well known that carcinogenic *N*-nitrosamines, which cause predominantly G:C to A:T base substitutions and comprise one of the candidates for carcinogens of the stomach carcinogenesis [30], are frequently contained in the foods noted above and can be produced from the amines with nitrates in the acidic environment of the stomach [31]. This point can be well applied to poorly differentiated adenocarcinoma of the stomach. On the other hand, in well differentiated adenocarcinoma, the main supply for nitroso compounds is supposed to be the abnormal anaerobic bacterial flora colonized on the mucosa with atrophic gastritis with a high pH environment [32]. The high incidence of mutation at the A:T pair may be explained by DNA depuration from irritants to

the mucosa, including ethanol or scalding temperatures and chemical carcinogens such as the urethane contained in alcoholic beverages as discussed for esophageal cancer by Hollstein et al. [33].

A susceptible tumor-suppressor gene for familial polyposis coli, *APC* has been isolated and characterized [34, 35]. Mutations in the *APC* gene also occur in sporadic colorectal and gastric cancers. Nakatsuru et al. [36] reported that more than 50% of well-differentiated gastric adenocarcinomas displayed somatic mutations of the *APC* gene, but no *APC* mutation was found in poorly differentiated gastric cancers. We identified *APC* gene alterations in three of eight gastric cancer cell lines [37]. In addition, there is a distinct difference in the nature of *APC* mutation between colorectum and stomach. That is, missense mutation of the *APC* gene is dominant in gastric cancer, whereas nonsense mutation and frameshift mutation frequently take place in colorectal cancers [36]. *APC* alteration is an early genetic event in stomach carcinogenesis, as has been characterized for colorectal carcinogenesis [38]. Somatic mutations of the *APC* gene were found in 20% to 42% of gastric adenomas [37, 39] and 6% of incomplete-type intestinal metaplasias of the stomach [37]. We observed a good corrlelation between the nature of *APC* gene mutations and histological atypia of adenomas of the stomach, as has also been discussed for *p53*. The adenomas with nonsense or frameshift mutations in the *APC* gene display high grade atypia, whereas the lesions with silent mutations show low grade atypia [37]. Therefore the nature of the mutations in the *APC* and *p53* tumor-suppressor genes can serve as a important biomarker for malignant potential of gastric lesions.

A tumor-suppressor gene located on the long arm of chromosome 18, *DCC* encodes a transmembrane protein with considerable homology to neural cell adhesion molecules [40]. LOH at the *DCC* locus is one of the characteristics of well-differentiated gastric carcinomas and is detected in 50% to 61% of gastric cancers [19, 41].

Several distinct chromosomal loci have been reported to be deleted in gastric carcinomas. LOH at 1q and 7q is frequently observed in well-differentiated lesions, loss of 1p is relatively common in advanced poorly differentiated gastric carcinomas [19], and LOH at 17q within the *BRCA1* locus is common in scirrhous gastric cancer, especially that affecting the young age group. Ezaki et al. [42] conducted an extensive deletion mapping study on 1q and defined the commonly deleted region between D1S201 and D1S197, which are 13 cM apart. Tamura et al. [43] described two distinct regions of deletion in well-differentiated gastric carcinomas on 5q apart from the *APC* locus. In addition, we reported LOH at the *bcl-2* gene locus was frequently associated with well-differentiated gastric cancers and colorectal cancer [44]. The results of our deletion mapping study on 7q [45], which is closely related to peritonal dissemination and a poor prognosis for gastric cancer, are discussed later in the chapter. From these assigned loci, candidates for the tumor-suppressor gene responsible for stomach carcinogenesis may be identified in the future.

Cell adhesion molecules also may function as tumor suppressors. The expression of E-cadherin, P-cadherin, and α-catenin is significantly lower in poorly differentiated or scirrhous gastric carcinomas compared with that in well differentiated cancers [46, 47]. Molecular biological analysis revealed that cell lines derived from scirrhous gastric cancers harbor gene abnormalities in either E-cadherin or catenins [48]. Mutations in the E-cadherin gene have been reported to occur preferentially in 50% of poorly differentiated gastric cancers [49]. These observations strongly suggest that gene alterations and reduced expression of cadherin and catenins are involved in the development and invasion of poorly differentiated or scirrhous gastric cancer.

Alterations of Cell Cycle Regulator Genes in Human Stomach Carcinogenesis

The molecular regulation of the cell cycle controls cell growth, differentiation, survival, and death through positive and negative regulators. The positive regulators cyclins and cyclin-dependent kinases (CDKs), which form complexes, regulate progression through key transitions in the cell cycle. Expression of the cyclin D family members is mediated by many growth factors, whereas expression of cyclin E and cyclins A and B is cell-cycle-dependent. Gene abnormalities and aberrant expressions of various cyclins may play a pivotal role in the pathogenesis of gastrointestinal cancers.

Studies have uncovered abnormalities in *cyclin E* gene expression in most gastric and colorectal carcinomas as well as breast cancers [50, 51]. The *cyclin E* gene was amplified 3- to 10-fold in 6 (13.3%) of 45 gastric carcinoma tissues [52]. The important additional finding is that all of the cases with *cyclin E* gene amplification had regional lymph node metastases. However, no gene amplification of the *cyclin D1* gene was found in any gastric and colorectal cancers. We have also found the concurrent amplification of *cyclin E* and *CDK2* genes in colorectal carcinomas [53]. Overexpression of *cyclin E* is more frequently detected in adenocarcinomas than in adenomas of the stomach, and *cyclin E* overexpression correlates well with tumor staging, invasiveness, histological grade, and proliferative activity measured by the Ki-67 antigen and the abnormal accumulation of *p53* protein [54]. These findings suggest that overexpression of *cyclin E* and subsequent deregulation of the cell cycle may control the development and progression of gastric and colorectal adenocarcinomas. *Cyclin E* expression may provide a biomarker for the detection of malignant transformations or high malignant phenotypes of gastric and colorectal cancers. Interestingly, this situation contrasts with the observations in esophageal squamous cell carcinoma that co-amplification of the *cyclin D1* gene together with the *hst*-1 and *int*-2 genes occurs in 50% of primary tumors and in 100% of metastatic tumors [55, 56]. Overall, these findings suggest that cyclins involved in the development and progression of gastric or colorectal adenocarcinomas and esophageal squamous cell carcinomas are different.

As for the negative regulators, five CDK inhibitor genes have been identified as attractive candidates for new tumor-suppressor genes: *p21* (SDI1/WAF1/CIP1) [57–59], *p27* (KIP1) [60], *p28* [61], *p16* (MTS1) [62], and *p15* (MTS2) [63] genes. Found among them is the mutation and allele loss of the gene encoding *p16*, the so-called multiple tumor-suppressor-1 (*MTS1*) gene. It has been found in diverse primary and cultured cancer cells, including esophageal cancer, breast cancer, astrocytoma, glioma, familial melanoma, and osteosarcoma [62]. The p16 protein binds to CDK4 and inhibits the cyclin D1–CDK4 complex that phosphorylates pRb [61]. The gene encoding *p15* (*MTS2*) is located adjacent to the *MTS1* gene in the short arm of human chromosome 9. The p15 protein also binds directly to CDK4 and CDK6

[63]. Although no somatic mutation of the *p16* gene is found in any of the gastric adenomas or carcinoma tissues [64], three of eight gastric cancer cell lines exhibit genetic alteration in the *p16* and *p15* genes, whereas no colorectal cancer cell lines have any change in either gene [65]. On the other hand, most esophageal cancer cell lines harbor homozygous deletions of the *p16* and *p15* genes, associated with overexpression of cyclin D1, CDK4, p27Kip1, and phosphorylated Rb protein, suggesting that loss of the *p16* gene and subsequent overexpression of cyclin D1 and CDK4 could confer an autonomous growth of esophageal cancer cells [66]. Merlo et al. reported that 5'CpG island methylation is associated with transcriptional block of *p16* in a variety of human cancers [67]. A question for further study is whether methylation of the 5'CpG island of the *p16* gene promoter region associated with tumor-suppressor gene inactivation occurs in primary gastrointestinal cancer tissues. Recently we reported that deeply invasive tumors showed a significantly higher incidence of p16 protein loss than did superficial tumors [67a].

The remaining CDK inhibitor, *p21*, which inhibits cyclins/CDK2 kinase, is induced by wild-type p53 and is expressed in senescent human fibroblasts at high levels [57, 68]. However, induction of *p21* by the p53-independent pathway has been demonstrated in muscle and fully differentiated epithelial cells of the gastrointestinal tract [69]. In fact, we found that transforming growth factor-β1 (TGF-β1) induced *p21* expression and consequently suppressed CDK2 kinase activity, followed by a reduction in cyclin A and phosphorylation of Rb protein in the gastric cancer cell line TMK-1 containing mutant p53 [70]. The expression of *p21* in tumor cells of the stomach may account for both the p53-dependent and *p53*-independent pathways, because most gastric adenoma and carcinoma tissues express p21 protein [71]. Our results indicate that the expression of *p21* in gastric cancer correlates with tumor aggressiveness as determined by immunohistochemical analysis and invasiveness. However, no remarkable alterations in the *p21* and *p27* genes have been uncovered [65], although interferon-α (IFN-α) dramatically induces expression of *p27* mRNA and protein by TMK-1 cells, indicating the existence of a TGF-β-independent expression of *p27*. What is more important is that *p27* reduction or loss correlates significantly with the advanced stage, the depth of tumor invasion, and lymph node metastasis [71a]. Moreover, the expression of *p27* shows an inverse correlation with the expression of *cyclin E*.

Concerning apoptotic cell death in gastric cancer cells, TGF-β1 causes apoptosis in some human gastric cancer cell lines [72]. Moreover, we found that IFN-α also induced expression of the *6–16* gene [73] in TMK-1 cells, followed by apoptosis. Therefore TGF-β and IFN-α, which may act as autocrine or paracrine growth regulators, are triggers for apoptotic cell death in gastric cancer cells. Kasagi et al. [74] reported an interesting observation that apoptotic indices (number of apoptotic cells/total number of tumor cells) measured by the terminal deoxynucleotidyl transferase (TdT)-mediated dUTP biotin nick end-labeling (TUNEL) method were significantly higher in well-differentiated than poorly differentiated adenocarcinomas. This finding indicates that poorly differentiated adenocarcinomas have a lower incidence of apoptosis. These results are compatible with our findings that LOH at the *bcl*-2 gene locus is frequently associated with well-differentiated gastric cancer, whereas *bcl*-2 overexpression is confined to poorly differentiated stomach cancer [44]. Evidence indicates that *bax* is directly induced by wild-type p53 and acts as an accelerator of apoptosis [75]. The bcl-2 and bax proteins can form heterodimers that regulate the ability of bcl-2 protein to block cell death. Alterations of the *bax* gene in gastric cancer should be examined in the future.

Alterations of Oncogenes, Growth Factors, and Growth Factor Receptors in Human Stomach Carcinogenesis

Proto-oncogenes are classified into four groups: growth factors, growth factor receptors, signal transducers, and nuclear proteins. Activation of proto-oncogenes was caused by amplification, rearrangement, point mutation, or translocation of the gene. Receptor tyrosine kinase mediates the mitogenic signal of growth factors through the phosphorylation cascade of signal transducers and nuclear proteins. Several receptor tyrosine kinases, especially c-*met*, K-*sam*, and c-*erb*B2, have been reported to be altered in human gastric cancer. Among these proto-oncogenes, alteration of c-*met* is most implicated in stomach carcinogenesis.

The c-*met* gene was isolated as a proto-oncogene corresponding to *met* oncogene activated by the rearrangement between the *TPR* locus and the *met* locus [76]. The c-*met* proto-oncogene encodes a receptor tyrosine kinase that has been identified as a receptor for hepatocyte growth factor/scatter factor (HGF/SF) [77]. Amplification of the c-*met* gene is frequently found with advanced gastric cancer, particularly scirrhous tumors [78]. This alteration is a rare event in esophageal or colorectal carcinomas. Most gastric cancers overexpress two c-*met* transcripts 7.0 and 6.0 kb in size. The 6.0 kb c-*met* transcript is expressed preferentially in cancer tissues and cancer cell lines of the stomach [79]. Expression of the 6.0 kb c-*met* transcript correlates well with tumor staging, lymph node metastasis, and depth of tumor invasion [79]. It is also known that c-*met* has several minor transcriptional variants [80, 81]. Yokozaki et al. [82] reported that gastric cancer cell lines, gastric carcinoma tissues, and their corresponding nonneoplastic gastric mucosa had the 54 bp$^-$ splice variant of c-*met*, which encodes mature 190 kDa heterodimeric protein as the major transcript population; the 54 bp$^+$ variant, which encodes 170 kDa protein (which is distinct from the met precursor protein), could not be detected. These findings provide a hypothesis that interaction between c-*met* overexpressed on gastric cancer cells and HGF/SF from stromal cells has implications for the morphogenesis and progression of gastric cancer in vivo. Stromal cells, especially fibroblasts, can secrete HGF with the stimulation of several growth factors, such as interleukin-1α (IL-1α), TGF-α, or TGF-β. All of these growth factors are well known to be produced by cancer cells and act in an autocrine or paracrine manner. On the other hand, gastric cancer cells so far analyzed do not have the ability to secrete HGF/SF. When the stromal cells activated by these tumor-derived growth factors and cytokines secrete HGF/SF, the HGF/SF could act as a morphogen and promote tubular formation of cancer cells in a clone maintaining expression of adhesion molecules such as cadherins and catenins, resulting in well differentiated adenocarcinoma histologically. Conversely, in the case of a clone exhibiting reduced expression of cell adhesion molecules, HGF/SF could act as a motogen and induce diffuse spreading or scattering of the cancer cells, resulting in poorly differentiated adenocarcinoma or scirrhous cancer of the stomach [83, 84]. This hypothesis is supported by the finding that there is cross-talk between E-cadherin/β-catenin and receptor tyrosine kinases including c-*met* and c-*erb*B2 [85].

K-*sam* (KATO-III cell-derived stomach cancer amplified gene) was isolated from KATO-III gastric signet ring cell carcinoma by the gel renaturation method [86–88]. K-*sam* has at least four transcription variants. Type I (brain type) and type II (KATO-III type) encode membrane-bound receptor tyrosine kinases, and other two species encode secreted receptors [89]. Type II transcript, encoding a receptor for keratinocyte growth factor (KGF), is expressed only in carcinoma cell lines, not in the cell lines derived from sarcomas. K-*sam* amplification takes place preferentially in poorly differentiated or scirrhous gastric carcinomas but not in well-differentiated gastric carcinomas [90]. Most of the gastric carcinomas with amplified K-*sam* gene are in the advanced stage, and some show K-*sam* amplification only in metastatic foci, suggesting that amplification of the K-*sam* gene is a late event during carcinogenesis of the stomach [90]. In addition, the amplification of K-*sam* is generally a phenomenon independent of c-*met* amplification.

The c-*erb*B2 gene is one of the members of the epidermal growth factor (EGF) receptor gene family. In contrast to the EGF receptor, which frequently displays amplification in squamous cell carcinomas, c-*erb*B2 is amplified in adenocarcinomas, including salivary gland [7], breast, and stomach [91, 92] cancers. The amplification of this tyrosine kinase receptor gene is preferentially found in well-differentiated but not poorly differentiated gastric carcinomas [91, 92]. Moreover, overexpression associated with amplification of c-*erb*B2 is closely related to a poor prognosis [93] including liver metastasis of gastric cancer [94, 95]. The amplification of c-*erb*B1 (EGF receptor) and c-*erb*B3 was found in 3% [96] and 0% of human gastric carcinomas, respectively.

Mutational activation of the Ki-*ras* oncogene is found in 9% to 18% of gastric cancers, especially the well differentiated ones [97]. The *hst*-1 gene, isolated from a surgical specimen of human gastric cancer by the NIH/3T3 transformation assay, rarely (2%) amplifies in gastric cancer [98].

Gastric cancer cells express a broad spectrum of growth factors, gut hormones, and cytokines, including TGF-α [99, 100], EGF [101, 100), amphiregulin [102, 103], cripto [104, 105], TGF-β1 [106], platelet-derived growth factor (PDGF) [107], insulin-like growth factor (IGF) II [108], basic fibroblast growth factor (bFGF) [109], IL-1α [110], IL-6 [108], and IL-8. Among them, the EGF family growth factors, including TGF-α, EGF, cripto, and amphiregulin are the common positive growth stimulators for gastric cancer. Synchronous overexpression of TGF-α and EGF receptor correlated well with the biological malignancy of stomach cancer. Overexpression of these growth factors and their receptors usually did not accompany gene amplifications [111]. Most of these genes have consensus sequence for GC factor (GCF), a negative regulator, as well as a sequence for Sp-1, a positive regulator for gene expression, in their promotor region. Our investigation revealed that the levels of the expression of positive growth factors and their receptors were well correlated with the relative expression levels of these two transcription factors [112]. In fact, an in vitro transfection study using GCF expression vector demonstrated repression of transcription of several growth factor/receptor genes and caused growth inhibition of gastric cancer cell lines [113].

The negative growth factor TGF-β1 is commonly overexpressed in gastric carcinomas [106]. With regard to the relation between the incidence of TGF-β1 overexpression and histological types, overexpression of this negative growth factor is frequently observed in poorly differentiated adenocarcinoma of the stomach. Although it is reasonable that TGF-β1 from cancer cells themselves may play a role in desmoplasia in scirrhous gastric cancer, there must be some escape mechanism from the growth inhibitory effect of TGF-β1 in cancer cells. Our study on the gastric cancer cell line TMK-1, which expresses TGF-β1, demonstrated that TGF-β1 inhibits DNA synthesis in TMK-1 and that the type I receptor for TGF-β is mainly linked to the growth-inhibitory signal by a

decrease in retinoblastoma protein phosphorylation by p34cdc2 without suppression of c-*myc* expression [114]. Interestingly, more than 80% of gastric carcinoma tissues display a reduction in TGF-β1 receptor regardless of histological type [115]. Moreover, Park et al. [116] reported that four of seven gastric cancer cell lines that were resistant to TGF-β1-mediated growth inhibition had a genetic alteration, including deletions and amplifications in the type II TGF-β receptor. Frequent alterations in the poly-adenine tract in the TGF-β type II receptor gene open reading frame were reported in the replication error-positive colorectal cancers and in gastric carcinomas [117]. Intensive study on the mutation of these complexed TGF-β receptor system is required to answer the question of why most the gastric cancer cells escape the growth inhibitory effect of TGF-β1.

In addition to these EGF-related growth factors and TGF-β, PDGF, IGF-II, and bFGF are commonly overexpressed in poorly differentiated gastric carcinomas including scirrhous cancers [108]. In particular, the development of scirrhous gastric carcinoma may require synchronous overexpression of TGF-β1, PDGF, IGF-II, and bFGF, all of which may function mainly as paracrine growth factors. This situation reflects the close interaction of tumor cells and stromal cells, including fibroblasts, endothelial cells, macrophages, and lymphocytes. In addition, we lately found that most of the gastric cancer cell lines and gastric cancer tissues produced vascular endothelial growth factor, whose expression was up-regulated by several stromal- and cancer-

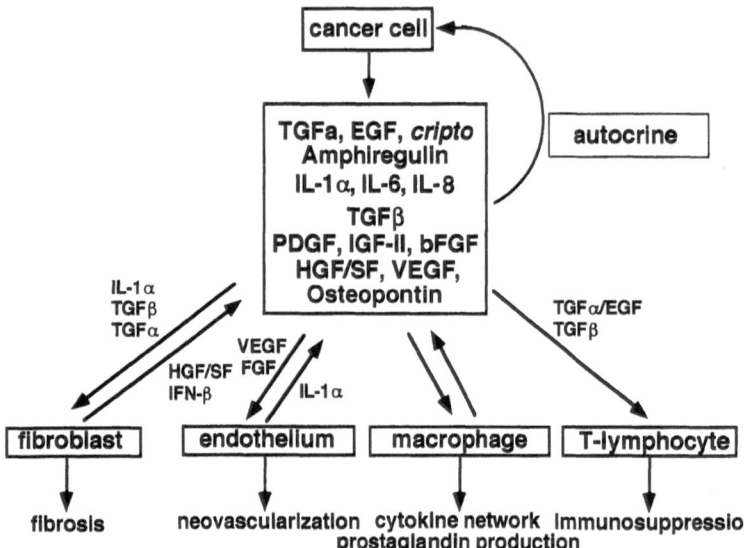

Fig. 1. Interaction of tumor-derived growth factors and cytokines with stromal cells of the microenvironment. *TGF*, transforming growth factor; *EGF*, epidermal growth factor; *PDGF*, platelet-derived growth factor; *IGF*, insulin-like growth factor; *bFGF*, basic fibroblast growth factor; *HGF/SF*, hepatocyte growth factor/scatter factor; *VEGF*, vascular endothelial growth factor; *IL-1*, interleukin-1

derived growth factors and cytokines (Yamamoto et al., unpublished data).

Gastric carcinomas can produce not only growth factors but cytokines as well. Surprisingly, IL-1α gene is expressed at various levels by most of the gastric carcinoma cell lines [110]. More than 60% of gastric carcinoma tissues reveal higher levels of IL-1α mRNA expression than normal mucosa. Moreover, we found that IL-1α acts as an autocrine or paracrine growth factor for some of the gastric cancer cell lines, and the expression of IL-1α was stimulated by TGF-α and EGF. We found that IL-6 was also overexpressed in some of the gastric cancer cell lines (Ito et al., unpublished data). Tumor-derived IL-1α may induce an increase in proteolytic enzyme activity, cell adhesion molecules, and cytokine production and a decrease in extracellulan matrix production by stromal cells. Recently, we found that IL-8 produced by tumor cells strongly correlated with neovascularization [110a]. Therefore cytokines and growth factors produced by tumor cells not only affect autocrine or paracrine growth and motility of tumor cells themselves, they may also have an effect on stromal cells' interaction with their receptors, leading to fibrosis, angiogenesis, activation of the cytokine network, and immunosuppression (Fig. 1).

Conversely, stromal cells stimulated by tumor-derived growth factors may induce secretion of multiple growth factors and cytokines, resulting in proliferation, enhanced motility, and sometimes apoptotic cell death or necrosis of tumor cells.

Alterations of Metastasis-Related Genes in Human Stomach Carcinogenesis

Alterations in multiple genes and multiple growth factors including cytokines may facilitate the development of metastasis of gastric cancer. Well differentiated gastric cancers frequently metastasize to liver, whereas poorly differentiated ones often display peritoneal dissemination.

CD44 was originally implicated as a "homing" receptor that directed the migration of recirculating lymphocytes across the high endothelial venular membranes of the lymph nodes and inflamed synovia [118]. It has been confirmed that CD44 is expressed not only in lymphocytes but in a wide variety of tissues. It is considered to be an important cell adhesion molecule for cell–cell in-

teraction [119]. Molecular cloning and analysis of the genetic structure have revealed that the CD44 gene contains at least 20 exons of which 12 exons can be alternatively spliced to make up a wide variety of molecular variants [120]. Expression of the CD44 splice variant(s) has been found in various human malignancies and is considered to be implicated in tumor progression and metastasis [121–123]. We also detected expression of abnormal CD44 transcript including exon 11 in all gastric cancer tissues and metastatic tumors [124]. In addition, the difference in the CD44 abnormal transcript pattern is observed between well-differentiated and poorly differentiated gastric cancers, suggesting that two types of gastric cancer may have different genetic pathways as well as different biological implications in the expression of CD44 [124]. What is more important is that CD44 variants found in cancer tissue frequently had retention of intronic sequences, especially that of intron 9 [125, 126]. Therefore overexpression of abnormal CD44 transcripts containing the intron 9 sequence is presumably a powerful indicator of the presence of adenocarcinoma in the gastrointestinal tract [127]. It has been confirmed that CD44 variants regulate adhesion, movement, and activation of normal and neoplastic cells through interaction with hyaluronic acid.

Osteopontin, also termed Eta-1 (early T lymphocyte activation-1), was reported to be a protein ligand for CD44 and to elicit a different cellular response with its ligation from that of the carbohydrate ligand [128]. Moreover, osteopontin has internal RGD consensus to interact with integrin family proteins [129]. Our experimental evidence showed that osteopontin is overexpressed in gastric cancer tissues, compared with corresponding normal gastric mucosa. It is of considerable interest that gastric cancer cells express the receptor adhesion molecule (CD44) and protein ligand (osteopontin) synchronously. Our recent study on the interaction between CD44 variants and osteopontin may provide some biological clues to the mechanisms of lymphogenous metastasis.

A candidate suppressor gene of metastasis, nm23 encodes nucleotide diphosphate kinase and c-myc transcription factor. LOH at the nm23 locus has been found in 85 primary gastric cancers, most of which tumors express nm23 mRNA at higher levels in primary tumor tissue than in the corresponding normal mucosa [130]. However, the reduction of nm23 expression is frequently associated with metastases of gastric cancer.

In addition to nm23, elevated levels of urokinase-type plasminogen activator and plasminogen activator inhibitor in tumor tissues are linked with metastasis of gastrointestinal cancer [131, 132]. Nekarda et al. [133] found that elevated iPA and PAI-1 levels were closely correlated with vascular invasion, lymph node metastases, and poor prognosis. Additionally, a 31-kDa lactoside lectin (L-31) is frequently overexpressed in primary tumors and liver metastases of well differentiated gastric cancers [134], suggesting that overexpression of this lectin may correlate with liver metastasis of gastric cancer.

Peritoneal invasion and dissemination may require not only abnormalities of cell adhesion molecules but also LOH of the long arm of chromosome 7. Our study on deletion mapping of 7q demonstrated that LOH at the D7S95 locus was correlated closely with poor prognosis and a high incidence of peritoneal dissemination in gastric cancer [45]. It is likely that the D7S95 locus contains a candidate suppressor gene for the progression and metastasis of gastric carcinoma.

Future Perspectives

Molecular dissections of human gastric cancers have revealed that multiple genetic alterations are involved in stomach carcinogenesis. The overall observations on this issue may provide supporting evidence for our working hypothesis that there are two distinctive major genetic pathways for stomach carcinogenesis (Fig. 2). K-ras mutation, APC inactivation, loss of DCC, and amplification of c-erbB2 are preferentially found in well-differentiated gastric carcinomas, whereas gene mutations, loss of the cadherin–catenin system, and amplification of K-sam are frequently observed in poorly differentiated cancers. In addition, the present findings support the use of some molecular biological approaches to the diagnosis and evaluation of gastric malignancy. Early genetic changes, such as microsatellite instability, not only serve as good biological markers for screening precancerous lesions that have malignant potential but also for the possible development of secondary cancer. Alterations preferentially occurring at the point of malignant transformation, such as reactivation of telomerase and p53 inactivation, may provide a powerful tool for the evaluation of malignancy. The late changes, including amplification of cyclin E gene, c-erbB2 amplification, and 7q LOH, are good indicators for biological malignancy. Applying these results to routine clinical practice, we are able to facilitate and improve cancer diagnosis and to predict grade of malignancy or patient prognosis and to discover novel types of therapeutic approaches.

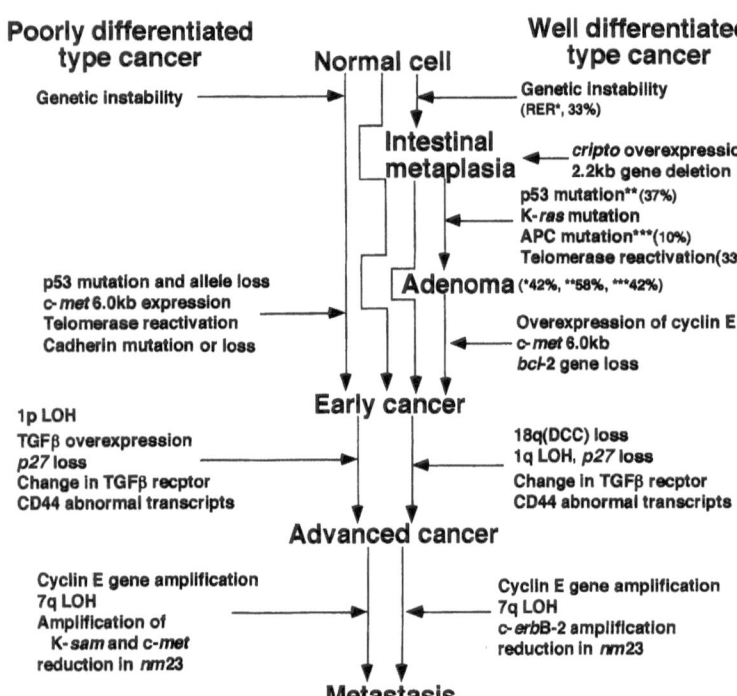

Fig. 2. Genetic pathway of two types of stomach cancer. *RER*, replication error; *LOH*, loss of heterozygosity; *TGF*, transforming growth factor

We have implemented and utilized a new strategy of molecular diagnosis of gastrointestinal tract cancers based on the above-mentioned overall findings as a routine service in the Hiroshima City Medical Association Clinical Laboratory since 1993 [135]. The detailed philosophy and description on this strategy appear in the chapter by W. Yasui and E. Tahara of this book. Finally, the major remaining work on this field is identification of the specific gene(s) responsible for stomach carcinogenesis.

References

1. Fearon ER, Vogelstein B (1990) A genetic model for colorectal tumorigenesis. Cell 61:759–767
2. Tahara E, Semba S, Tahara H (1996) Molecular biological observations in gastric cancer. Semin Oncol 23:307–315
3. Han HJ, Yanagisawa A, Kato Y, Park JG, Nakamura Y (1993) Genetic instability in pancreatic cancer and poorly differentiated type of gastric cancer. Cancer Res 53:5087–5089
4. Rhyu MG, Park WS, Meltzer SJ (1994) Microsatellite instability occurs frequently in human gastric carcinoma. Oncogene 9:29–32
5. Strickler JG, Zheng J, Shu Q, Burgart LJ, Alberts SR, Shibata D (1994) *p53* mutations and microsatellite instability in sporadic gastric cancer: when guardians fail. Cancer Res 54:4750–4755
6. Chong JM, Fukayama M, Hayashi Y, Takizawa T, Koike M, Konishi M, Kikuchi Yanoshita R, Miyaki M (1994) Microsatellite instability in the progression of gastric carcinoma. Cancer Res 54:4595–4597
7. Semba S, Yokozaki H, Yamamoto S, Yasui W, Tahara E (1996) Microsatellite instability in precancerous lesions and adenocarcinomas of the stomach. Cancer 77:1620–1627
8. Seruca R, Santos NR, David L, Constancia M, Barroca H, Carneiro F, Seixas M, Peltomaki P, Lothe R, Sobrinho Simoes M (1995) Sporadic gastric carcinomas with microsatellite instability display a particular clinicopathologic profile. Int J Cancer 64:32–36
9. Horii A, Han HJ, Shimada M, Yanagisawa A, Kato Y, Ohta H, Yasui W, Tahara E, Nakamura Y (1994) Frequent replication errors at microsatellite loci in tumors of patients with multiple primary cancers. Cancer Res 54:3373–3375
10. Counter CM, Avilion AA, LeFeuvre CE, Stewart NG, Greider CW, Harley CB, Bacchetti S (1992) Telomere shortening associated with chromosome instability is arrested in immortal cells which express telomerase activity. EMBO J 11:1921–1929
11. Hastie ND, Dempster M, Dunlop MG, Thompson AM, Green DK, Allshire RC (1990) Telomere re-

duction in human colorectal carcinoma and with ageing. Nature 346:866–868
12. Tahara E, Kuniyasu H, Yasui W, Yokozaki H (1994) Gene alterations in intestinal metaplasia and gastric cancer. Eur J Gastroenterol Hepatol 6(suppl 1):S97–S101
13. Tahara H, Kuniyasu H, Yokozaki H, Yasui W, Shay JW, Ide T, Tahara E (1995) Telomerase activity in preneoplastic and neoplastic gastric and colorectal lesions. Clin Cancer Res 1:1245–1251
14. Hiyama E, Yokoyama T, Tatsumoto N, Hiyama K, Imamura Y, Murakami Y, Kodama T, Piatyszek MA, Shay JW, Matsuura Y (1995) Telomerase activity in gastric cancer. Cancer Res 55:3258–3262
15. Feng J, Funk WD, Wang SS, Weinrich SL, Avilion AA, Chiu CP, Adams RR, Chang E, Allsopp RC, Yu J, Le S, West MD, Harley CB, Andrews WH, Greider CW, Villeponteau B (1995) The RNA component of human telomerase. Science 269:1236–1241
16. Avilion AA, Piatyszek MA, Gupta J, Shay JW, Bacchetti S, Greider CW (1996) Human telomerase RNA and telomerase activity in immortal cell lines and tumor tissues. Cancer Res 56:645–650
17. Blasco MA, Rizen M, Greider CW, Hanahan D (1996) Differential regulation of telomerase activity and telomerase RNA during multi-stage tumorigensis. Nat Genet 12:200–204
18. Kuniyasu H, Domen T, Hamamoto T, Yokozaki H, Yasui W, Tahara H, Tahara E (1997) Expression of human telomerase RNA is an early event of stomach carcinogenesis. Jpn J Cancer Res 88:103–107
19. Sano T, Tsujino T, Yoshida K, Nakayama H, Haruma K, Ito H, Nakamura Y, Kajiyama G, Tahara E (1991) Frequent loss of heterozygosity on chromosomes 1q, 5q, and 17p in human gastric carcinomas. Cancer Res 51:2926–2931
20. Yokozaki H, Kuniyasu H, Kitadai Y, Nishimura K, Todo H, Ayhan A, Yasui W, Ito H, Tahara E (1992) *p53* point mutations in primary human gastric carcinomas. J Cancer Res Clin Oncol 119:67–70
21. Tamura G, Kihana T, Nomura K, Terada M, Sugimura T, Hirohashi S (1991) Detection of frequent *p53* gene mutations in primary gastric cancer by cell sorting and polymerase chain reaction single-strand conformation polymorphism analysis. Cancer Res 51:3056–3058
22. Mattar R, Yokozaki H, Yasui W, Ito H, Tahara E (1992) *p53* gene mutations in gastric cancer cell lines. Oncology (Life Sci Adv) 11:7–12
23. Tohdo H, Yokozaki H, Haruma K, Kajiyama G, Tahara E (1993) *p53* gene mutations in gastric adenomas. Virchows Arch B Cell Pathol 63:191–195

66   H. Yokozaki et al.

24. Sakurai S, Sano T, Nakajima T (1995) Clinicopathological and molecular biological studies of gastric adenomas with special reference to p53 abnormality. Pathol Int 45:51–57

25. Ochiai A, Yamauchi Y, Hirohashi S (1996) *p53* mutations in the non-neoplastic mucosa of the human stomach showing intestinal metaplasia. Int J Cancer 69:28–33

26. Maesawa C, Tamura G, Suzuki Y, Ogasawara S, Sakata K, Kashiwaba M, Satodate R (1995) The sequential accumulation of genetic alterations characteristic of the colorectal adenoma-carcinoma sequence does not occur between gastric adenoma and adenocarcinoma. J Pathol 176:249–258

27. Harris CC (1991) Chemical and physical carcinogenesis: advances and perspectives for the 1990s. Cancer Res 51:5023s–5044s

28. Uchino S, Noguchi M, Ochiai A, Saito T, Kobayashi M, Hirohashi S (1993) *p53* mutation in gastric cancer: a genetic model for carcinogenesis is common to gastric and colorectal cancer. Int J Cancer 54:759–764

29. Poremba C, Yandell DW, Huang Q, Little JB, Mellin W, Schmid KW, Bocker W, Dockhorn Dworniczak B (1995) Frequency and spectrum of *p53* mutations in gastric cancer—a molecular genetic and immunohistochemical study. Virchows Arch 426:447–455

30. Sugimura T, Fujimura S, Baba T (1970) Tumor production in the glandular stomach and alimentary tract of the rat by N-methyl-N'-nitro-N-nitrosoguanidine. Cancer Res 30:455–465

31. Mirvish S (1971) Kinetics of nitrosamine formation from alkylureas, N-alkylurethanes, and alkylguanidines: possible implications for the etiology of human gastric cancer. J Natl Cancer Inst 46:1183–1193

32. Correa P (1991) The new era of cancer epidemiology. Cancer Epidemiol Biomarkers Prev 1:5–11

33. Hollstein MC, Metcalf RA, Welsh JA, Montesano R, Harris CC (1990) Frequent mutation of the *p53* gene in human esophageal cancer. Proc Natl Acad Sci USA 87:9958–9961

34. Nishisho I, Nakamura Y, Miyoshi Y, Miki Y, Ando H, Horii A, Koyama K, Utsunomiya J, Baba S, Hedge P (1991) Mutations of chromosome 5q21 genes in FAP and colorectal cancer patients. Science 253:665–669

35. Kinzler KW, Nilbert MC, Su LK, Vogelstein B, Bryan TM, Levy DB, Smith KJ, Preisinger AC, Hedge P, McKechnie D, Finniear R, Markham A, Groffen J, Boguski MS, Altschul SF, Horii A, Ando H, Miyoshi Y, Miki Y, Nishisho I, Nakamura Y (1991) Identification of FAP locus genes from chromosome 5q21. Science 253:661–665

36. Nakatsuru S, Yanagisawa A, Ichii S, Tahara E, Kato Y, Nakamura Y, Horii A (1992) Somatic mutation of the *APC* gene in gastric cancer: frequent mutations in very well differentiated adenocarcinoma and signet-ring cell carcinoma. Hum Mol Genet 1:559–563

37. Nishimura K, Yokozaki H, Haruma K, Kajiyama G, Tahara E (1995) Alterations of the *APC* gene in carcinoma cell lines and precancerous lesions of the stomach. Int J Oncol 7:587–592

38. Nakatsuru S, Yanagisawa A, Furukawa Y, Ichii S, Kato Y, Nakamura Y, Horii A (1993) Somatic mutations of the *APC* gene in precancerous lesion of the stomach. Hum Mol Genet 2:1463–1465

39. Tamura G, Maesawa C, Suzuki Y, Tamada H, Satoh M, Ogasawara S, Kashiwaba M, Satodate R (1994) Mutations of the *APC* gene occur during early stages of gastric adenoma development. Cancer Res 54:1149–1151

40. Fearon ER, Cho KR, Nigro JM, Kern SE, Simons JW, Ruppert JM, Hamilton SR, Preisinger AC, Thomas G, Kinzler KW, Vogelstein B (1990) Identification of a chromosome 18q gene that is altered in colorectal cancers. Science 247:49–56

41. Uchino S, Tsuda H, Noguchi M, Yokota J, Terada M, Saito T, Kobayashi M, Sugimura T, Hirohashi S (1992) Frequent loss of heterozygosity at the DCC locus in gastric cancer. Cancer Res 52:3099–3102

42. Ezaki T, Yanagisawa A, Ohta K, Aiso S, Watanabe M, Hibi T, Kato Y, Nakajima T, Ariyama T, Inazawa J, Nakamura Y, Horii A (1996) Deletion mapping on chromosome 1p in well-differentiated gastric cancer. Br J Cancer 73:424–428

43. Tamura G, Ogasawara S, Nishizuka S, Sakata K, Maesawa C, Suzuki Y, Terashima M, Saito K, Satodate R (1996) Two distinct regions of deletion on the long arm of chromosome 5 in differentiated adenocarcinomas of the stomach. Cancer Res 56:612–615

44. Ayhan A, Yasui W, Yokozaki H, Seto M, Ueda R, Tahara E (1994) Loss of heterozygosity at the *bcl-*2 gene locus and expression of *bcl-*2 in human gastric and colorectal carcinomas. Jpn J Cancer Res 85:584–591

45. Kuniyasu H, Yasui W, Yokozaki H, Akagi M, Akama Y, Kitahara K, Fujii K, Tahara E (1994) Frequent loss of heterozygosity of the long arm of chromosome 7 is closely associated with progression of human gastric carcinomas. Int J Cancer 59:597–600

46. Ochiai A, Akimoto S, Shimoyama Y, Nagafuchi A, Tsukita S, Hirohashi S (1994) Frequent loss of alpha catenin expression in scirrhous carcinomas with scattered cell growth. Jpn J Cancer Res 85:266–273

47. Yasui W, Kuniyasu H, Akama Y, Kitahara K, Nagafuchi A, Tsukita S, Tahara E (1995) Expression of E-cadherin, alpha- and beta-catenins in

human gastric carcinomas: correlation with histology and tumor progression. Oncol Rep 2:111–117

48. Shimoyama Y, Nagafuchi A, Fujita S, Gotoh M, Takeichi M, Tsukita S, Hirohashi S (1992) Cadherin dysfunction in a human cancer cell line: possible involvement of loss of alpha-catenin expression in reduced cell-cell adhesiveness. Cancer Res 52:5770–5774

49. Becker KF, Atkinson MJ, Reich U, Becker I, Nekarda H, Siewert JR, Hofler H (1994) E-Cadherin gene mutations provide clues to diffuse type gastric carcinomas. Cancer Res 54:3845–3852

50. Keyomarsi K, Pardee AB (1993) Redundant *cyclin* overexpression and gene amplification in breast cancer. Proc Natl Acad Sci USA 90:1112–1116

51. Keyomarsi K, O'Leary N, Molnar G, Lees E, Fingert HJ, Pardee AB (1994) Cyclin E, a potential prognostic marker for breast cancer. Cancer Res 54:380–385

52. Akama Y, Yasui W, Yokozaki H, Kuniyasu H, Kitahara K, Ishikawa T, Tahara E (1995) Frequent amplification of the *cyclin* E gene in human gastric carcinomas. Jpn J Cancer Res 86:617–621

53. Kitahara K, Yasui W, Kuniyasu H, Yokozaki H, Akama Y, Yunotani S, Hisatsugu T, Tahara E (1995) Concurrent amplification of *cyclin E* and *CDK2* genes in colorectal carcinomas. Int J Cancer 62:25–28

54. Yasui W, Akama Y, Kuniyasu H, Yokozaki H, Semba S, Shimamoto F, Tahara E (1996) Expression of *cyclin E* in human gastric adenomas and adenocarcinomas: correlation with proliferative activity and *p53* status. J Exp Ther Oncol 1:88–94

55. Tsuda T, Nakatani H, Matsumura T, Yoshida K, Tahara E, Nishihira T, Sakamoto H, Yoshida T, Terada M, Sugimura T (1988) Amplification of the *hst*-1 gene in human esophageal carcinomas. Jpn J Cancer Res 79:584–588

56. Yoshida K, Kawami H, Kuniyasu H, Nishiyama M, Yasui W, Hirai T, Toge T, Tahara E (1994) Coamplification of *cyclin* D, *hst*-1 and *int*-2 genes is a good biological marker of high malignancy for human esophageal carcinomas. Oncol Rep 1:493–496

57. Noda A, Ning Y, Venable SF, Percira-Smith OM, Smith JR (1994) Cloning of senescent cell derived inhibitors of DNA synthesis using an expression screen. Exp Cell Res 11:90–98

58. El Deiry WS, Tokino T, Velculescu VE, Levy DB, Parsons R, Trent JM, Lin D, Mercer WE, Kinzler KW, Vogelstein B (1993) WAF1, a potential mediator of *p53* tumor suppression. Cell 75:817–825

59. Harper JW, Adami GR, Wei N, Keyomarsi K, Elledge SJ (1993) The *p21* Cdk-interacting protein Cip1 is a potent inhibitor of G1 *cyclin*-dependent kinases. Cell 75:805–816

60. Toyoshima H, Hunter T (1994) *p27*, novel inhibitor of G1 cdk protein kinase activity, is related to *p21*. Cell 78:67–74

61. Hengst L, Dulic V, Slingerland JM, Lees E, Reed SI (1994) A cell cycle-regulated inhibitor of *cyclin*-dependent kinases. Proc Natl Acad Sci USA 91:5291–5295

62. Serrano M, Hannon GJ, Beach D (1993) A new regulatory motif in cell-cycle control causing specific inhibition of *cyclin* D/*CDK4*. Nature 366:704–707

63. Hammon GJ, Beach D (1994) p15INK4B is a potential effector of TGF-β induced cell cycle arrest. Nature 371:257–261

64. Sakata K, Tamura G, Maesawa C, Suzuki Y, Terashima M, Satoh K, Eda Y, Suzuki A, Sekiyama S, Satodate R (1995) Loss of heterozygosity on the short arm of chromosome 9 without *p16* gene mutation in gastric carcinomas. Jpn J Cancer Res 86:333–335

65. Akama Y, Yasui W, Kuniyasu H, Yokozaki H, Akagi M, Tahara H, Ishikawa T, Tahara E (1996) Genetic status and expression of the *cyclin*-dependent kinase inhibitors in human gastric carcinoma cell lines. Jpn J Cancer Res 87:824–830

66. Kitahara K, Yasui W, Yokozaki H, Semba S, Hamamoto T, Hisatsugu T, Tahara E (1996) Expression of *cyclin* D1, *CDK4* and *p27*[KIP1] is associated with the *p16*[MTS1] gene status in human esophageal carcinoma cell lines. J Exp Ther Oncol 1:7–12

67. Merlo A, Herman JG, Mao L, Lee DJ, Gabrielson E, Burger PC, Baylin SB, Sidransky D (1995) 5'CpG island methylation is associated with transcriptional silencing of the tumour suppressor *p16*/*CDKN2*/*MTS1* in human cancers. Nat Med 1:686–692

67a. Yasui W, Yokozaki H, Kuniyasu F, Shimamoto R, Tahara E (1996) Expression of CDK inhibitor p16 in human gastric carcinomas. In: Tahara E, Sugimachi K, Oohara T (eds) Recent advances in gastroenterological carcinogenesis I. Monduzzi Editore, Bologna, pp 765–769

68. Tahara H, Sato E, Noda A, Ide T (1995) Increase in expression level of *p21*[sdi1]/*cip1*/*waf1* with increasing division age in both normal and SV40-transformed human fibroblasts. Oncogene 10:835–840

69. Parker SB, Eichele G, Zhang P, Rawls A, Sands AT, Bradley A, Olson EN, Harper JW, Elledge SJ (1995) *p53*-Independent expression of *p21*[cip1] in muscle and other terminally differentiating cells. Science 267:1024–1027

70. Akagi M, Yasui W, Akama Y, Yokozaki H, Tahara H, Haruma K, Kajiyama G, Tahara E (1996) Inhibition of cell growth by transforming growth factor β1 is associated with *p53*-independ-

ent induction of *p21* in gastric carcinoma cells. Jpn J Cancer Res 87:377–384

71. Yasui W, Akama Y, Kuniyasu H, Semba S, Shimamoto F, Tahara E (1996) Expression of *cyclin*-dependent kinase inhibitor *p21*^{WAFI}/*CIP1* in non-neoplastic mucosa and neoplasia of the stomach: relation with *p53* status and proliferative activity. J Pathol 180:122–128

71a. Yasui W, Kudo Y, Semba S, Yokozaki H, Tahara E (1997) Reduced expression of cyclin-dependent kinase inhibitor *p27*^{KIP1} is associated with advanced stage and invasiveness of gastric carcinomas. Jpn J Canser Res (in press)

72. Yanagihara K, Tsumuraya M (1992) Transforming growth factor beta 1 induces apoptotic cell death in cultured human gastric carcinoma cells. Cancer Res 52:4042–4045

73. Tahara H, Kamada K, Sato E, Tsuyama N, Kim JK, Hara E, Oda K, Ide T (1995) Increase in expression levels of interferon-inducible genes in senescent human diploid fibroblasts and in SV40-transformed human fibroblasts with extended lifespan. Oncogene 11:1125–1132

74. Kasagi N, Gomyo Y, Shirai H, Tsujitani S, Ito H (1994) Apoptotic cell death in human gastric carcinoma: analysis by terminal deoxynucleotidyl transferase-mediated dUTP-biotin nick end labeling. Jpn J Cancer Res 85:939–945

75. Miyashita T, Reed JC (1995) Tumor suppressor *p53* is a direct transcriptional activator of the human *bax* gene. Cell 80:293–299

76. Park M, Dean M, Kaul K, Braun MJ, Gonda MA, Vande Woude G (1987) Sequence of MET protooncogene cDNA has features characteristic of the tyrosine kinase family of growth-factor receptors. Proc Natl Acad Sci USA 84:6379–6383

77. Bottaro DP, Rubin JS, Faletto DL, Chan AM, Kmiecik TE, Vande Woude GF, Aaronson SA (1991) Identification of the hepatocyte growth factor receptor as the c-*met* proto-oncogene product. Science 251:802–804

78. Kuniyasu H, Yasui W, Kitadai Y, Yokozaki H, Ito H, Tahara E (1992) Frequent amplification of the c-*met* gene in scirrhous type stomach cancer. Biochem Biophys Res Commun 189:227–232

79. Kuniyasu H, Yasui W, Yokozaki H, Kitadai Y, Tahara E (1993) Aberrant expression of c-*met* mRNA in human gastric carcinomas. Int J Cancer 55:72–75

80. Rodrigues GA, Naujokas MA, Park M (1991) Alternative splicing generates isoforms of the met receptor tyrosine kinase which undergo differential processing. Mol Cell Biol 11:2962–2970

81. Rodrigues GA, Park M (1993) Isoforms of the met receptor tyrosine kinase. EXS 65:167–179

82. Yokozaki H, Semba S, Yamamoto S, Tahara E (1996) A splice variant of the c-*met* protooncogene is the predominant population ex-

pressed in human gastric mucosa and carcinoma. Oncol Rep 3:425–428

83. Yokozaki H, Ito M, Yasui W, Kyo E, Kuniyasu H, Kitadai Y, Tsubouchi H, Daikuhara Y, Tahara E (1993) Biologic effect of human hepatocyte growth factor on human gastric carcinoma cell lines. Int J Oncol 3:89–93

84. Tannapfel A, Wittekind C, Tahara E (1994) Effect of hepatocyte growth factor (HGF)/scatter factor (SF) on cell adhesion in gastric cancer. Z Gastroenterol 32:91–93

85. Ochiai A, Akimoto S, Kanai Y, Shibata T, Oyama T, Hirohashi S (1994) c-*erb*B-2 gene product associates with catenins in human cancer cells. Biochem Biophys Res Commun 205:73–78

86. Nakatani H, Tahara E, Sakamoto H, Terada M, Sugimura T (1985) Amplified DNA sequences in cancers. Biochem Biophys Res Commun 130:508–514

87. Nakatani H, Tahara E, Yoshida T, Sakamoto H, Suzuki T, Watanabe H, Sekiguchi M, Kaneko Y, Sakurai M, Terada M, Sugimura T (1986) Detection of amplified DNA sequences in gastric cancers by a DNA renaturation method in gel. Jpn J Cancer Res 77:849–853

88. Nakatani H, Sakamoto H, Yoshida T, Yokota J, Tahara E, Sugimura T, Terada M (1990) Isolation of an amplified DNA sequence in stomach cancer. Jpn J Cancer Res 81:707–710

89. Katoh M, Hattori Y, Sasaki H, Tanaka M, Sugano K, Yazaki Y, Sugimura T, Terada M (1992) K-*sam* gene encodes secreted as well as transmembrane receptor tyrosine kinase. Proc Natl Acad Sci USA 89:2960–2964

90. Hattori Y, Odagiri H, Nakatani H, Miyagawa K, Naito K, Sakamoto H, Katoh O, Yoshida T, Sugimura T, Terada M (1990) K-*sam*, an amplified gene in stomach cancer, is a member of the heparin-binding growth factor receptor genes. Proc Natl Acad Sci USA 87:5983–5987

91. Yokota J, Yamamoto T, Miyajima N, Toyoshima K, Nomura N, Sakamoto H, Yoshida T, Terada M, Sugimura T (1988) Genetic alterations of the c-*erb*B-2 oncogene occur frequently in tubular adenocarcinoma of the stomach and are often accompanied by amplification of the v-*erb*A homologue. Oncogene 2:283–287

92. Kameda T, Yasui W, Yoshida K, Tsujino T, Nakayama H, Ito M, Ito H, Tahara E (1990) Expression of *ERBB2* in human gastric carcinomas: relationship between *p185ERBB2* expression and the gene amplification. Cancer Res 50:8002–8009

93. Yonemura Y, Ninomiya I, Ohoyama S, Kimura H, Yamaguchi A, Fushida S, Kosaka T, Miwa K, Miyazaki I, Endou Y, Tanaka M, Sasaki T (1991) Expression of c-*erb*B-2 oncoprotein in gastric carcinoma: immunoreactivity for c-*erb*B-2 protein is an independent indicator of poor short-term prog-

nosis is patients with gastric carcinoma. Cancer 67:2914–2918

94. Oda N, Tsujino T, Tsuda T, Yoshida K, Nakayama H, Yasui W, Tahara E (1990) DNA ploidy pattern and amplification of *ERBB* and *ERBB2* genes in human gastric carcinomas. Virchows Arch B Cell Pathol 58:273–277

95. Tsujino T, Yoshida K, Nakayama H, Ito H, Shimosato T, Tahara E (1990) Alterations of oncogenes in metastatic tumours of human gastric carcinomas. Br J Cancer 62:226–230

96. Yoshida K, Tsuda T, Matsumura T, Tsujino T, Hattori T, Ito H, Tahara E (1989) Amplification of epidermal growth factor receptor (EGFR) gene and oncogenes in human gastric carcinomas. Virchows Arch B Cell Pathol 57:285–290

97. Tahara E (1993) Molecular mechanism of stomach carcinogenesis. J Cancer Res Clin Oncol 119:265–272 (editorial)

98. Yoshida MC, Wada M, Satoh H, Yoshida T, Sakamoto H, Miyagawa K, Yokota J, Koda T, Kakinuma M, Sugimura T, Terada M (1988) Human *hst*-1 (*HSTF*-1) gene maps to chromosome band 11q13 and coamplifies with the *int*-2 gene in human cancer. Proc Natl Acad Sci USA 85:4861–4864

99. Yamamoto T, Hattori T, Tahara E (1988) Interaction between transforming growth factor-alpha and c-Ha-*ras* p21 in progression of human gastric carcinoma. Pathol Res Pract 183:663–669

100. Yoshida K, Kyo E, Tsuda T, Tsujino T, Ito M, Niimoto M, Tahara E (1990) EGF and TGF-alpha, the ligands of hyperproduced EGFR in human esophageal carcinoma cells, act as autocrine growth factors. Int J Cancer 45:131–135

101. Tahara E, Sumiyoshi H, Hata J, Yasui W, Taniyama K, Hayashi T, Nagae S, Sakamoto S (1986) Human epidermal growth factor in gastric carcinoma as a biologic marker of high malignancy. Jpn J Cancer Res 77:145–152

102. Kitadai Y, Yasui W, Yokozaki H, Kuniyasu H, Ayhan A, Haruma K, Kajiyama G, Johnson GR, Tahara E (1993) Expression of amphiregulin, a novel gene of the epidermal growth factor family, in human gastric carcinomas. Jpn J Cancer Res 84:879–884

103. Akagi M, Yokozaki H, Kitadai Y, Ito R, Yasui W, Haruma K, Kajiyama G, Tahara E (1995) Expression of amphiregulin in human gastric cancer cell lines. Cancer 75:1460–1466

104. Kuniyasu H, Yoshida K, Yokozaki H, Yasui W, Ito H, Toge T, Ciardiello F, Persico MG, Saeki T, Salomon DS, Tahara E (1991) Expression of *cripto*, a novel gene of the epidermal growth factor family, in human gastrointestinal carcinomas. Jpn J Cancer Res 82:969–973

105. Kuniyasu H, Yasui W, Akama Y, Akagi M, Tohdo H, Ji Z-Q, Kitadai Y, Yokozaki H, Tahara E (1994) Expression of *cripto* in human gastric carcinomas: an association with tumor stage and prognosis. J Exp Clin Cancer Res 13:151–157

106. Yoshida K, Yokozaki H, Niimoto M, Ito H, Ito M, Tahara E (1989) Expression of TGF-beta and procollagen type I and type III in human gastric carcinomas. Int J Cancer 44:394–398

107. Tsuda T, Yoshida K, Tsujino T, Nakayama H, Kajiyama G, Tahara E (1989) Coexpression of platelet-derived growth factor (PDGF) A-chain and PDGF receptor genes in human gastric carcinomas. Jpn J Cancer Res 80:813–817

108. Tahara E, Kuniyasu H, Yasui W, Yokozaki H (1994) Abnormal expression of growth factors and their receptors in stomach cancer. In: Nishi M, Ichikawa H, Nakajima T, Maruyama K, Tahara E (eds) Gastric cancer. Springer, Tokyo, pp 163–173

109. Tanimoto H, Yoshida K, Yokozaki H, Yasui W, Nakayama H, Ito H, Ohama K, Tahara E (1991) Expression of basic fibroblast growth factor in human gastric carcinomas. Virchows Arch B Cell Pathol 61:263–267

110. Ito R, Kitadai Y, Kyo E, Yokozaki H, Yasui W, Yamashita U, Nikai H, Tahara E (1993) Interleukin 1 alpha acts as an autocrine growth stimulator for human gastric carcinoma cells. Cancer Res 53:4102–4106

110a. Kitadai Y, Haruma K, Yamamoto S, Ue T, Omoto Y, Fridler IJ, Tahara E, Kajiyama G (1997) Inter leukin 8 (IL-8) acts as an angiogenic factor in human gastric carcinomas. Proceedings of the 88th Annual Meeting of the American Association for Cancer Research 38:53

111. Yoshida K, Yasui W, Ito H, Tahara E (1990) Growth factors in progression of human esophageal and gastric carcinomas. Exp Pathol 40:291–300

112. Kitadai Y, Yasui W, Yokozaki H, Kuniyasu H, Haruma K, Kajiyama G, Tahara E (1992) The level of a transcription factor Sp1 is correlated with the expression of EGF receptor in human gastric carcinomas. Biochem Biophys Res Commun 189:1342–1348

113. Kitadai Y, Yamazaki H, Yasui W, Kyo E, Yokozaki H, Kajiyama G, Johnson AC, Pastan I, Tahara E (1993) GC factor represses transcription of several growth factor/receptor genes and causes growth inhibition of human gastric carcinoma cell lines. Cell Growth Differ 4:291–296

114. Ito M, Yasui W, Kyo E, Yokozaki H, Nakayama H, Ito H, Tahara E (1992) Growth inhibition of transforming growth factor beta on human gastric carcinoma cells: receptor and postreceptor signaling. Cancer Res 52:295–300

115. Ito M, Yasui W, Nakayama H, Yokozaki H, Ito H, Tahara E (1992) Reduced levels of transforming growth factor-beta type I receptor in human gastric carcinomas. Jpn J Cancer Res 83:86–92

116. Park K, Kim SJ, Bang YJ, Park JG, Kim NK, Roberts AB, Sporn MB (1994) Genetic changes in the transforming growth factor beta (TGF-beta) type II receptor gene in human gastric cancer cells: correlation with sensitivity to growth inhibition by TGF-beta. Proc Natl Acad Sci USA 91:8772–8776

117. Myeroff LL, Parsons R, Kim SJ, Hedrick L, Cho KR, Orth K, Mathis M, Kinzler KW, Lutterbaugh J, Park K, Bang Y-J, Lee H, Park J-G, Lynch HT, Roberts AB, Vogelstein B, Markowitz SD (1995) A transforming growth factor beta receptor type II gene mutation common in colon and gastric but rare in endometrial cancers with microsatellite instability. Cancer Res 55:5545–5547

118. Stamenkovic I, Aruffo A, Amiot M, Seed B (1991) The hematopoietic and epithelial forms of CD44 are distinct polypeptides with different adhesion potentials for hyaluronate-bearing cells. EMBO J 10:343–348

119. Jackson DG, Buckley J, Bell JI (1992) Multiple variants of the human lymphocyte homing receptor CD44 generated by insertions at a single site in the extracellular domain. J Biol Chem 267:4732–4739

120. Cooper DL, Dougherty G, Harn HJ, Jackson S, Baptist EW, Byers J, Datta A, Phillips G, Isola NR (1992) The complex CD44 transcriptional unit; alternative splicing of three internal exons generates the epithelial form of CD44. Biochem Biophys Res Commun 182:569–578

121. Matsumura Y, Tarin D (1992) Significance of CD44 gene products for cancer diagnosis and disease evaluation. Lancet 340:1053–1058

122. Tanabe KK, Ellis LM, Saya H (1993) Expression of CD44R1 adhesion molecule in colon carcinomas and metastases. Lancet 341:725–726

123. Heider K-H, Hofmann M, Hors E, van den Berg F, Ponta H, Herrlich P, Pals ST (1993) A human homologue of the rat metastasis-associated variant of CD44 is expressed in colorectal carcinomas and adenomatous polyps. J Cell Biol 120:227–233

124. Yokozaki H, Ito R, Nakayama H, Kuniyasu H, Taniyama K, Tahara E (1994) Expression of CD44 abnormal transcripts in human gastric carcinomas. Cancer Lett 83:229–234

125. Matsumura Y, Sugiyama M, Matsumura S, Hayle AJ, Robinson P, Smith JC, Tarin D (1995) Unusual retention of introns in CD44 gene transcripts in bladder cancer provides new diagnostic and clinical oncological opportunities. J Pathol 177:11–20

126. Yoshida K, Bolodeoku J, Sugino T, Goodison S, Matsumura Y, Warren BF, Toge T, Tahara E, Tarin D (1995) Abnormal retention of intron 9 in CD44 gene transcripts in human gastrointestinal tumors. Cancer Res 55:4273–4277

127. Higashikawa K, Yokozaki H, Ue T, Taniyama K, Ishikawa T, Tarin D, Tahara E (1996) Evaluation of CD44 transcription variants in human digestive tract carcinomas and normal tissues. Int J Cancer 66:11–17

128. Weber GF, Ashkar S, Glimcher MJ, Cantor H (1996) Receptor–ligand interaction between CD44 and osteopontin (Eta-1). Science 271:509–512

129. Ruoslahti E, Pierschbacher MD (1987) New perspectives in cell adhesion: RGD and integrins. Science 238:491–497

130. Nakayama H, Yasui W, Yokozaki H, Tahara E (1993) Reduced expression of nm23 is associated with metastasis of human gastric carcinomas. Jpn J Cancer Res 84:184–190

131. Sier CF, Verspaget HW, Griffioen G, Ganesh S, Vloedgraven HJ, Lamers CB (1993) Plasminogen activators in normal tissue and carcinomas of the human oesophagus and stomach. Gut 34:80–85

132. Tanaka N, Fukao H, Ueshima S, Okada K, Yasutomi M, Matsuo O (1991) Plasminogen activator inhibitor 1 in human carcinoma tissues. Int J Cancer 48:481–484

133. Nekarda H, Schmitt M, Ulm K, Wenninger A, Vogelsang H, Becker K, Roder JD, Fink U, Siewert JR (1994) Prognostic impact of urokinase-type plasminogen activator and its inhibitor PAI-1 in completely resected gastric cancer. Cancer Res 54:2900–2907

134. Lotan R, Ito H, Yasui W, Yokozaki H, Lotan D, Tahara E (1994) Expression of a 31-kDa lactoside-binding lectin in normal human gastric mucosa and in primary and metastatic gastric carcinomas. Int J Cancer 56:474–480

135. Tahara E (1995) Genetic alterations in human gastrointestinal cancers: the application to molecular diagnosis. Cancer 75:1410–1417

Galectins in Gastric and Colorectal Cancers: Implications for Tumor Progression and Metastasis

Reuben Lotan[1] and Eiichi Tahara[2]

Summary. Galectins 1 and 3, galactoside-binding proteins, have been implicated in cellular interactions, growth, apoptosis, differentiation, transformation, and metastasis. Galectins' expression was detected in normal mucosa and in primary and metastatic colorectal and gastric carcinomas by Western blotting of extracts from cultured tumor cells and surgical specimens and by immunohistochemistry using histological sections of fixed tissues. Galectin-1 was detected in only 7 of 21 cultured human colon carcinoma cell lines, whereas galectin-3 was found in 20 of 21. In gastric cancer cell lines, galectin-1 was detected in most (six of eight) and galectin-3 in all of eight cell lines. Most of the cell lines expressed carcinoembryonic antigen and lysosome-associated membrane proteins, which can serve as endogenous ligands for galectins. Immunoblotting of extracts of malignant colorectal tissues from 48 patients revealed that the galectin-3 level was higher in tumor specimens from patients classified as Dukes' stage D than in those in other stages. Immunoblotting of extracts of normal and malignant gastric tissues from 26 patients revealed that the galectin-3 level was higher in tumor tissue than in normal tissue in 9 of 26 cases but lower than that in normal tissue in only 3 of 26 cases. An immunohistochemical analysis revealed that galectin-3 expression increased in gastric cancers relative to normal mucosa and in some metastatic lesions relative to primary tumors. These results implicate galectin-3 in the progression of certain types of colorectal and gastric cancers to the metastatic phenotype.

Introduction

Normal development, cell growth and differentiation, and tumor invasion and metastasis involve various types of cellular interactions among cells and between cells and exogenous soluble or insoluble macromolecules. Although most of these interactions are mediated by a variety of specific cell surface components that are involved in protein–protein interactions, such as integrins, selectins, or members of the immunoglobulin superfamily, some interactions are mediated by carbohydrate-recognition mechanisms. Such interactions occur during embryonic development [1–3], cell growth and differentiation, and cancer metastasis [4–8].

The expression of cellular glycoconjugates, including mucins, glycoproteins, glycolipids, and blood group-associated carbohydrate antigens, has been found to change during normal differentiation, after malignant transformation, and during progression to metastatic stages in a variety of cell types including gastrointestinal neoplasms [1, 9–13]. The various monosaccharides present in vertebrate oligosaccharides can be linked in specific sequences and types of anomeric linkages, and it has been suggested that they form specific recognition codes that can specify intercellular recognition and adhesion [1, 6, 14]. Complementary molecules capable of binding specific carbohydrates would be required for recognition and for mediating the functional consequences of such recognition. Lectin-like proteins endowed with the ability to bind different types of saccharides have been found in various animal tissues [15] and malignant cells [16–18]. The binding of neoglycoproteins to tissue sections revealed that the expression of several endogenous lectins was different in primary and metastatic lesions of human colon and lung carcinoma, which suggests a role for lectins in metastasis [19–21]. Some lectins have been implicated in mediating the adhesion of

[1] Department of Tumor Biology, Box 108, The University of Texas M. D. Anderson Cancer Center, 1515 Holcombe Boulevard, Houston, TX 77030, USA
[2] First Department of Pathology, Hiroshima University School of Medicine, 1-2-3 Kasumi, Minami-ku, Hiroshima 734, Japan

metastatic tumor cells to target organ cells (i.e., lung) [22–24].

Galectins: A family of Galactoside-Binding Proteins

The most prevalent vertebrate lectins bind β-galactosides [6, 8, 25, 26]. These lectins constitute a family of proteins called galectins, which are related by sharing amino acid sequences [25, 27]. The best studied among the galectins are galectin-1 (13.0–14.5 kDa) [26, 28] and galectin-3 (29–35 kDa) [5, 6, 28–32].

Galectin-1 is developmentally regulated in several vertebrate tissues including intestine, skin, lung, muscle, and nervous system [27, 33–36]. In most cell types this lectin is present in the cytoplasm with a lower but detectable level of expression on the cell surface. The latter localization is also supported by the presence of carbohydrate-binding activity at the cell surface [18, 37]. Galectin-1 is also secreted by some cells [38].

Galectin-3 [5], a 35 kDa lactose-binding lectin, shares regions of complete homology with galectin-1, including a 39-amino-acid residue sequence in which there are 15 invariant amino acids [6, 25, 27, 32]. These residues are located in the carbohydrate recognition domain. Site-directed mutagenesis of galectin-1 revealed that sequences conserved in this region between galectin-1 and galectin-3 are critical for the carbohydrate-binding activity of galectin-1 [39, 40]. Galectin-3 is identical to the murine macrophage cell surface antigen Mac-2 [30]. Mouse galectin-2 also exhibits amino acid sequence homology at its amino-terminus with heterogeneous nuclear ribonucleo-proteins (hnRNPs) and can be localized in the cell nucleus [32].

Functions of Galectins

The developmental regulation of galectin-1 expression has led to speculation that this protein may be involved in the control of cellular proliferation and differentiation, and there are indications for a role of this lectin in cell adhesion as well [24, 41]. The ability of galectin-1 to stimulate DNA synthesis in a lactose-inhibitable process was demonstrated in aortic smooth muscle cells and pulmonary endothelial cells [42]. Galectin-1

has been implicated in malignant transformation by the demonstration that BALB3T3 fibroblasts that had been transfected with the galectin's cDNA became transformed as evidenced by their ability to form colonies in soft agar, and they were tumorigenic when injected into nude mice [43]. In contrast, in mouse embryo fibroblasts galectin-1 was found to act as an autocrine negative growth inhibitor, which is endogenously produced and secreted by these cells [44]. Because the latter two activities could not be inhibited by galactosides, they may be unrelated to the carbohydrate-binding function of the galectin. The rapid induction of galectin-1 in cells induced to undergo apoptosis and its ability to mediate apoptosis of T cells have implicated this galectin in programmed cell death [45, 46].

The secretion of galectin-1 suggests that it may possess an extracellular function [38]. Binding of the secreted galectin to the cell surface or to extracellular matrix (ECM) stabilizes the protein and protects it from inactivation [47]. Furthermore, once bound to the ECM, the secreted galectin-1 can mediate attachment of tumor cells via cell surface lysosomal-associated membrane proteins (LAMPs) [41].

In addition to its possible role in cell adhesion, it has been proposed that galectin-3 may function in the nucleus in the transport of mRNA to the cytosol [32], and it may be involved in pre-mRNA splicing [48]. Furthermore, galectin-3 may play a role in cell proliferation, as the levels of galectin-3 protein and mRNA are low in quiescent mouse fibroblasts and increase rapidly after mitogenic stimulation [49]. The transfection of galectin-3 into immortalized fibroblastic cells increased their ability to form colonies in agar, to form tumors, and to colonize the lungs in mice [50]. Thus galectin-3 may also be involved in transformation and metastasis.

Galectins in Gastrointestinal Tumors

Colorectal Cancers

A high level of binding of the Mac-2 antibody, which recognizes galectin-3 [35, 36], has been detected in small intestinal epithelial cells located at the tips of villi, whereas only a low level of reactivity was found in cells at the base of the villi [46]. The expression of galectin-3 increases along the crypt–surface axis in normal colonic epithelium, suggesting a relation with differentiation. Furthermore, nonmalignant colonic mucosa cells adjacent to colon carcinomas were found to contain the galectin-3 mRNA and protein [47, 48].

There have been several reports on the presence of lactose-binding lectins in human colon carcinoma [20, 51–58]. Most of these studies detected the presence of galectin-1 in primary colon tissue and tumor samples after affinity chromatography on immobilized lactose. Organ-dependent differences in lectin profiles in metastatic lesions to either lung or liver from primary colon carcinomas have been demonstrated [20].

Other studies have identified the expression of galectins in cultured colon carcinoma cells. Galectin-3 expression was detected in six of seven hepatocellular carcinoma (HCC) cell lines [57]. We found that galectin-3 was present in 20 of 21 colon carcinoma cell lines [37] and in surgical specimens of colorectal cancers [56]. This expression was related to progression to metastatic stages in cancer patients [56]. Specifically, the levels of galectin-3 in primary tumors of patients having distant metastases (dukes' stage D) were significantly higher than in those from patients without detectable metastases (Dukes' stages B1 and B2). Likewise, the level of galectin-3 correlated significantly with the serum carcinembryonic antigen (CEA) level in the same patients. In contrast, the variation in the level of galectin-1 among the varirus specimens was smaller, and there was no correlation between the amount of galectin-1 and cancer stage or CEA level. The results indicated that the relative amount of galectin-3 increases as the colorectal cancer progresses to the more malignant stage. However, galectin-3 has been reported to be found primarily in the cytoplasm of human colon carcinoma in tissue sections where staining of adjacent normal colonic epithelium shows most of the lectin localized in the nucleus [59]. The intensity of staining for galectin-3 was also more pronounced in normal colonic epithelium than it was in colon carcinomas. The reason for the differences between results obtained in different laboratories is not clear but may be related to the small sample size of the study. This contention is based on the findings of a large study in which galectin-3 was analyzed in 153 tissue specimens, including 29 adenomas containing premalignant lesions, 66 colon carcinomas of known Dukes' stage, and 23 other primary carcinomas with 35 associated metastases [58]. This study has demonstrated that galectin-3 expression was sig-

nificantly elevated in high-grade dysplasia and early invasive cancers relative to adenomatous tissues from which they derived. The expression of galectin-3 increased with Dukes' stage and was higher in metastases than in the corresponding primary tumors, thereby confirming with immunohistochemical data the immunoblotting data of Irimura et al. [56]. Furthermore, enhanced galectin-3 expression correlated with decreased long-term patient survival [58]. In conclusion, the study indicated that galectin-3 expression is related to neoplastic transformation and metastatic progression in colon cancer in vivo.

Gastric Cancers

To determine whether galectins also play a role in the progression of gastric cancer, we analyzed the expression of galectin-3 by Western immunoblotting in extracts prepared from surgical specimens from 26 patients with gastric cancer and adjacent nonneoplastic mucosa and from 7 specimens of normal mucosa [60]. The level of galectin-3 was higher in the tumor samples than in the normal specimens in 34.6% (9/26) of cases, similar to the normal specimens in 53.8% (14/26) of cases, and lower than the normal specimens in 11.5% (3/26) of cases. The difference in lectin level was not related to the histological type of the tumor.

We next used formalin-fixed paraffin-embedded tissue sections from 39 patients with various types of primary gastric carcinoma and adjacent "normal" mucosa, as well as specimens from primary gastric carcinomas and their metastases to lymph nodes, liver, lungs, kidney, or ovaries from 74 cases. The galectin-3 level was higher in tubular gastric carcinoma specimens than in normal mucosa specimens in 55% of the cases, and the mean staining index was higher in the carcinoma specimens than in the normal tissue specimens. The difference between the galectin-3 level in the tumor and the corresponding normal mucosa in 11 cases was statistically significant ($P < 0.05$). Galectin-3 levels were not significantly different between tumor tissue and normal tissue in cases of well differentiated papillary carcinomas or poorly differentiated carcinomas. Likewise, there was no significant difference between galectin-3 levels in tumors at different stages of disease, although galectin-3 levels tended to be higher in state III cancer than in normal mucosa [60].

There were distinct patterns of galectin-3 staining in different tumors. In some cases the staining appeared to be associated with the cell surface membrane, whereas in others the staining was cytoplasmic [60]. These patterns of localization were observed previously in cultured cells [61].

A comparison of galectin-3 lectin levels in primary gastric carcinomas and their metastases was also performed using immunohistochemical methods on specimens from 74 patients, including primary gastric carcinoma and metastases to at least one distant organ (lymph node, liver, lung, kidney, or ovary) isolated from the same patient. The results were analyzed according to the histology and differentiation of the tumors and the site of metastasis. The galectin-3 level in lymph node metastases was similar to that of the corresponding primary carcinoma in about 50% of the 51 cases analyzed. A trend ($P = 0.1$) for a higher level of galectin-3 in lymph node metastases than in poorly differentiated primary carcinomas from which they dervied was indicated by the finding of such a relation in 38% of the cases, whereas only 6% of the cases showed a higher galectin-3 level in primary cancers compared to their corresponding metastases. Furthermore, a higher galectin-3 level in liver metastases than in well-differentiated tubular primary cancers ($P = 0.02$) was indicated by the finding of such a relation in 31% of the cases, whereas only 11% of cases showed a higher level of galectin-3 in primary carcinomas than in their liver metastases. In contrast, no such trend could be detected when lymph node metastases were compared with their well differentiated primary carcinomas or when liver or lung metastases were compared with their corresponding well-differentiated papillary or poorly differentiated primary cancers. The higher expression of galectin-3 in certain types of primary gastric cancers and metastases implicates this lectin in the metastatic phenotype [60].

Endogenous Ligands for Galectins in Gastrointestinal Mucosa

Glycoconjugates containing terminal or penultimate lactosyl residues may play a role in cellular interactions by serving as complementary molecules for endogenous lactoside-binding proteins [6, 8, 24, 31, 62]. Important interactions of lectins may be mediated by glycoconjugates that are expressed on the surface of adjacent cells or are present in the ECM and contain mono- or oligosaccharides that are recognized by the complementary binding site in the lectin molecule. The ECM is composed mainly of laminin, fibronectin, type IV collagen, and various proteoglycans, many of which are heavily glycosylated and whose oligosaccharide side chains can provide recognition determinants for lectins. Although the functions of galectin-3 are not clearly established, this lectin is thought to play a role in cellular recognition and adhesion. Galectin-3 isolated from a human lung exhibited a higer affinity for blood group A-related structures and for polylactosaminoglycan chains than for lactose [31, 63]. The ability of galectin-3, which is present on the surface of hepatocellular carcinoma (HCC) cells to bind laminin is well established [37, 64–66]. This activity may play a role in cell binding to ECM, an important event in cancer cell invasion and metastasis [67]. However, the mere expression of galectin-3 on the surface of a cell may not be sufficient to mediate carbohydrate-specific adhesion to laminin [66]. The binding of recombinant human galectin-3 to mouse EHS laminin has also been reported [66, 68]. A number of cellular interactions with laminin have been shown to be dependent on the state of glycosylation of this glycoprotein [69]. Whether it is related to important interactions of laminin and galectins remains to be elucidated. It is noteworthy in this regard that one report demonstrated that galectin-1 may be involved in the adhesion of cells to laminin [70]

Carcinoembryonic antigen (CD66e), a 180 kDa member of the immunoglobulin superfamily, is more than 50% carbohydrate by weight, and some of its oligosaccharides are lactosaminoglycans [71], the preferred complementary structure for galectin-3 [5, 6, 8, 62, 72]. Increased CEA expression is characteristic of metastatic colon carcinoma cells [73]. We have demonstrated that galectin-3 is capable of binding to immobilized CEA in a carbohydrate-dependent manner. More importantly, we found that galectin-3 and CEA appeared to be co-localized on the cell surface, suggesting that galectin-3 may interact with CEA at the cell surface. If such interactions can occur between galectin-3 and CEA on adjacent cells, they may mediate cell–cell adhesion. In addition, interactions between galectin-3 and CEA on the same cell could modulate the distribution of CEA in the membrane and its efficiency as a cell adhesion molecule because microclustered CEA–lectin complexes would likely participate in multivalent interactions. Our data suggest that another member of the immunoglobulin superfamily, most probably nonspecific cross-reacting antigen (NCA) (CD66c) or a related family member, is also recognized by galectin-3. CEA and NCA have been found to be involved in calcium-independent homotypic and heterotypic adhesion in colon carcinoma cells [73–75]. Whether galectin-3 plays a role in these effects of CEA and NCA remains to be established.

Another class of cellular glycoconjugates we examined for their ability to bind to galectin-3 was the lysosome-associated membrane glycoproteins (LAMP) [76, 77]. LAMP-1 and LAMP-2 were shown to be heavily glycosylated, with more than 50% of their molecular weights being contributed by carbohydrate side chains. They are the major sialoglycoproteins in a variety of cell types and the major carriers of poly-N-acetyllactosamine [77, 78]. LAMP-1 and LAMP-2, although predominantly intracellular, are present on the surface of some cells including the KM12 cell line [79]. Cell surface LAMPs have been implicated in cell adhesion and metastasis of KM12 cells by several studies [79, 80]. The ability of galectin-3 to bind LAMP-1 and LAMP-2 suggests that these molecules may also be functional ligands for this lectin. Previously, it was reported that galectin-1 was able to bind LAMPs from Chinese hamster ovary and ovarian carcinoma cells [41, 81]. We found that human galectin-3 can also interact with LAMPs.

To be able to mediate cell–cell and cell–ECM interactions, galectin-3 should be present on the cell surface; it should be able to bind exogenous glycoconjugates; and the cells should express complementary glycoconjugates that could serve as binding sites for galectin. The presence of various carbohydrate-binding proteins on the surface of HCC cells has been shown previously [53]. That galectin-3 is present on the cell surface was demonstrated by several methods, including cell surface radioiodination, immunofluorescence microscopy, and flow cytofluorimetry; that galactoside-specific, lectin-like activity is present on the surface of intact KM12 cells was indicated by the binding of thiodigalactoside-containing neoglycoproteins; that exogenous biotinylated galectin-3 can bind in a lactoside-inhibitable fashion to the surface of KM12 cells was shown by flow cytofluorimetry. The co-localization of galectin-3 and CEA, observed by double indirect immunofluorescence, suggests that CEA is one of the cell surface ligands for galectin-3. Preliminary identification of additional potential cell surface galectin-3 ligands was achieved by analysis of radioiodinated molecules that were co-immunoprecipitated with galectin-3 from extracts of cell surface radiolabeled cells. Some of these surface molecules are distinct from those labeled metabolically with sugars (e.g. 120 kDa). In this regard, it is interesting to note that galectin-1 has been shown to bind to the surface of mouse embryo fibroblasts by means of a carbohydrate-independent mechanism [44]. Our finding that only 50% of exogenously added galectin-3 can be removed from the KM12 cell surface by lactose also supports the possibility of the existence of carbohydrate-independent interactions of the lectin with cell surface components.

Thus we have demonstrated that galectin-3 is expressed in a large number of HCC cell lines, whereas the expression of galectin-1 seems to be restricted to more poorly differentiated HCC cell lines. Focusing on galectin-3, we determined that this protein can bind in a carbohydrate-dependent manner to several endogenous and exogenous glycoproteins shown previously to be involved in cellular interactions in colon carcinoma cells, including CEA, LAMPs 1 and 2, and laminin. Furthermore, the presence of cognate ligands for galectin-3 on the cell surface suggests that such proteins may play a role in the function of the lectin at this location.

The potential complementary glycoconjugates for galectin-3 in gastric cancer have not been characterized, although some reports (described below) suggest the expression of potential cognate molecules for galectin-3 on the surface of gastric carcinoma cells. The patterns of binding of plant lectins indicated that glycoconjugates are altered during differentiation of normal gastric mucosa, in metaplastic lesions, and in gastric carcinomas [82]. Furthermore, several reports suggest that glycoproteins play an important role in determining the malignant behavior of gastric carcinoma and that such molecules might be promising biochemical markers of tumor progression [83–87]. For example, the binding of Helix pomatia agglutinin, a blood group A-specific lectin, has been detected in 59% of primary gastric carcinomas; this binding was significantly correlated with tumor invasiveness and metastasis and was inversely related to survival [86]. Similarly, the pattern of binding of several plant lectins (Con A, WGA, PNA, UEA-

1, and DBA) to tissue specimens from normal and metaplastic gastric mucosa and in adenomas and carcinomas revealed changes that were related to tumor progression [87]. Changes in glycocojugate structure between primary and metastatic gastric cancer have been found by the binding of monoclonal antibodies generated against glycoproteins isolated from gastric carcinoma by lectin-affinity chromatography. The expression of this glycoprotein was lower in liver metastases than in primary cancers [88]. Lastly, one report described the increased expression of *N*-acetyllactosamine moiety detected by binding of plant lectins in gastrointestinal neoplasms relative to normal mucosal cells [9]. Among gastric carcinomas, tubular (intestinal type) carcinomas expressed a higher level of the carbohydrate than the diffuse-type, signet-ring, and poorly differentiated carcinomas [9]. Some of these glycoproteins could be bound by galectin-3 via their carbohydrate side chains. We found that galectin-3 binds CEA isolated from a liver metastasis of a colon carcinoma [37]. This glycoprotein antigen is expressed on the surface of gastric carcinomas [89–91], and we found by immunoblotting that it is also expressed in gastric cancer surgical specimens and cell lines that contain galectin-3 (unpublished observations). Thus galectin-3 could bind CEA on adjacent cells and mediate cell–cell adhesion. Likewise, galectin-3 could bind an asialoglycoprotein antigen that was detected on gastric cancer cells [83] or blood group A-containing glycoproteins expressed by invasive primary gastric tumors [86].

Potential Clinical Relevance of Galectin Analysis in Gastrointestinal Cancer

Gastric carcinoma is one of the major causes of cancer mortality in Japan and is still a frequent disease in Western countries [92]. The prognosis of a patient with gastric cancer is related directly to the disease stage at the time of initial diagnosis. Thus the pathological type of the lesion, its location in the stomach, and most importantly the presence or absence of lymph node metastases are the most significant indicators of prognosis [93]. Surgery and adjuvant chemotherapy of gastric cancer before it has metastasized to lymph nodes seem to improve survival. Specific cellular and biochemical markers that change during the pro-

gression of localized premalignant and malignant gastric lesions to metastatic stages may provide a means with which to detect highly metastatic cells within a heterogeneous primary tumor. Such markers could lead to the design of sensitive diagnostic methods to identify patients at risk for the development of metastases (i.e., methods that would indicate to the clinician that an aggressive treatment may be appropriate for improving the patient's prognosis). Our findings revealed a higher level of galectin-3 in lymph node metastases than in primary poorly differentiated gastric carcinomas and a higher galectin-3 level in liver metastases than in primary well-differentiated tubular carcinomas. These results suggest that galectins, in particular galectin-3, can serve as a marker of tumor progression and metastasis in gastrointestinal carcinomas.

References

1. Feizi T (1991) Carbohydrate differentiation antigens: probable ligands for cell adhesion molecules. Trends Biochem Sci 16:84–86
2. Kimber SJ (1990) Glycoconjugates and cell surface interactions in pre- and peri-implantation mammalian embryonic development. Int Rev Cytol 120:53–167
3. Thorpe SJ, Bellairs R, Feizi T (1988) Developmental patterning of carbohydrate antigens during early embryogenesis of the chick: expression of antigens of the poly-N-acetyllactosamine series. Development 102:193–210
4. Harrison FL, Wilson TJ (1992) The 14kDa beta-galactoside binding lectin in myoblast and myotube cultures: localization by confocal microscopy. J Cell Sci 101:635–646
5. Hughes RC (1994) Mac-2: a versatile galactose-binding protein of mammalian tissues. Glycobiology 4:5–12
6. Lotan R (1992) β-Galactoside-binding vertebrate lectins: synthesis, molecular biology, function. In: Allen H, Kisailus E (eds) Glycoconjugates: composition, structure, and function. Dekker, New York, pp 635–671
7. Raz A, Lotan R (1987) Endogenous galactoside-binding lectin: a new class of functional tumor cell surface molecules related to metastasis. Cancer Metastasis Rev 6:433–452
8. Zhou Q, Cummings RD (1992) Animal lectins: a distinct group of carbohydrate binding proteins involved in cell adhesion, molecular recognition, and development. In: Fukuda M (ed) Cell surface carbohydrates and cell development. CRC, Boca Raton, pp 99–126

9. Baldus SE, Park Y-O, Kotlarek GM, Hell K, Fischer R (1996) Expression of Galβ-1-4GlcNAc sequences by human gastrointestinal neoplasms and their precursors as detected by *Erythrina cristagalli* and *Erythrina corallodendron* lectins. Int J Oncol 9:43–48

10. Alhadeff JA (1989) Malignant cell glycoproteins and glycolipids. Crit Rev Oncol Hematol 9:37–107

11. Hakomori S-I (1989) Aberrant glycosylation in tumors and tumor associated carbohydrate antigens. Adv Cancer Res 52:257–331

12. Dennis JW, Laferte S, Yagel S, Breitman ML (1989) Asparagine-linked oligosaccharides associated with metastatic cancer. Cancer Cells 1:87–92

13. Fernandes B, Sagman U, Auger M, Demetrio M, Dennis JW (1991) Beta 1–6 branched oligosaccharides as a marker of tumor progression in human breast and colon neoplasia. Cancer Res 51:718–723

14. Paulson JC (1991) Glycoproteins; what are the sugar chains for? Trends Biochem Sci 14:272–276

15. Barondes SH (1986) Vertebrate lectins: properties and functions. In: Liener IE, Sharon N, Goldstein IJ (eds) The lectins. Academic, New York, pp 437–466

16. Raz A, Lotan R (1987) Endogenous galactoside-binding lectins: a new class of functional tumor cell surface molecules related to metastasis. Cancer Metastasis Rev 6:433–452

17. Monsigny M, Roche AC, Kieda C, Midoux P, Oberenovitch A (1988) Characterization and biological implications of membrane lectins in tumor, lymphoid and myeloid cells. Biochimie 70:1633–1649

18. Gabius HJ (1991) Detection and functions of mammalian lectins—with emphasis on membrane lectins. Biochim Biophys Acta 1071:1–18

19. Gabius HJ, Engelhardt R (1988) Sugar receptors of different types in human metastases to lung and liver. Tumor Biol 9:21–36

20. Gabius HJ, Ciesiolka T, Kunze E, Vehmeyer K (1989) Detection of metastasis-associated differences for receptors of glycoconjugates (lectins) in histomorphologically unchanged xenotransplants from primary and metastatic lesions of human colon adenocarcinomas. Clin Exp Met 7:571–584

21. Glaves D, Gabius HJ, Weiss L (1989) Site-associated expression of endogenous tumor lectins. Int J Cancer 44:506–511

22. Kieda C, Monsigny M (1986) Involvement of membrane sugar receptors and membrane glycoconjugates in the adhesion of 3LL cell subpopulations to cultured pulmonary cells. Invasion Metastasis 6:347–366

23. Meromsky L, Lotan R, Raz A (1986) Implications of endogenous tumor cell surface lectins as mediators of cellular interactions and lung colonization. Cancer Res 46:5270–5275

24. Lotan R, Raz A (1988) Endogenous lectins as mediators of tumor cell adhesion. J Cell Biochem 37:107–117

25. Barondes SH, Castronovo V, Cooper DNW, Cummings RD, Drickamer K, Feizi T, Gitt MA, Hirabayashi J, Hughes C, Kasai K, Leffler H, Liu F-T, Lotan R, Mercurio AM, Monsigny M, Pillai S, Poirier F, Raz A, Rigby PWJ, Rini JM, Wang JL (1994) Galectins: a family of animal β-galactoside-binding lectins. Cell 76:597–598

26. Harrison FL (1991) Soluble vertebrate lectins: ubiquitous but inscrutable proteins. J Cell Sci 100:9–14

27. Barondes SH, Cooper DNW, Gitt MA, Leffler H (1994) Galectins: structure and function of a large family of animal lectins. J Biol Chem 269:20807–20810

28. Raz A, Meromsky L, Zvibel I, Lotan R (1987) Transformation-related changes in the expression of endogenous cell lectins. Int J Cancer 39:353–360

29. Albrandt K, Orida NK, Liu FT (1987) An IgE-binding protein with a distinctive repetitive sequence and homology with an IgG receptor. Proc Natl Acad Sci USA 84:6859–6863

30. Cherayil BJ, Weiner SJ, Pillai S (1989) The Mac-2 antigen is a galactose-specific lectin that binds IgE. J Exp Med 170:1959–1972

31. Leffler H, Barondes SH (1986) Specificity of binding of three soluble rat lung lectins to substituted and unsubstituted mammalian β-galactosides. J Biol Chem 261:10119–10126

32. Wang JL, Werner EA, Laing JG, Patterson RJ (1992) Nuclear and cytoplasmic localization of a lectin–ribonucleoprotein complex. Biochem Soc Trans 20:269–272

33. Akimoto Y, Kawakami H, Oda Y, Obinata A, Endo H, Kasai K-I, Hirano H (1992) Changes in expression of the endogenous β-galactoside-binding 14-kDa lectin of chick embryonic skin during epidermal differentiation. Exp Cell Res 199:297–304

34. Oda N, Tsujino T, Tsuda T, Yoshida K, Nakayama H, Yasui W, Tahara E (1990) DNA ploidy pattern and amplification of ERBB and ERBB2 genes in human gastric carcinomas. Virchows Arch B Cell Pathol 58:273–277

35. Powell JT, Whitney PL (1984) Endogenous ligands of rat lung β-galactoside-binding protein (galaptin) isolated by affinity chromatography on carboxyamidomethylated-galaptin-Sepharose. Biochem J 223:769–774

36. Regan LJ, Dodd J, Barondes SH, Jessell TM (1986) Selective expression of endogenous lactose-binding lectins and lactoseries glycoconjugates in subsets of rat sensory neurons. Proc Natl Acad Sci USA 83:2248–2252

37. Ohannesian DW, Lotan D, Thomas P, Jessup JM, Fukuda M, Gabius H-J, Lotan R (1995) Carcinoembryonic antigen and other glycoconjugates act as ligands for galectin-3 in human colon carcinoma cells. Cancer Res 55:2191–2199

38. Cooper DN, Barondes SH (1990) Evidence for export of a muscle lectin from cytosol to extracellular matrix and for a novel secretory mechanism. J Cell Biol 110:1681–1691

39. Hirabayashi J, Kasai K (1991) Effect of amino acid substitution by site-directed mutagenesis on the carbohydrate recognition and stability of human 14-kDa β-galactoside-binding lectin. J Biol Chem 266:23648–23653

40. Kasai K-I, Hirabayashi J (1996) Galectins: a family of animal lectins that decipher glycocodes. J Biochem 119:1–8

41. Skrincosky DM, Allen HJ, Bernacki RJ (1993) Galaptin-mediated adhesion of human ovarian carcinoma A121 cells and detection of cellular galaptin-binding glycoproteins. Cancer Res 53:2667–2675

42. Sanford GL, Harris-Hooker S (1990) Stimulation of vascular cell proliferation by β-galactoside specific lectins. FASEB J 4:2912–2918

43. Yamaoka K, Ohno S, Kawasaki H, Suzuki K (1991) Overexpression of a β-galactoside binding protein causes transformation of BALB3T3 fibroblast cells. Biochem Biophys Res Commun 179:272–279

44. Wells V, Mallucci L (1991) Identification of an autocrine negative growth factor: mouse β-galactoside-binding protein is a cytostatic factor and cell growth regulator. Cell 64:91–97

45. Goldstone SD, Lavin MF (1991) Isolation of a cDNA clone, encoding a human beta-galactoside binding protein, overexpressed during glucocorticoid-induced cell death. Biochem Biophys Res Commun 178:746–750

46. Perillo NL, Pace KE, Seilhamer JJ, Baum LG (1995) Apoptosis of T cells mediated by galectin-1. Nature 378:736–738

47. Zhou Q, Cummings RD (1993) L-14 lectin recognition of laminin and its promotion of in vitro cell adhesion. Arch Biochem Biophys 300:6–17

48. Dagher SF, Wang JJ, Patterson RJ (1995) Identification of galectin-3 as a factor in pre-mRNA splicing. Proc Natl Acad Sci USA 92:1213–1217

49. Agrwal N, Wang JL, Voss P (1989) Carbohydrate-binding protein 35: levels of transcription and mRNA accumulation in quiescent and proliferating cells. J Biol Chem 264:17236–17242

50. Raz A, Zhu D, Hogan V, Shah N, Raz T, Karkash R, Pazerini G, Carmi P (1990) Evidence for the role of 34-kDa galactoside-binding lectin in transformation and metastasis. Int J Cancer 46:871–877

51. Allen HJ, Karakousis C, Piver MS, Gamarra M, Nava H, Forsyth B, Matecki B, Jazayeri A, Sucato D, Kisailus E, DiCioccio R (1987) Galactoside-binding lectin in human tissues. Tumor Biol 8:218–229

52. Castronovo V, Campo E, van den Brule FA, Claysmith AP, Cioce V, Liu F-T, Fernandez PL, Sobel ME (1992) Inverse modulation of steady state messenger RNA levels of two non-integrin laminin-binding proteins in human colon carcinoma. J Natl Cancer Inst 84:1161–1169

53. Gabius H-J, Engelhardt R, Hellmann T, Midoux P, Monsigny M, Nagel GA, Vehmeyer K (1987) Characterization of membrane lectins in human colon carcinoma cells by flow cytometry, drug targeting and affinity chromatography. Anticancer Res 7:109–112

54. Gabius S, Schirrmacher V, Franz H, Joshi SS, Gabius H-J (1990) Analysis of cell-surface sugar receptor expression by neoglycoenzyme binding and adhesion to plastic-immobilized neoglycoproteins for related weakly and strongly metastatic cell lines of murine tumor model systems. Int J Cancer 46:500–507

55. Lee EC, Woo H-J, Korzelius CA, Steele GD, Mercurio AM (1991) Carbohydrate-binding protein 35 is the major cell-surface laminin-binding protein in colon carcinoma. Arch Surg 126:1498–1502

56. Irimura T, Matsushita Y, Sutton RC, Carralero D, Ohannesian DW, Cleary KR, Ota DM, Nicolson GL, Lotan R (1991) Increased content of an endogenous lactose-binding lectin in human colorectal carcinoma progressed to metastatic stages. Cancer Res 51:387–393

57. Rosenberg I, Cherayil BJ, Isselbacher KJ, Pillai S (1991) Mac-2 binding glycoproteins: putative ligands for a cytosolic β-galactoside lectin. J Biol Chem 266:18731–18736

58. Schoeppner HL, Raz A, Ho SB, Bresalier RS (1995) Expression of an endogenous galactose-binding lectin correlates with neoplastic progression in the colon. Cancer 75:2818–2826

59. Lotz MM, Andrews CW, Korzelius CA, Lee EC, Steele GD, Clarke A, Mercurio A (1993) Decreased expression of Mac-2 (carbohydrate binding protein 35) and loss of its nuclear localization are associated with the neoplastic progression of colon carcinoma. Proc Natl Acad Sci USA 90:3466–3470

60. Lotan R, Ito H, Yasui W, Yokozaki H, Lotan D, Tahara E (1994) Expression of a 31-kDa lactoside-binding lectin in normal human gastric mucosa and in primary and metastatic gastric carcinomas. Int J Cancer 56:474–480

61. Moutsatsos IK, Davis JM, Wang JL (1986) Endogenous lectins from cultured cells: subcellular localization of carbohydrate-binding protein 35 in 3T3 fibroblasts. J Cell Biol 102:477–483

62. Barondes SH (1988) Bifunctional properties of lectins: lectins redefined. Trends Biochem Sci 13:480–482

63. Sparrow CP, Leffler H, Barondes SH (1987) Multiple soluble β-galactoside-binding lectins from human lung. J Biol Chem 262:7383–7390

64. Woo H-J, Shaw LM, Messier JM, Mercurio AM (1990) The major non-integrin laminin binding protein of macrophages is identical to carbohydrate binding protein 35 (Mac-2). J Biol Chem 265:7097–7099

65. Lee EC, Woo H-J, Korzelius CA, Steele GD Jr, Mercurio AM (1991) Carbohydrate-binding protein 35 is the major cell-surface laminin-binding protein in colon carcinoma. Arch Surg 126:1498–1502

66. Ochieng J, Gerold M, Raz A (1992) Dichotomy in the laminin-binding properties of soluble and membrane-bound human galactoside-binding protein. Biochem Biophys Res Commun 186:1674–1680

67. Liotta LA, Rao CN, Wewer UM (1986) Biochemical interactions of tumor cells with the basement membrane. Annu Rev Cell Biol 55:1037–1057

68. Massa SM, Cooper DNW, Leffler H, Barondes S (1993) L-29, an endogenous lectin, binds to glycoconjugate ligands with positive cooperativity. Biochemistry 32:260–267

69. Chandrasekaran S, Dean JW, Giniger MS, Tanzer ML (1991) Laminin carbohydrates are implicated in cell signaling. J Cell Biochem 46:115–124

70. Mahanthapa NK, Cooper DNW, Barondes SH, Schwarting GA (1994) Rat olfactory neurons can utilize the endogenous lectin, L-14, in a novel adhesion mechanism. Development 120:1373–1384

71. Yamashita K, Totani K, Kuroki M, Mastuoka Y, Ueda I, Kobata A (1987) Structural studies of the carbohydrate moieties of carcinoembryonic antigens. Cancer Res 47:3451–3459

72. Knibbs RN, Agrwal N, Wang JL, Goldstein IJ (1993) Carbohydrate-binding protein 35: analysis of the interaction of the recombinant polypeptide with saccharides. J Biol Chem 268:14940–14947

73. Jessup JM, Thomas P (1989) Carcinoembryonic antigen: function in metastasis by human colorectal carcinoma. Cancer Metastasis Rev 8:263–280

74. Benchimol S, Fuks A, Jothy S, Beauchemin N, Shirota K, Stanners CP (1989) Carcinoembryonic antigen, a human tumor marker, functions as an intercellular adhesion molecule. Cell 57:327–334

75. Zhou H, Fuks A, Stanners CP (1990) Specificity of intercellular adhesion mediated by various members of the immunoglobulin supergene family. Cell Growth Differ 1:209–215

76. Dennis JW (1991) N-Linked oligosaccharide processing and tumor cell biology. Semin Cancer Biol 2:411–420

77. Fukuda M (1991) Lysosomal membrane glycoproteins: structure, biosynthesis, and intracellular trafficking. J Biol Chem 266:21327–21330

78. Carlsson SR, Roth J, Piller F, Fukuda M (1988) Isolation and characterization of human lysosomal membrane glycoproteins, h-LAMP-1 and h-LAMP-2: major sialoglycoproteins carrying polylactosaminoglycan. J Biol Chem 263:18911–18919

79. Saitoh O, Wang W-C, Lotan R, Fukuda M (1992) Differential glycosylation and cell surface expression of lysosomal membrane glycoproteins in sublines of a human colon cancer exhibiting distinct metastatic potentials. J Biol Chem 267:5700–5711

80. Sawada R, Tsuboi S, Fukuda M (1994) Differential E-selectin-dependent adhesion efficiency in sublines of a human colon cancer exhibiting distinct metastatic potentials. J Biol Chem 269:1425–1431

81. Do KY, Smith DF, Cummings RD (1990) LAMP-1 in CHO cells is a primary carrier of poly-N-acetyllactosamine chains and is bound preferentially by a mammalian S-type lectin. Biochem Biophys Res Commun 173:1123–1128

82. Skutta B, Klein PJ, Fischer J, Stark W (1988) Lectin binding sites as a parameter of cell differentiation in normal gastric mucosa, intestinal metaplasia, and gastric carcinoma. Verh Dtsch Ges Pathol 72:299–303

83. Adachi M, Sekine T, Imai K, Sato S (1987) Serological and immunohistochemical detection of a gastrointestinal cancer-associated asialoglycoprotein antigen of human with a murine monoclonal antibody. Jpn J Cancer Res 78:1370–1377

84. Ogasawara M, Takebe T, Ishii K (1988) Tumor-associated antigen defined by a monoclonal antibody against neuraminidase-treated human cancer cells. Cancer Res 48:412–417

85. Mori M, Ambe K, adachi Y, Yakeishi Y, Nakamura K, Hachitanda Y, Enjoji M, Sugimachi K (1988) Prognostic value of immunohistochemically identified CEA, SC, AFP, and S-100 protein positive cells in gastric carcinoma. Cancer 62:534–540

86. Kakeji Y, Tsujitani S, Mori M, Maehara Y, Sugimachi K (1991) Helix pomatia agglutinin binding activity is a predictor of survival time for patients with gastric carcinoma. Cancer 68:2438–2442

87. Narita T, Numao H (1992) Lectin binding patterns in normal, metaplastic, and neoplastic gastric mucosa. J Histochem Cytochem 40:681–687

88. Hokita S, Takao S, Muramatsu T, Shimazu H (1992) Monoclonal antibodies against a human gastric cancer cell line with lung metastatic potential in nude mice define antigens with different expression between the primary and metastatic liver lesions. J Cancer Res Clin Oncol 118:228–234

89. Ochiai A, Yokozaki H, Kyo E, Hozumi T, Tahara E (1985) A monoclonal antibody reacting with various human carcinomas and fetal colon and esophagus. Jpn J Cancer Res 76:915–918

90. Ohuchi N, Wunderlich D, Fujita J, Colcher D, Muraro R, Nose M, Schlom J (1987) Differential expression of carcinoembryonic antigen in early gastric adenocarcinomas versus benign gastric lesions defined by monoclonal antibodies reactive with restricted antigen epitopes. Cancer Res 47:3565–3571

91. Fukuyama R, Minoshima S, Ochiai A, Tahara E, Shimizu N (1991) Flow cytometric analysis of the expression of 9A3 antigen, E-cadherin, and EGF receptor in TMK-1 stomach cancer cells. Int J Cancer 48:81–84

92. Parkin DM, Stjernward J, Muir CS (1984) Estimates of the worldwide frequency of twelve major cancers. Bull World Health Organ 62:163–182

93. Lawrence W (1986) Gastric cancer. In: American Caner Society Professional Education Publication. American Cancer Society, Atlanta, pp 5–25

Stomach Cancer and Apoptosis: A Review*

Hisao Ito, Masato Ishida, Satoshi Ohfuji, Mitsuhiko Osaki, Hisae Hayashi, and Shigeru Tatebe

Summary. Apoptosis is a distinct form of cell death, distinguishable from necrosis. It is a natural, active process by which cells are eliminated from normal or neoplastic tissue. We describe apoptotic cells in human gastric mucosa, adenomas, and carcinomas with special reference to the role of the *p53* gene. Apoptosis plays a role in the morphogenesis of gastritis mucosa, including intestinal metaplasia to eliminate unnecessary or possibly DNA-damaged cells. The frequent occurrence of apoptosis in gastric adenomas may reflect their rather static nature. Apoptosis correlates with proliferative activity and tumorigenesis of gastric carcinoma, in which the apoptotic index (AI) correlates with the histologic type and depth of invasion. Gastric carcinoma with lymphoid stroma (GCLS) demonstrated the lowest AI among the histologic types. This fact might partly correlate with their favorable postoperative prognosis of GCLS compared with ordinary gastric carcinomas. Although the mutated *p53* gene attenuates apoptotic cell death, apoptosis of gastric cancer cells occurs in a cell cycle-dependent and a cell cycle-independent manner in vivo. Anticancer agents, transforming growth factor beta, and anti-Fas antibody variably induce apoptosis in the various human gastric cancer cell lines. In fact, preoperative administration of 5-fluorouracil significantly increased the number of apoptotic cancer cells. Thus apoptosis plays a crucial role in the tumorigenesis and progression of human gastric carcinoma. Selective induction of apoptosis of cancer cells is undoubtedly the best way to treat gastric cancer patients. Further studies should be conducted to clarify variable pathways of signal transduction, which might show a diverse spectrum of biologic effects depending on the apoptosis-inducible agents.

Introduction

Knowledge about cell death has greatly increased and even changed since the mid-1970s [1–5]. During the course of this rapid advance, a new concept of cell death, apoptosis, has been extensively analyzed in the field of basic cell biology and pathology, resulting in confusion about definitions and terminology [4, 5].

Apoptosis refers to energy-dependent cell death in which individual cells participate in their own fragmentation and deletion from living tissue [1, 3, 4]. It has distinct morphologic features, including compacting of chromatin against the nuclear membrane, cell shrinkage with the preservation of organelles, loss of cell–cell contact, and finally nuclear and cytoplasmic budding to form membrane-bound fragments known as apoptotic bodies, which are rapidly phagocytosed by adjacent parenchymal cells or macrophages [1, 3–5]. Increased endogenous nuclease activity causes fragmentation of DNA, showing a "ladder" appearance on electrophoresis that is known to be a biochemical feature of apoptosis [2].

Advances in molecular biology have disclosed the roles of a variety of protein molecules or oncogenes and suppressor genes in the process and regulation of apoptosis. They include *p53*, *c-myc*, *ras*, *c-fos*, *bcl-2*, *bax*, and *p21* genes [3]. Many studies have focused on *p53* and *bcl-2* expression [6–8]. For example, the expression of nuclear *p53* almost tallies with that of the mutant [9], which suppresses apoptosis. Thus apoptosis is now defined as a mode of cell death that exhibits distinct morphologic, biochemical, and molecular biologic properties (Table 1).

Apoptosis is a basic biologic phenomenon of critical importance in the regulation of cell populations in situations as diverse as metamor-

First Department of Pathology, Faculty of Medicine, Tottori University, Nishi-machi 86, Yonago, Tottori 683, Japan
*This chapter is dedicated to Professor Eiichi Tahara on the occasion of his 60th birthday

phosis, embryogenetic growth and modeling, hormone-induced organ involution, and neoplasia. Because of the short duration of the process [10] and seemingly low incidence, apoptosis can be difficult to detect on routine histologic sections, which is why pathologists have generally paid little attention to this process in a variety of human tumors including gastric cancer. Given the considerable evidence that proliferation indices of gastric cancer cells may be of prognostic significance and that parameters of cell loss are biologically relevant, enhanced apoptosis may be of considerable clinical significance. Tumor progression should be analyzed on the basis of both proliferation and apoptotic cell death (cell loss). The comparative rates of cell proliferation and cell

death determine how fast cancers can grow. In fact, studies indicate that estimates of cells showing apoptosis may have prognostic significance in non-Hodgkin's lymphomas [11, 12] and prostatic cancers [13–15]. The apoptotic index becomes higher with progression of colorectal cancers, with even higher values detected in metastatic foci [16]. Thus apoptosis might be correlated with a higher proliferative activity of various human tumors.

The purpose of this chapter is to offer the results of our investigations and a review of the literature on apoptosis of human gastric cancer. Special attention is given to the role of the *p53* gene and related molecules.

Apoptosis in Gastric Mucosa, Adenomatous Dysplasia, and Carcinoma

Table 1. Definition of apoptosis

Parameter	Apoptosis
Morphology	Karyorrhexis, membrane blebbing, and cell shrinkage, followed by formation of apoptotic bodies
Biochemistry	DNA ladder formation on agarose gel due to naturally occurring DNA strand breaks caused by endogenous nuclease activity
Molecular biology	Cell death accompanying the expression of various oncogenes and suppressor genes

Apoptotic cells can be confirmed on routinely prepared hematoxylin and eosin (H&E) sections and by terminal deoxynucleotidyl transferase (TdT)-mediated dUTP-biotin nick end labeling (TUNEL) (Figs. 1–3) [17–21]. This method is based on detecting naturally occurring DNA strand breaks caused by endogeneous nuclease activity in formalin-fixed, paraffin-embedded tissue sections. The histology of TUNEL-positive apoptotic cells found in gastritis mucosa (Fig. 1), tubular adenoma (Fig. 2), and carcinoma (Fig. 3)

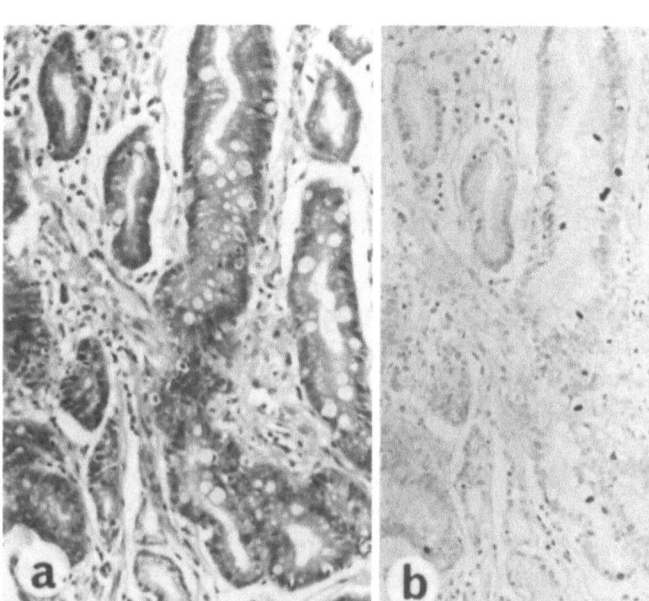

Fig. 1a,b. Serial section of gastric-intestinal metaplasia, incomplete type. **a** A few apoptotic cells distribute mainly in the deep portion of metaplastic glands. (H&E, ×140) **b** Apoptotic cells obviously demonstrate a TUNEL signal in their nuclei. (TUNEL, ×140)

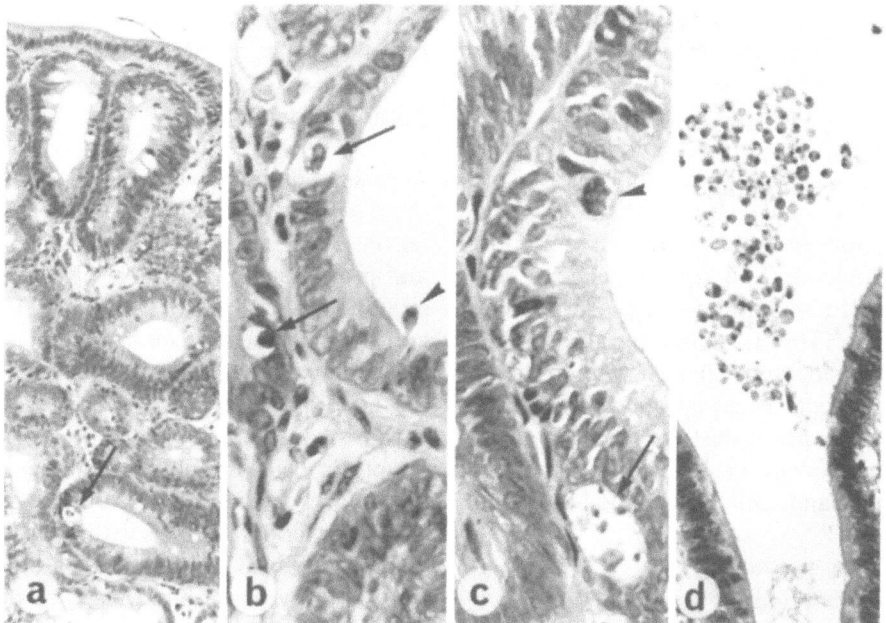

Fig. 2a–d. Histology of apoptosis in tubular adenoma of the stomach. **a** Tubular adenoma with low-grade dysplasia. The location of the nuclei in the cells is regular at the basal portion. A few goblet cells are evident. Apoptotic adenoma cell is recognizable even at this magnification (*arrow*). (H&E, ×150) **b** Apoptotic cells with condensed, nonfragmented chromatin having a clear halo (*arrows*). Note the apoptotic cell shedding into the glandular lumen (*arrowhead*). (H&E, ×600) **c** Apoptotic cell with fragments of condensed chromatin, corresponding to apoptotic bodies (*arrow*). A mitotic figure is noted at the luminal portion of the gland (*arrowhead*). (H&E, ×600) **d** Accumulation of apoptotic bodies in the lumen of the adenoma gland, a rare occurrence. Usually only a few apoptotic bodies are detected in the lumen. (H&E, ×300)

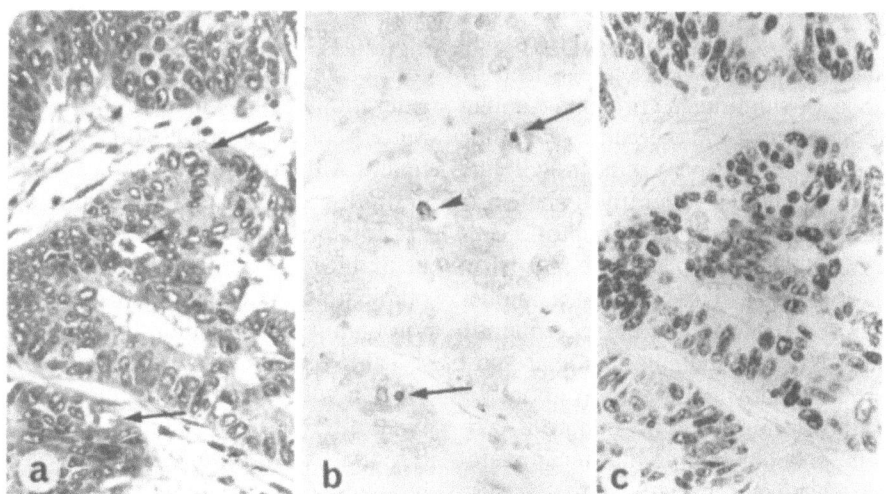

Fig. 3a–c. Serial sections of P53-positive gastric carcinoma, well-differentiated type. **a** A few apoptotic cells (*arrows*) are noted. Apoptotic cancer cells are shedding into the glandular lumen (*arrowhead*). (H&E, ×260) **b** Cancer cells showing apoptosis demonstrate an obvious positive signal for the TUNEL procedure. (TUNEL, ×260) **c** Most of the cancer cells contain P53 immunoreactivity in their nuclei. (Immunostaining for P53, ×260)

is as follows [21–25]: (1) a single structure with fragments of condensed chromatin, separated from the surrounding intact cells by a clear halo; (2) cells with a single nucleus containing condensed chromatin and eosinophilic cytoplasm. The latter has a superficial resemblance to small lymphocytes but could be differentiated by noting their scant, noneosinophilic cytoplasm, uniform pattern of chromatin, and lack of leukocyte common antigen (LCA) immunoreactivity. We have confirmed that TUNEL signals are also found in seemingly nonapoptotic cells that were in the initial phase of apoptosis. Apoptotic bodies known as nuclear fragments or dust are occasionally detected in the lumens of a few cancerous and noncancerous glands and even in the interstitium of tumor tissue.

Normal Gastric Mucosa, Gastritis Mucosa, Intestinal Metaplasia

Apoptotic cells are rare in normal gastric mucosa without atrophy. They exist in the neck zone of the mucosa, where Ki-67 antigen-positive, proliferative cells are located (generative zone). With increasing degree of severity of atrophic gastritis, apoptotic cells move downward and are frequently detected in the basal zone of the mucosa [22].

Intestinal metaplasia can be classified into two types: complete and incomplete [26]. The complete type is characterized by the absence of sulfomucin-containing goblet cells and the presence of Paneth cells, as in the mucosa of the small intestine. The incomplete type is categorized by the appearance of sulfomucin-containing goblet cells and the absence of Paneth cells. Apoptotic cells are present in deeper portions of the metaplastic glands where a generative zone exists (Fig. 1). The average number of apoptotic cells per gland is 2.2 in the incomplete type and 1.1 in the complete type [22]. This difference implies that DNA-damaged cells appear more frequently in the incomplete type of metaplasia and are presumably more frequently eliminated by apoptosis to avoid cell transformation. This finding is consistent with the previous finding that incomplete-type metaplasia has a closer relationship to gastric cancer than the complete type [26]. In fact, we found P53-immunoreactive cells, and even *p53* gene mutation, in cells of the incomplete type but not in complete-type metaplasia [27–29]. Moreover, the existence of apoptotic cells in the gen-

erative cell zone suggests a cell cycle-dependent type process in nonneoplastic gastric mucosa.

Tubular Adenoma

Tubular adenoma showing various grades of dysplasia is now considered to be a precancerous lesion [30–32]. Although its slow-growing nature and proliferative activity have been well demonstrated [33–35], no attention has been paid to apoptotic cell death (cell loss) until now.

Tubular adenoma is suitable for exemplifying the histology of apoptotic cells (Fig. 2a–d). The authors have initially compared the number of apoptotic cells in tubular adenomas with low-grade and high-grade dysplasia. The average number of apoptotic cells within a 10×20 magnification field was 4.5 ± 1.7 in 25 adenomas with low-grade dysplasia and 6.4 ± 2.2 in high-grade dysplasias, the number being significantly higher ($P < 0.01$) in the latter [23]. The apoptotic cells showed a relatively uniform pattern of distribution with no significant regional (field-to-field) variation. On the other hand, there was no significant difference in the number of mitotic figures between the two categories. Mitotic figures can be detected, most commonly in the luminal portion of the glands (Fig. 2c), especially with high-grade dysplasia. Although they are distributed throughout the entire gland, there is a tendency to find them more frequently at the upper portion of adenomatous glands. This finding might be a seeming paradox, as frequent cell loss by apoptosis may reflect a slow-growing or static nature of gastric adenomas. However, careful consideration of the kinetics of both apoptosis and mitosis partly resolves this apparent inconsistency. Although the mechanisms responsible for apoptosis and its significance in neoplastic lesions are still incompletely understood, apoptosis might be induced in gastric dysplasias as a means of eliminating nonproliferative or unnecessary cells to obtain higher proliferative activity.

Table 2 summarizes our results on the apoptotic cells in tubular adenoma and gastric carcinoma (well-differentiated adenocarcinoma, poorly differentiated type, and gastric carcinoma with lymphoid stroma) [23–25]. Of these lesions, 15 gastric adenomas and 15 well-differentiated adenocarcinomas existed simultaneously in the same stomach. The apoptotic index (AI) was determined by counting the number of TUNEL signal-positive nuclei in at least 1000 cells; it is

Table 2. Frequency of apoptotic cells and Ki-67$^+$ cells in gastric adenoma and carcinoma

Histologic type	No. of lesions	Apoptotic index^a (%)	Ki-67 index (%)
Tubular adenoma			
Low-grade dysplasia	7	4.6 ± 1.4^b	29.3 ± 11.4
High-grade dysplasia	8	5.2 ± 2.7	29.6 ± 7.7
Gastric carcinoma			
Well differentiated			
Early	7	3.6 ± 1.1	45.1 ± 13.4
Advanced	8	4.1 ± 1.2	53.6 ± 13.4
Poorly differentiated: advanced	11	2.2 ± 1.1	43.1 ± 9.2
Gastric carcinoma with lymphoid stroma	19	1.8 ± 0.6	40.0 ± 10.8

^{a} Apoptotic and Ki-67 indices are expressed as a percentage of TUNEL signal-positive cells and Ki-67 immunoreactive cells in all the tumor cells, respectively.
^{b} Values are means ± SD.

expressed as the number of positive nuclei per 100 tumor cells. Of interest is that the AI is significantly ($P < 0.05$) higher in tubular adenomas than in gastric carcinomas of any type. On the other hand, the percentage of Ki-67-positive tumor cells (Ki-67 index) is higher in gastric carcinomas than in tubular adenomas. Thus the gastric tubular adenoma is characterized as having relatively higher AI and lower Ki-67 index than gastric carcinomas, which may partly explain the slow-growing nature of gastric tubular adenomas.

Gastric Carcinoma

The progression of human gastric cancer is slower than generally considered. Fujita [36] analyzed clinical observations and proposed a model for the natural history of human gastric carcinoma. The total duration of the disease had been estimated at 16.5 to 33.0 years for average cases, with possible variations ranging from 2.0 years to several decades. He also pointed out that there was a discrepancy between the generation times (cell level) and doubling times (tissue level) of human gastric carcinomas. The latter was longer than the former. This discrepancy might be partly explained by cell loss rates, including apoptosis. In fact, apoptosis frequently occurs in gastric carcinomas.

The number of apoptotic cells, or AI, correlates with several factors, including histologic type, depth of invasion, preoperative chemotherapy, and gene alterations of the tumor cells. Among the histologic types, the AI is significantly highest ($P < 0.05$) in well-differentiated adenocarcinomas, followed by poorly differentiated

adenocarcinomas and gastric carcinomas with lymphoid stroma (GCLS) [24], in the order given (Table 2). Of the well-differentiated adenocarcinomas, the AI is higher in the advanced carcinomas than in the early ones, although there is no significant difference.

The GCLS has been demonstrated to be associated with Epstein-Barr virus [37–39]. These carcinomas are characterized by a marked degree of lymphoid stroma with minimal fibrosis, a predominance in males, relatively preferential occurrence in the fundic gland area, less marked cellular pleomorphism, and rare mitotic figures. Moreover, several authors have reported a favorable postoperative prognosis for GCLS compared to that for ordinary gastric carcinomas [40, 41]. The mechanism underlying the rather static nature of GCLS has not been elucidated. Apoptosis was noted less frequently in GCLS than in ordinary carcinomas (Table 2). The Ki-67 index is also lower. Thus GCLSs might be characterized as tumors with a lower cell elimination rate and lower proliferation activity.

Moreover, there is a tendency for the AI to be directly proportional to the Ki-67 index (Table 2), implying cell cycle-dependent apoptosis in gastric cancer cells.

In summary, apoptosis plays a role in the morphogenesis of gastritis mucosa including intestinal metaplasia to eliminate unnecessary or possibly DNA-damaged cells. The frequent occurrence of apoptosis in gastric adenoma might reflect the rather static nature of these tumors. In addition, apoptosis is correlated with proliferative activity as well as tumorigenesis of gastric carcinoma to obtain higher proliferative activity.

Apoptosis and *p53* Gene

Alterations and overexpression of the *p53* gene are the most common events in various human tumors, including gastric cancer, which involves mutation and deletion of the gene [42]. Gastric cancer has been shown to involve *p53* mutation at a high frequency (20–58%) [42–47]; Sano et al. [48] found a loss of heterozygosity at the *p53* locus in 13 (68%) of 19 informative cases, regardless of the histologic type. We found the gene deletion in 10 (77%) of 13 well-differentiated carcinomas by interphase cytogenetics using fluorescence in situ hybridization (FISH) [29]. The precise role in gastric tumorigenesis and biologic significance of the gene, however, is not well understood. Some authors have pointed out that *p53* mutations correlate with depth of invasion, stage, and poor clinical outcome [49–52].

The *p53* gene product has been shown to be required for induction of the apoptotic pathway triggered by oncogenous activation and cytotoxic genes [53, 54]. The product may sensitize damaged cells to apoptosis, acting to prevent the propagation of transforming mutations. P21$^{CIP1/WAF1}$, induced by the wild-type *p53* gene, might play a crucial role in the process of apoptosis [6]. These results, however, have been obtained only in primary cell culture and a transgenic mouse model.

Table 3 summarizes the status of *p53* gene mutation, the average AI (percentage of TUNEL-positive cells in all the tumor cells), and the proliferating cell nuclear antigen (PCNA) index (PI) in 18 nuclear P53-positive cases (category A) and 17 negative cases (category B). The polymerase chain reaction–single strand conformation polymorphism analysis (PCR-SSCP) showed a shifted band, indicating the point muta-

tion in 13 (72%) of category A and in 3 (18%) of category B, the frequency being significantly higher in the former ($P < 0.05$). These results are in good agreement with previous findings wherein the mutated *p53* gene is coincident with the gene expression in a variety of human carcinomas [55–58]. The mutated gene product has been demonstrated to be accumulated in the nucleus through binding to oncogenous proteins or by a prolonged half-life [9, 59]. Thus it might be roughly considered that nuclear P53-positive tumor cells are involved in point mutation. Carcinomas showing P53 expression without a shifted band imply possible false-negative results, which might occur during analysis by PCR-SSCP. A nonshifted band does not necessarily imply the existence of the wild-type *p53* gene. On the other hand, the cases showing no P53 expression with an abnormal band might indicate the existence of silent mutation, or non-sense mutation.

As shown in Table 3, the AI was 3.8 ± 1.4 in category A and 4.9 ± 1.2 in category B, the value being significantly higher in the latter ($P < 0.05$). The PI was 56.4 ± 16.3 in category A and 42.8 ± 17.6 in category B, the value being significantly higher in the former. Moreover, the PI was higher in advanced carcinomas than in early carcinomas in both categories. Thus human gastric cancers with *p53* gene mutation might be characterized as having a lower apoptotic incidence and higher proliferative activity, reflecting their possibly aggressive nature. This finding is in good agreement with clinical observations wherein *p53* mutations correlate with depth of invasion, stage, and poor clinical outcome [49–52].

Apoptosis can occur in a cell cycle dependent or independent manner [60, 61]. With the former, apoptosis is induced in cells at the late G1 or G2 phase but not in cells at G0 or M. Thus

Table 3. Relations among *p53* gene status, expression of *p21* and *bax*, and apoptotic index in human gastric carcinomas

p53 expression	No. of cases	Cases with mutation[a]	Average AI (%)	Average PI (%)	No. of cases with cancer cells	
					p21	*bax*
Positive	18	13 (72%)	3.8 ± 1.4	56.4 ± 16.3	7 (39%)	11 (61%)
Negative	17	3 (18%)	4.9 ± 1.2	42.8 ± 17.6	5 (29%)	5 (29%)

AI, apoptotic index; PI, PCNA index.
[a] Point mutation was analyzed by PCR-SSCP.
*There is a significant difference by Student's *t*-test ($P < 0.05$).

hyperproliferative cells might be more subject to apoptosis, resulting in a higher AI. Overexpression of wild-type P53 has been shown to sensitize transformed cells to apoptosis. Moreover, cells with DNA damage cannot undergo apoptosis when the *p53* gene is inactive [62, 63]. On the other hand, defects in the *p53* gene were associated with attenuated apoptosis and chemo- and radioresistance in a mouse sarcoma model [64]. Our results might partly support these observations. The mutated-type *p53* fails to lead to G1 arrest, resulting in increasing survival rate and attenuating apoptosis, and it may offer a selective advantage for the DNA-damaged cancer cells. A similar result was obtained by Kobayashi et al. [65], who examined the correlation of P53 expression and apoptosis in human colonic adenomas and carcinomas without analysis of *p53* gene status. They found that the apoptotic incidence was significantly less frequent in colonic tumors with diffuse P53 expression than in those with sporadic expression.

Attention should be paid, however, to the mean AI of the category without nuclear P53 protein. Despite a statistical difference, the AIs between the two categories were not as different as we had initially expected, implying that apoptotic cell death occurs via the *p53* gene in a cell cycle-dependent or cell cycle-independent manner in gastric cancer in vivo. It is likely that apoptosis is not induced solely by overexpression of the wild-type P53 and may require accumulation of additional oncogenous insults to actuate the process of cell death.

The growth-inhibitory protein P21$^{WAF1/CIP1}$ is a potent inhibitor of various cyclin-dependent kinase, the expression of which is regulated at the transcriptional level in both a *p53*-dependent and *p53*-independent manner [66]. The *p21* gene is induced by DNA-damaging agents that trigger G1 arrest in *p53* wild-type cells but not in *p53* mutated cells [67]. Immunohistochemistry showed a difference of P21 expression between the two categories. P21-positive tumor cells were detected in eight of category A and five of category B tumors, suggesting that *p21* expression is triggered by a *p53*-independent pathway in human gastric carcinoma. In fact, studies indicate that the existence of *p53*-independent pathways induce *p21* expression [68–70]. The *bax* gene has been shown to be activated by the *p53* gene. The Bax protein promotes apoptosis, in contrast to Bcl-2, which prevents apoptosis [71]. We have found that Bax-positive tumor cells were more frequently detected in the carcinomas with nuclear P53, which showed less frequent apoptosis.

Thus the mechanisms of apoptosis induction in gastric carcinomas are diverse. Other pathways of apoptosis not involving the *p53* gene remain to be elucidated.

Apoptosis in Human Gastric Carcinoma Cell Lines

Apoptosis might be induced in the various cultured cell lines by a variety of events or agents, such as anticancer agents, radiation, growth factor deprivation, cytokines, and hormones. Only a few reports, however, are available on the induction of apoptosis in the gastric cancer cell lines.

That anticancer agents can induce apoptosis of the various gastric cancer cell lines in our laboratory has been confirmed. For example, DNA fragmentation was detected in HSC-39 after 6h of incubation with Adriamycin (ADR) 50ng/ml or after 24h with 100ng/ml [72]. On the other hand, the cell line MKN-28 did not show DNA fragmentation after 6h of incubation with ADR 100ng/ml. 5-Fluorouracil (5FU) 1mM induces apoptosis in MKN-74 but not in MKN-28 or KATO-III [73]. Thus the sensitivity of gastric cancer to anticancer agents is diverse, and induction of apoptosis depends on the dose and mechanism of the antitumor action of the agents, as well as the cell line involved, each of which possesses different biologic properties. In fact, we have confirmed that preoperative administration of 5FU increased apoptosis in gastric and colonic cancer cells in vivo [74, 75].

Transforming growth factor beta (TGF-β) is a polypeptide homodimer with a molecular weight of 25kDa that is present in platelets and other normal and tumor cells. TGF-β has been shown to act as a growth-inhibitory factor for certain carcinoma cell lines, including gastric carcinoma. Yanagihara et al. [76] reported that exogenous TGF-β strongly inhibited proliferation of cell lines HSC-39 and HSC-43, followed by induction of apoptosis in a dose-dependent manner. The other five cell lines (MKN-1, MKN-7, MKN-28, MKN-45, MKN-74) were unresponsive. On the other hand, Yamamoto et al. [77] found that TGF-β induced apoptosis in KATO-III but not in other cell lines, such as MKN-1, MKN-28, MKN-45,

Table 4. *p53* Gene alteration and expression of apoptosis-related protein in human gastric cancer cell lines

Cell line	Histology	*p53* gene status (codon)	Expression of antigen[a] P53	Fas	Bcl-2
MKN-1	As	143, 147	++	+	++
MKN-7	Well	278	+	+	+
MKN-28	Well	251	++	++	++
MKN-74	Well	Wild type	−	+	+
MKN-45	Poorly	Wild type	+	+	+
TMK-1	Poorly	173	+	++	−/+
KATO-III	Scirrhous	Complete deletion	−	+	++
HSC-39	Scirrhous	245	++	++	++

[a] Expressions of P53, Fas antigen, and Bcl-2 protein were examined by Western blot.

MKN-74, SCH, and AZ521. It is of interest that exogenous TGF-β induced apoptosis in all three cell lines derived from scirrhous-type gastric carcinoma (Table 4). The growth inhibition effect of TGF-β is mediated by its receptor, especially type I [78], with the *p53* gene not likely participating in the process [77].

The transmembrane receptor protein Fas was originally identified on the basis of its ability to trigger apoptosis, a response similar to that mediated by TNF-R1, upon specific antibody binding [79]. Fas is expressed in thymocytes, activated B and T cells, normal liver, heart, lung, ovary, and several tumors [80]. Anti-Fas antibody has been reported to induce apoptosis in many leukemia/lymphoma cell lines in vitro [81]. Fas-mediated apoptosis has been shown to be induced within a few hours after anti-Fas antibody treatment. This mode of apoptosis occurs in a cell cycle-independent manner and might be affected by Bcl-2 protein [82].

We confirmed the expression of Fas antigen in the human gastric cancer cell lines, among which MKN-74, MKN-45, and HSC-39 demonstrated the higher expression of the antigen at levels comparable to those previously reported for lymphoid cells, in contrast to lower expression in KATO-III, HSC-43, and MKN-7 (Fig. 4, Table 4). Simultaneous treatment of anti-Fas antigen and interferon gamma (INF-γ) 50 IU/ml induces apoptosis on the cultured cell lines to variable degrees (Fig. 5). At 72 h after treatment, approximately 60% of MKN-74, 33% of MKN-45, 25% of KATO-III, and 20% of TMK-1 cells demonstrated apoptosis (Fig. 6); MKN-28 was resistant to the antibody-induced apoptosis. These preliminary results indicate that: (1) Fas is expressed on cultured human gastric

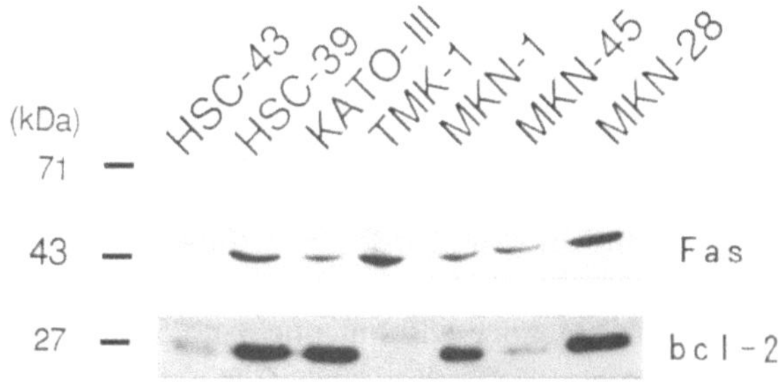

Fig. 4. Expression of Fas antigen and bcl-2 protein in the seven gastric carcinoma cell lines by Western blotting

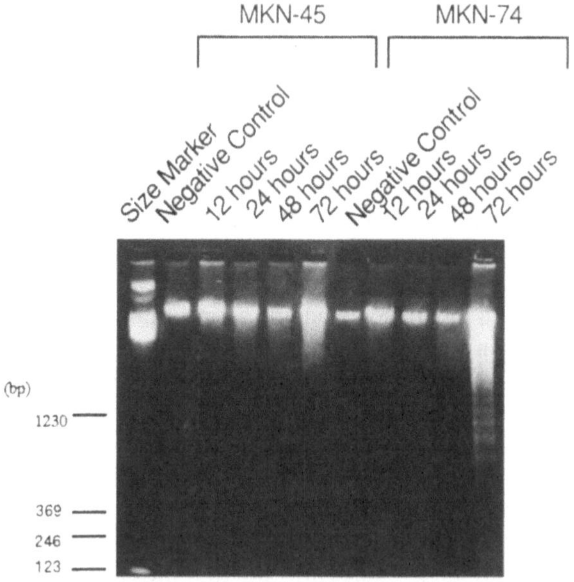

Fig. 5. Induction of apoptosis in MKN-45 and MKN-74 by simultaneous treatment of anti-Fas antibody and interferon. Both of the cells demonstrate the DNA ladder at 72 h after treatment. The negative control was not treated with anti-Fas antibody

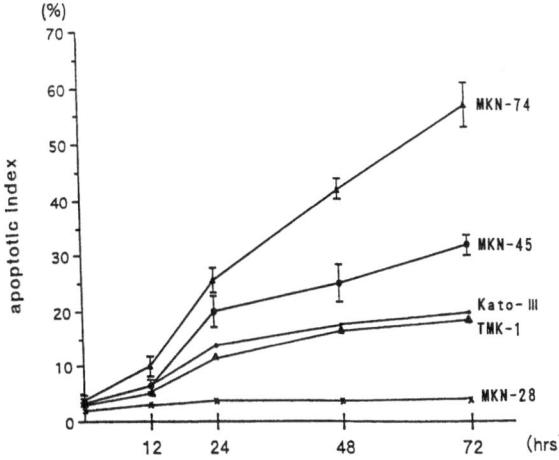

Fig. 6. Apoptotic index after simultaneous treatment of anti-Fas antibody and interferon (INF-γ), which induces apoptosis on the cultured cell line to variable degrees. MKN-28 is resistant to the antibody-induced apoptosis

carcinoma cells at variable levels; (2) anti-Fas-induced apoptosis occurs gradually and is prolonged compared to that in hematopoietic tumors; (3) the inherent susceptibility to anti-Fas antibody is not necessarily correlated with expression of Fas; and (4) the wild-type *p53* gene may promote the process of anti-Fas antibody-mediated apoptosis. There might exist a diverse spectrum of biologic effects induced by anti-Fas engagement of the Fas protein.

Vollmers et al. successfully induced apoptosis in stomach carcinoma cells by a human monoclonal antibody, SC-1, which was isolated from a patient with signet ring cell carcinoma and identifies a membrane glycoprotein of 49 kDa [83]. SC-1 antibody 1 μg/ml dispersed the cultured cells of gastric carcinoma cell line 23132, followed by induction of apoptosis, which was confirmed by the DNA ladder formation and typical morphology of apoptosis after 24 h of treatment. In vivo growth of the cells in nu-nu mice was also reduced when the antibody was injected. The pathway of signal transduction for apoptosis was not investigated in this model.

Further studies should be conducted to elucidate the spontaneously triggered signal transduction pathways as well as the various agents that mediate apoptosis of gastric cancer cells, which have remained obscure up to now.

Acknowledgments. This work was supported in part by a Grant-in-Aid for Cancer Research from the Ministry of Education, Science, and Culture and the Ministry of Health and Welfare of Japan. The authors thank Mr. N. Itaki for his skillful technical assistance.

References

1. Kerr JFR, Wyllie AH, Currie AR (1972) Apoptosis: a basic biological phenomenon with wide-ranging implications in tissue kinetics. Br J Cancer 26:239–257
2. Wyllie AH, Morris RG, Smith AL, Dunlop D (1984) Chromatin cleavage in apoptosis: association with condensed chromatin morphology and dependence on macromolecular synthesis. J Pathol 142:67–77
3. Kerr JFR, Winterford CM, Harmon BV (1994) Apoptosis: its significance in cancer and cancer therapy. Cancer 73:2013–2026
4. Payne CM, Bernstein H, Bernstein C, Garewal H (1995) Role of apoptosis and pathology: resistance to apoptosis in colon carcinogenesis. Ultrastruct Pathol 19:221–248
5. Majno G, Joris I (1995) Apoptosis, oncosis, and necrosis: an overview of cell death. Am J Pathol 146:3–15
6. Clarke AR, Purdie CA, Harrison DJ, Morris RG, Bird CC, Hooper ML, Wyllie AH (1993) Thymocyte apoptosis induced by *p53*-dependent and -independent pathways. Nature 362:849–852
7. Sierra A, Lloveras B, Castellsague X, Moreno L, Garcia-Ramirez M, Fabra A (1995) *bcl-2* expression is associated with lymph-node metastasis in human ductal breast carcinoma. Int J Cancer 60:54–60
8. Sincrope FA, Ruan SB, Cleary KR, Stephens LC, Lee JJ, Levin B (1995) *bcl-2* and *p53* oncoprotein expression during colorectal tumorigenesis. Cancer Res 55:237–241
9. Finlay CA, Hinds PW, Tan TH, Eliyahu D, Oren M, Levine AJ (1988) Activating mutations for transformation by *p53* produce a gene product that forms an *hsc70–p53* complex with an altered half-life. Mol Cell Biol 8:531–539
10. Bursch W, Paffe S, Putz B, Barthel G, Schulte-Hermann R (1990) Determination of the length of the histological stages of apoptosis in normal liver and in altered hepatic foci of rats. Carcinogenesis 11:847–853
11. Del Vecchio MT, Leoncini L, Buerki K, Kraft R, Megha T, Barbini P, Tosi P, Cottier H (1991) Diffuse centrocytic and/or centroblastic malignant non-Hodgkin's lymphomas: comparison of mitotic and pyknotic (apoptotic) indices. Int J Cancer 47:38–43
12. Leoncini L, Del Vecchio MT, Megha T, Barbini P, Galieni P, Pileri S, Sabattini E, Gherlinzoni F, Tosi P, Kraft R, Cottier H (1993) Correlations between

apoptotic and proliferative indices in malignant non-Hodgkin's lymphomas. Am J Pathol 142:755–763

13. Montironi R, Galluzzi CM, Scarpelli M, Giannulis I, Diamanti L (1993) Occurrence of cell death (apoptosis) in prostatic intraepithelial neoplasia. Virchows Arch [Pathol Anat] 423:351–357

14. Aihara M, Truong LD, Dunn JK, Wheeler TM, Scardino PT, Thompson TC (1994) Frequency of apoptotic bodies positively correlates with Gleason grade in prostate cancer. Hum Pathol 25:797–801

15. Gaffney EF (1994) The extent of apoptosis in different types of high grade prostatic carcinoma. Histopathology 25:269–273

16. Tatebe S, Ishida M, Kasagi N, Tsujitani S, Kaibara N, Ito H (1996) Apoptosis occurs more frequently in metastatic foci than in primary lesions of human colorectal carcinomas: analysis by terminal-deoxynucleotidyl-transferase-mediated dUTP-biotin nick end labeling. Int J Cancer 65:173–177

17. Gavrieli Y, Sherman Y, Ben-Sasson SA (1992) Identification of programmed cell death in situ via specific labeling of nuclear DNA fragmentation. J Cell Biol 119:493–501

18. Ansari B, Coates PJ, Greenstein BD, Hall PA (1993) In situ end-labelling detects DNA strand breaks in apoptosis and other physiological and pathological states. J Pathol 170:1–8

19. Wijsman JH, Jonker RR, Keijzer R, Van De Velde CJH, Cornelisse CJ, Van Dierendonck JH (1993) A new method to detect apoptosis in paraffin sections: in situ end-labeling of fragmented DNA. J Histochem Cytochem 41:7–12

20. Gorczyca W, Gong J, Darzynkiewicz Z (1993) Detection of DNA strand breaks in individual apoptotic cells by the in situ terminal deoxynucleotidyl transferase and nick translation assays. Cancer Res 53:1945–1951

21. Kasagi N, Gomyo Y, Shirai H, Tsujitani S, Ito H (1994) Apoptotic cell death in human gastric carcinoma. Jpn J Cancer Res 85:939–945

22. Ishida M, Gomyo Y, Tatebe S, Ohfuji S, Ito H (1996) Apoptosis in human gastric mucosa, chronic gastritis, dysplasia and carcinoma: analysis by terminal deoxynucleotidyl transferase (TdT)-mediated dUTP-biotin nick end labeling (TUNEL). Virchows Arch 428:229–235

23. Gomyo Y, Osaki M, Ito H (1996) Frequent occurrence of cell death in gastric adenomas: comparison between apoptosis and mitosis. Yonago Acta Med 39:49–58

24. Ohfuji S, Osaki M, Tsujitani S, Ikeguchi M, Kaibara N, Sairenji T, Ito H (1996) Low frequency of apoptosis in Epstein-Barr virus-associated gastric carcinoma with lymphoid stroma. Int J Cancer 68:710–715

25. Ishida M, Gomyo Y, Ohfuji S, Ikeda M, Ito H (1997) In vivo evidence that mutated p53 gene expression attenuates apoptotic cell death in human gastric carcinoma. Jpn J Cancer Res (in press)

26. Matsukura N, Suzuki K, Kawachi T, Aoyagi M, Sugimura T, Kiraoka H, Nakajima H, Shirota A, Itabashi M, Hirota T (1980) Distribution of marker enzymes and mucin in intestinal metaplasia to minute gastric carcinomas. J Natl Cancer Inst 65:231–240

27. Shiao YH, Rugge M, Correa P, Lehmann HP, Scheer WD (1994) p53 alteration in gastric precancerous lesions. Am J Pathol 144:511–517

28. Ochiai A, Yamauchi Y, Hirohashi S (1996) p53 mutations in the non-neoplastic mucosa of the human stomach. Int J Cancer 69:28–33

29. Gomyo Y, Osaki M, Kaibara N, Ito H (1996) Numerical aberration and point mutation of p53 gene in human gastric intestinal metaplasia and well-differentiated adenocarcinoma: analysis by fluorescence in situ hybridization (FISH) and PCR-SSCP. Int J Cancer 66:594–599

30. Morson BC, Sobin LH, Grundmann E, Johansen A, Nagayo T, Serck-Hanssen A (1980) Precancerous conditions and epithelial dysplasia in the stomach. J Clin Pathol 33:711–721

31. Ming S-C, Bajtai A, Correa P, Elster K, Jarvi OH, Munoz N, Nagayo T, Stemmerman GN (1984) Gastric dysplasia: significance and pathologic criteria. Cancer 54:1794–1801

32. Ito H, Hata J, Yokozaki H, Nakatani H, Oda N, Tahara E (1986) Tubular adenoma of the human stomach: an immunohistochemical analysis of gut hormones, serotonin, carcinoembryonic antigen, secretory component, and lysozyme. Cancer 58:2264–2272

33. Oehlert W, Keller P, Henke M, Strauch M (1979) Gastric mucosal dysplasia: what is its clinical significance? Front Gastrointest Res 4:173–182

34. Kamiya T, Morishita T, Asakura H, Miura S, Munakata Y, Tsuchiya M (1982) Long-term follow-up study on gastric adenoma and its relation to gastric protruded carcinoma. Cancer 50:2496–2503

35. Saraga E-P, Gardiol D, Costa J (1988) Gastric dysplasia: a histological follow-up study. Am J Surg Pathol 11:788–796

36. Fujita S (1978) Biology of early gastric carcinoma. Pathol Res Pract 163:297–309

37. Tokunaga M, Uemura Y, Tokudome T, Ishidate T, Masuda H, Okazaki E, Kaneko C, Naoe S, Ito M, Okamura A, Shimada A, Sato E, Land CE (1993) Epstein-Barr virus related gastric cancer in Japan: a molecular patho-epidemiological study. Acta Pathol Jpn 43:574–581

38. Takano Y, Kato Y, Sugano H (1994) Epstein-Barr virus-associated medullary carcinomas with lymphoid infiltration of the stomach. J Cancer Res Clin Oncol 120:303–308

39. Nakamura S, Ueki T, Yao T, Ueyama T, Tsuneyoshi M (1994) Epstein-Barr virus in gastric

carcinoma with lymphoid stroma. Cancer 73:2239–2249

40. Ito H, Masuda H, Shimamoto F, Inokuchi C, Tahara E (1990) Gastric carcinoma with lymphoid stroma: pathological and immunohistochemical analysis. Hiroshima J Med Sci 39:29–37

41. Nakamura K, Ueyama T, Yao T, Xuan ZX, Ambe K, Adachi Y, Yakeishi Y, Matsukura A, Enjoji M (1992) Pathology and prognosis of gastric carcinoma: findings in 10000 patients who underwent primary gastrectomy. Cancer 70:1030–1037

42. Stemmermann G, Heffelfinger SC, Noffsinger A, Hui YZ, Miller MA, Fenoglio-Preiser CM (1994) The molecular biology of esophageal and gastric cancer and their precursors: oncogenes, tumor suppressor genes, and growth factors. Hum Pathol 25:968–981

43. Yokozaki H, Kuniyasu H, Kitadai Y, Nishimura K, Todo H, Ayhan A, Yasui W, Ito H, Tahara E (1992) p53 point mutations in primary human gastric carcinomas. J Cancer Res Clin Oncol 119:67–70

44. Tamura G, Kihana T, Nomura K, Terada M, Sugimura T, Hirohashi S (1991) Detection of frequent p53 gene mutations in primary gastric cancer by cell sorting and polymerase chain reaction single-strand conformation polymorphism analysis. Cancer Res 51:3056–3058

45. Kim JH, Takahashi T, Chiba I, Park JG, Birrer MJ, Roh JK, Lee HD, Kim J-P, Minna JD, Gazdar AF (1991) Occurrence of p53 gene abnormalities in gastric carcinoma tumors and cell line. J Natl Cancer Inst 83:938–943

46. Matozaki T, Sakamoto C, Matsuda K, Suzuki T, Konda Y, Nakano O, Wada K, Ucida T, Nishisaki H, Nagao M, Kasuga M (1993) Missense mutations and a deletion of the p53 gene in human gastric cancer. Biochem Biophys Res Commun 182:215–223

47. Uchino S, Noguchi M, Ochiai A, Saito T, Kobayashi M, Hirohashi S (1993) p53 mutation in gastric cancer: a genetic mode for carcinogenesis is common to gastric and colorectal cancer. Int J Cancer 54:759–764

48. Sano T, Tsujino T, Yoshida K, Nakayama H, Haruma K, Ito H, Nakamura Y, Kajiyama G, Tahara E (1991) Frequent loss of heterozygosity on chromosomes 1q, 5q, and 17p in human gastric carcinomas. Cancer Res 51:2926–2931

49. Yamada Y, Yoshida T, Hayashi K, Sekiya T, Yokota J, Hirohashi S, Nakatani K, Nakano H, Sugimura T, Terada M (1991) p53 gene mutations in gastric cancer metastases and in gastric cancer cell lines derived from metastases. Cancer Res 51:5800–5805

50. Uchino S, Tsuda H, Noguchi M, Yokota J, Terada M, Saito T, Kobayshi M, Sugimura T, Hirohashi S (1992) Frequent loss of heterozygosity at the DCC locus in gastric cancer. Cancer Res 52:3099–3102

51. Starzynska T, Bromly M, Ghosh A, Stern PL (1992) Prognostic significance of p53 overexpression in gastric and colorectal carcinoma. Br J Cancer 66:558–562

52. Kakeji Y, Korenaga D, Tsujitani S, Baba H, Anai H, Maehara Y, Sugimachi K (1993) Gastric cancer with p53 overexpression in gastric and colorectal carcinoma. Br J Cancer 67:589–593

53. Lowe SW, Schmitt EM, Smith SW, Osborne BA, Kacks T (1993) p53 is required for radiation-induced apoptosis in mouse thymocytes. Nature 362:847–849

54. Lowe SW, Ruley HE, Jack T, Housman DE (1993) p53-dependent apoptosis modulates the cytotoxicity of anticancer agents. Cell 74:957–967

55. Kikuchi-Yanoshita R, Konishi M, Ito S, Seki M, Tanaka K, Maeda Y, Iino H, Fukuyama M, Koike M, Mori T (1992) Genetic changes of both p53 alleles associated with the conversion from colorectal adenoma to early carcinoma in familial adenomatous polyposis and non-familial adenomatous polyposis patients. Cancer Res 52:3965–3971

56. Esrig D, Spruck CHIII, Nichols PW, Chaiwun B, Steven K, Groshen S, Chen SC, Skinner DG, Jones PA, Cote RJ (1993) p53 nuclear protein accumulation correlates with mutations in the p53 gene, tumor grade, and stage in bladder cancer. Am J Pathol 143:1389–1397

57. Baas IO, Mulder J-WR, Offerhaus GJA, Vogelstein B, Hamilton S (1994) An evaluation of six antibodies for immunohistochemistry of mutant p53 gene product in archival colorectal neoplasms. J Pathol 172:5–12

58. Tsuda H, Hirohashi S (1994) Association among p53 gene mutation, nuclear accumulation of the P53 protein and aggressive phenotypes in breast cancer. Int J Cancer 57:498–503

59. Lane DP, Benchimol S (1990) p53: oncogene or antioncogene? Genes Dev 4:1–8

60. Zhan Q, Lord KA, Alamo I Jr, Hollander MC, Carrier F, Ron D, Kohn KW, Hoffman B, Lieberman DA, Fornace AJ Jr (1994) The gadd and MyD genes define a novel set of mammalian genes encoding acidic protein that synergistically suppress cell growth. Mol Cell Biol 14:2361–2371

61. Canman CE, Gilmer TM, Coutts SB, Kastan MB (1995) Growth factor modulation of p53-mediated growth arrest versus apoptosis. Genes Dev 9:600–611

62. Lowe SW, Jacks T, Housman DE, Ruley HE (1994) Abrogation of oncogene-associated apoptosis allows transformation of p53-deficient cells. Proc Natl Acad Sci USA 91:2026–2030

63. Lane DP (1992) p53, guardian of the genome. Nature 358:15–16

64. Lowe SW, Bodia S, McClatchey A, Remington L, Ruley HE, Fisher DE, Housman DE, Jacks T

92   H. Ito et al.

(1994) *p53* status and the efficacy of cancer therapy in vivo. Science 266:807–810

65. Kobayashi M, Watanabe H, Ajioka Y, Yoshida M, Hitomi Y, Asakura H (1995) Correlation of *p53* protein expression with apoptotic incidence in colorectal neoplasia. Virchows Arch 427:27–32

66. Waldmann T, Kinzler KW, Vogelstein B (1995) *p21* necessary for the *p53*-mediated G1 arrest in human cancer cells. Cancer Res 55:5187–5190

67. El-Deiry WS, Harper JW, O'Connor PM, Veolculescu VE, Canman CE, Jackman J, Pietenpol JA, Burrell M, Hill DE, Wang Y, Wiman KG, Mercer WE, Kastan MB, Kohn KW, Elledge SJ, Kinzler KW, Vogelstein B (1994) WAF1/CIP1 is induced in *p53*-mediated G1 arrest and apoptosis. Cancer Res 54:1169–1174

68. Steinman RA, Hoffman B, Iro A, Guillouf C, Lieberman DA, El-Houseini ME (1994) Induction of *p21* (WAF1/CIP1) during differentiation. Oncogene 9:3389–3396

69. Michieli P, Chedid M, Lin D, Pierce JH, Mercer WE, Givol D (1994) Induction of WAF1/CIP1 by a *p53*-independent pathway. Cancer Res 54:3391–3395

70. Jiang H, Kin J, Su ZZ, Collart FR, Huberman E, Fisher PB (1994) Induction of differentiation in human promyelocytic HL-60 leukemia cells activates *p21*, WAF1/CIP1, expression in the absence of *p53*. Oncogene 9:3397–3406

71. Miyashita T, Krajewski S, Krajewska M, Wang HG, Lin HK, Libermann DA, Hoffman B, Reed JC (1994) Tumor suppressor *p53* is a regulator of *bcl-2* and *bax* gene expression in vitro and in vivo. Oncogene 9:1799–1805

72. Ikeguchi M, Kaibara N, Horikawa H, Ito H (1995) Adriamycin induces apoptosis in human gastric cancer cell lines. Presented at the First International Gastric Cancer Congress, pp 1611–1616

73. Osaki M, Tatebe S, Goto A, Hayashi H, Oshimura M, Ito H (1997) 5-Fluorouracil (5-FU) induced apoptosis in gastric cancer cell lines; Role of the *p53* gene. Apoptosis (in press)

74. Makino M, Shirai H, Sugamura K, Kimura O, Maeta M, Ito H, Kaibara N (1996) Increased induc-

tion of apoptosis of human colorectal cancer cells after preoperative treatment with 5-fluorouracil. Oncol Rep 3:281–285

75. Sugamura K, Makino M, Shirai H, Kimura O, Maeta M, Ito H, Kaibara N (1997) Increased induction of apoptosis of human gastric cancer cells after preoperative treatment with 5-fluorouracil. Cancer 79:12–17

76. Yanagihara K, Tsumuraya M (1992) Transforming growth factor 1 induces apoptotic cell death in cultured human gastric carcinoma cells. Cancer Res 52:4042–4045

77. Yamamoto M, Maehara Y, Sakaguchi Y, Oda S, Kusumoto T, Ichiyoshi Y, Sugimachi K (1996) Transforming growth factor-β1 induces apoptosis in gastric cancer cells through a *p53*-independent pathway. Cancer 77(8 Suppl):1628–1633

78. Ito M, Yasui W, Kyo E, Yokozaki H, Nakayama H, Ito H, Tahara E (1992) Growth inhibition of transforming growth on human gastric carcinoma cells: receptor and postreceptor signaling. Cancer Res 52:295–300

79. Yonehara S, Ishii A, Yonehara M (1989) A cell-killing monoclonal antibody (anti-Fas) to a cell surface antigen co-downregulated with the receptor of tumor necrosis factor. J Exp Med 169:1747–1756

80. Owen-Schaub LB, Randinsky R, Kruzel E, Berry K, Yonehara S (1994) Anti-Fas on nonhematopoietic tumors: levels of Fas/Apo-1 and *bcl-2* are not predictive of biological responsiveness. Cancer Res 54:1580–1586

81. Weis M, Schlegel J, Kass GEN, Holmstrom TH, Peters I, Eriksson J, Orrenius S, Chow SC (1995) Cellular events in FAS/APO-1-mediated apoptosis in JURKAT T lymphocytes. Exp Cell Res 219:699–708

82. Itoh N, Tsujimoto Y, Nagata S (1993) Effect of *bcl-2* on Fas antigen-mediated cell death. J Immunol 151:621–627

83. Vollmers HP, Dammrich J, Ribbert H, Wozniak E, Muller-Hermelink H-K (1995) Apoptosis of stomach carcinoma cells induced by a human monoclonal antibody. Cancer 76:550–558

Pathogenesis of Serrated Adenoma of the Colorectum: Implication for Malignant Progression

Fumio Shimamoto[1], Shinji Tanaka[2], and Eiichi Tahara[3]

Summary. Hyperplastic polyps of the colorectum are known to show dysplastic changes and may be mixed hyperplastic adenomatous polyps. It is proposed that these polyps are serrated adenomas and represent a morphologically unique variant of adenoma. The serrated adenoma, characteristically containing proliferative activity in the lower portion of the crypts, is distinctly different from ordinary adenomas, which are found in the upper portion of the crypts. In proliferative lesions of the crypts, abnormal accumulation of P53 protein is frequently associated with serrated adenomas that display severe dysplasia and microinvasive serrated adenocarcinomas, regarded as hyperplastic polyps with pseudoinvasive glands. Some of the superficial-type serrated adenocarcinomas arising from serrated adenomas or hyperplastic polyps are small and display aggressive behavior, manifesting as liver metastasis. The changes found in both hyperplastic polyps and carcinoma—including increased secretion of carcinoembryonic antigen, altered blood antigen expression, and reduced secretion of sialomucin—which were found in hyperplastic polyps, cannot explained unless serrated adenomas arising in hyperplastic polyps are recognized as true neoplasia. Here we describe the relations among hyperplastic nodules, hyperplastic polyps, serrated adenomas, and traditional carcinomas with the hope of understanding this distinct neoplastic lesion of the colorectum. Recent data are reviewed.

[1] Department of Pathology, Hiroshima University Hospital, 1-2-3 Kasumi, Minami-ku, Hiroshima 734, Japan
[2] First Department of Internal Medicine, Hiroshima University School of Medicine, 1-2-3 Kasumi, Minami-ku, Hiroshima 734, Japan
[3] First Department of Pathology, Hiroshima University School of Medicine, 1-2-3 Kasumi, Minami-ku, Hiroshima 734, Japan

Introduction

Hyperplastic polyps are the most common polyps of the large intestine after age 40 and are often found in the rectosigmoid area, where colorectal cancers develop most frequently in Japan. It is also generally accepted that the hyperplastic polyp rarely progresses to malignancy, although epidemiological evidence reveals that the hyperplastic polyp is an indicator of high risk for colorectal carcinoma [1]. Hyperplastic and adenomatous polyps have been reported to occur in the same area [2–8], and hyperplastic polyps with foci of intramucosal carcinoma have been reported [9–11].

Hyperplastic polyps in an adenomatous lesion or mixed hyperplastic adenomatous polyps (MHAPs), which combine the morphologic features of hyperplastic and adenomatous epithelium, are not new forms of colorectal neoplasias, as they have been already described by pathologists for about 25 years [2–11]. MHAPs have not been defined as precancerous lesions.

Mixed hyperplastic adenomatous polyps are rare and are probably overdiagnosed. Moreover, hyperplastic polyps exhibit pseudoinvasion across the muscularis mucosa, which often misleads pathologist to regard them as malignant [12]. Furthermore, no convincing evidence of transition from a hyperplastic polyp to a traditional adenoma has been seen even among large numbers of hyperplastic polyps of the colorectum [13, 14]. The colorectal hyperplastic polyps examined came largely from autopsy or surgical specimens, not from resected tissue removed using improved colonoscopic procedures, by which the new entity of colonic tumor seen as a flat neoplastic lesion (flat adenomas and flat adenocarcinomas) had been found [15, 16].

Longacre and Fenoglio-Preiser investigated in detail the histologic features, classification, and histogenesis of MAHPs, comparing them with hyperplastic polyps and traditional adenomas. They proposed the term "serrated adenoma," which reflects a morphologically unique variant of adenoma. This variant exhibits incomplete mucinous differentiation, dysplastic serrated glands, and surface mitoses extended into the upper zone of the crypt. These authors also indicated that an adenoma-to-carcinoma sequence similar to that seen with ordinary adenomas occurred in these lesions; 37% of serrated adenomas contained foci of significant dysplasia, and 11% had areas of intramucosal carcinoma [17]. Our present aim is to emphasize the importance of understanding and diagnosing serrated adenomas of the large intestine to clarify the relation between serrated adenoma and malignancy.

Serrated Adenomas

Clinical and Macroscopic Features

The incidence of serrated adenomas of the colorectum is unknown, although it is reported that these lesions constituted about 0.5% of all colonic polyps reviewed [17]. It is difficult for endoscopists to differentiate between hyperplastic polyps and serrated adenomas.

Histologically, there are two distinct serrated adenomas: polypoid-type serrated adenomas [17] and superficial-type (flat type) serrated adenomas [18–20]. In brief, polypoid-type adenomas exhibit exophytic polypoid growth with infolding fibrous or fibromuscular stroma within the tumor. The superficial type has flat, elevated or simply flat mucosa, which is never more than two times the thickness of the adjacent normal mucosa of the colon without the stroma [16].

Table 1 shows the clinicopathological features for 27 polypoid-type (Fig. 1a) and 24 superficial-type (Fig. 2a) serrated adenomas, including adenocarcinoma (serrated adenocarcinoma) [18]. Of the patients with polypoid-type serrated adenomas, 14 were men and 13 women (M/F = 1.1:1.0). They ranged in age from 40 to 84 years (mean 61.7 years). In contrast, among patients with the superficial-type adenoma, 21 were men and 3 women (M/F = 7:1). The age range was 36 to 81 years (mean 57.9 years). The two major sites for both types were the sigmoid colon and rectum. Other, somewhat less common sites of the super-

Table 1. Clinical and macroscopic features of polypoid type and superficial type serrated adenomas

Feature	Polypoid type	Superficial type
No.	27	24
Sex (M:F)	1.1:1.0	7:1
Age (years)	40–84 (mean 61.7)	36–81 (mean 57.9)
Location		
Cecum	0	1 (4.2%)
Ascending colon	1 (3.7%)	3 (12.5%)
Transverse colon	2 (7.4%)	4 (16.7%)
Descending colon	1 (3.7%)	1 (4.2%)
Sigmoid colon	14 (51.9%)	6 (25.0%)
Rectum	9 (33.3%)	9 (37.5%)
Macroscopic classification		
Ip	10 (37.0%)	0
Isp	12 (44.4%)	3 (12.5%)
Is	5 (18.5%)	18 (75.0%)
IIa	0	3 (12.5%)
Size (mm)	4–30 (mean 10.6)	2–12 (mean 4.8)

Ip, pedunculated; Isp, subpedunculated; Is, sessile; IIa, flat and elevated.

ficial type in particular were the ascending (12.5%) and transverse (16.7%) colon [17, 18]. Macroscopically, the polypoid type was protruded, or pedunculated (37.5%), subpedunculated (44.4%), or sessile (18.5%), whereas the superficial types were subpedunculated (12.5%), sessile (75%), or flat and elevated (12.5%).

The superficial type, ranging in size from 2 to 12mm in diameter (mean 4.8mm), was significantly smaller than the polypoid type (4–30mm; mean 10.6mm). All of the large adenomas (>15mm) displayed the polypoid growth pattern, and more than 50% of adenomas contained intramucosal carcinoma. In contrast, most of the small adenomas (≤4mm) were predominantly the superficial type.

Histology

Serrated adenomas are characterized by varying degrees of serrated glandular patterns and dysplastic epithelium, which can be classified as mild, moderate, or severe atypia [18] according to the grade of epithelial atypia (structure atypia of serrated glands, nuclear configuration, nuclear

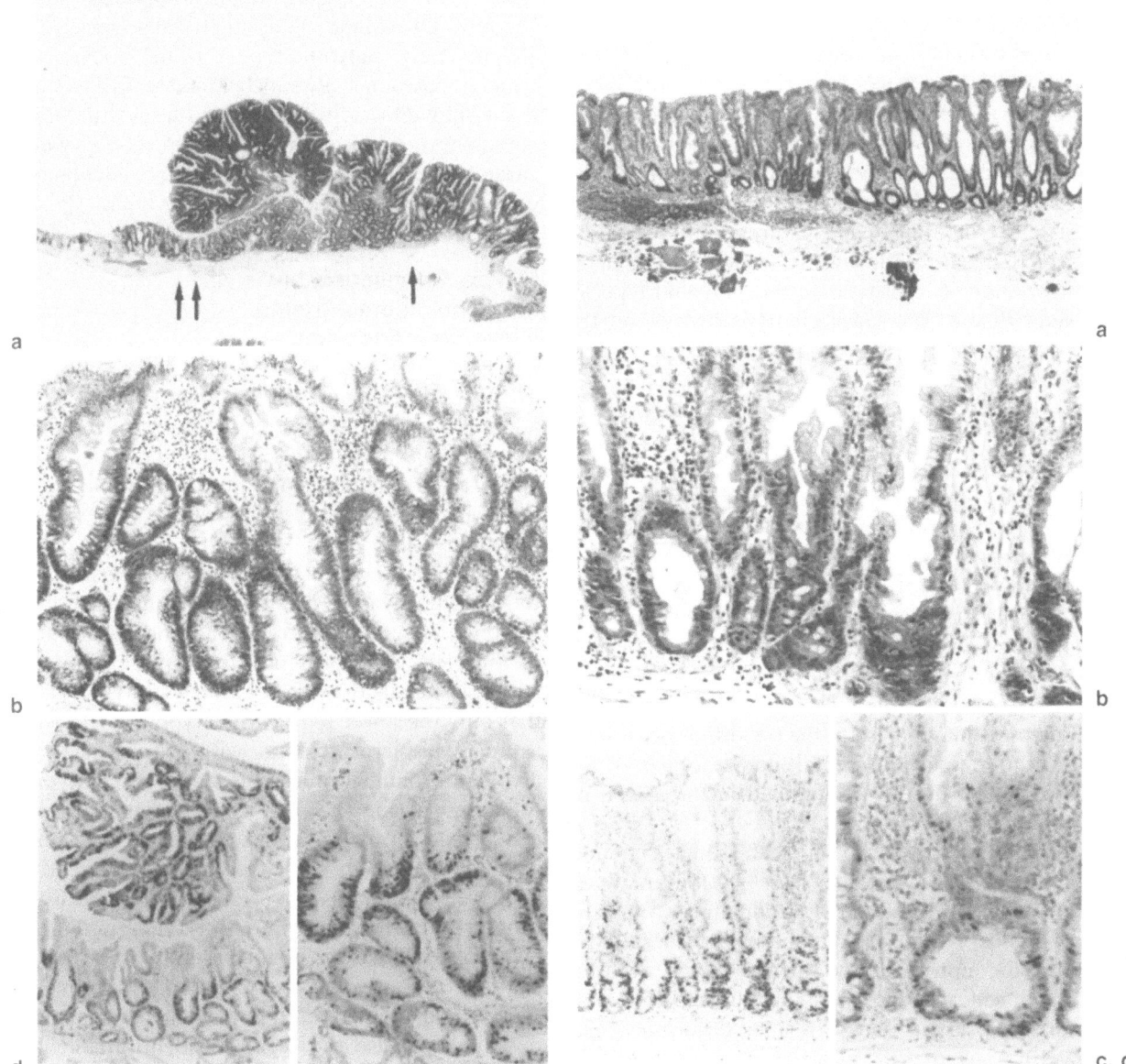

Fig. 1a–d. Polypoid-type serrated adenoma (sigmoid colon, 1.5 cm in diameter). **a** This subpedunculated polyp, composed of both polypoid (*single arrow*) and flat lesions (*double arrows*), has a tubulovillous appearance. (H&E, ×10) **b** Flat lesion of a polypoid-type serrated adenoma shows mild atypia. (H&E, ×100) **c** Ki-67-immunoreactive cells are found in the lower half of a flat lesion and in the tubulovillous glands of a polypoid lesion. (×40) **d** Main proliferative zone of a flat lesion of the polypoid type occupies more of the upper lesion of the lower crypt than that of superficial serrated adenoma. (×100)

Fig. 2a–d. Superficial-type serrated adenoma of the cecum, 9 mm in diameter. **a** Lesion is composed of mucosal dysplasia without an exophytic polypoid configuration and has a submucosal lymphoid follicle. (H&E, ×40) **b** Higher magnification of **a**. The lesion with severe atypia shows dysplastic glands with a prominent nucleolus and complicating branching. (H&E, ×200) **c** Ki-67-positive staining is localized in the lower one-third of the crypts. (×100) **d** P53-positive staining. Note P53 overexpression in the base of the crypts, which almost corresponds to the Ki-67-positive proliferative zone. (×200)

pseudostratification, nuclear/cytoplasmic ratio, and prominent nucleoli) [17].

In the superficial- and polypoid-type serrated adenomas, the tumor cells are more dysplastic in the lower portion of the crypt (which corresponds with the proliferative zone) than in the upper portion; and they have a tendency to extend to the upper portion of the crypts with increasing atypia [20]. Serrated glandular features—differentiation from the cells of the lower crypt and less atypia—were more conspicuous in the polypoid-type lesions than in the superficial type because of the difference in their growth patterns.

With mild atypia of both the superficial and polypoid types, the nuclei are ovoid or elongated, crowded, and mildly stratified; they also contain less prominent nucleoli. The nuclear/cytoplasmic ratio is slightly increased. Varying degrees of mature and immature goblet cells are usually preserved in the upper crypts. The overall architecture is not greatly altered from that of the hyperplastic polyp, showing serrated glands without complicated branching (Fig. 1b). Although it is sometimes difficult to discriminate between serrated adenomas with mild atypia and hyperplastic polyps, it may be useful for the differential diagnosis to examine the cryptal endocrine cells, which can almost always be identified in the glands of hyperplastic polyps [21].

With severe atypia in both superficial and polypoid types, the nuclei are greatly enlarged, are ovoid or round, and often contain a prominent nucleolus. Mitoses are numerous and extended into the upper portion of the crypts. Mature goblet cells decrease markedly but remain immature. The crypts show irregular branching (Fig. 2a,b).

On the other hand, depending on the degree of cellular dysplasia within the epithelium, Rubio and Rodensjoe categorized flat (superficial) serrated adenomas into (1) those with low-grade dysplasia (LGD) when the dysplastic cells are present in the deeper half of the epithelium, and (2) those with high-grade dysplasia (HGD) when the dysplastic cells are found in the upper half of the epithelium. Moreover, depending on the topographic distribution of the dysplastic cells within the crypts, flat serrated adenomas can be divided into type I when the dysplastic epithelium is limited to the lower half of the serrated crypts and type II when the dysplastic epithelium is present in the superficial half of the serrated crypts [22].

Serrated adenomas are histologically subclassified into tubulovillous and tubular types [23]. In our study, polypoid-type serrated adenomas could be histologically subclassified as 10 cases of the tubulovillous type (including 3 cases with focal carcinoma) and 17 of the tubular type (1 case with carcinoma). Superficial-type serrated adenomas could be subclassified as the tubular type.

Minute Submucosal Invasive Adenocarcinoma Arising in Serrated Adenomas

There are few data on small submucosal invasive adenocarcinomas arising in serrated adenomas [20, 24]. This lesion may be crucial to understanding serrated adenomas and adenocarcinomas and might be diagnosed as a hyperplastic polyp with pseudoinvasion.

In our study, the histological characteristics of the minute invasive carcinoma arising in a serrated adenoma demonstrated that the upper part of the crypts is represented by typical serrated hyperplastic glands with mild nuclear atypia, and that only the lower part of the crypts is regarded as invasive microcarcinoma with distinct nuclear atypia, a prominent nucleolus, and a fused atypical structure (Fig. 3a–c). It is interesting that five of six small serrated adenocarcinomas 3 to 12 mm in diameter and of the superficial type, already displayed submucosal invasion. Four of the five submucosal carcinomas were only 4 mm in diameter, so, these lesions might be easily missed on routine colonoscopic examination. Moreover, they should be recognized to have high malignant potential because the serrated adenocarcinoma develops above the thin muscularis mucosa, and they can invade the submucosa directly, similar to the traditional small, flat adenoma [16, 25, 26]. Moreover, Kasumi et al. reported that 8-mm and 12-mm flat invasive colon cancers, which derived from serrated adenoma and serrated hyperplastic epithelium, respectively, had infiltrated the subserosa and metastasized to the liver [27].

p53 Gene Mutation

To our knowledge, only a few studies of *p53* expression and mutations in serrated adenomas have been reported [22, 28, 29]. It is now widely accepted that overexpression of P53 nuclear protein correlates with mutation in the *p53* gene and

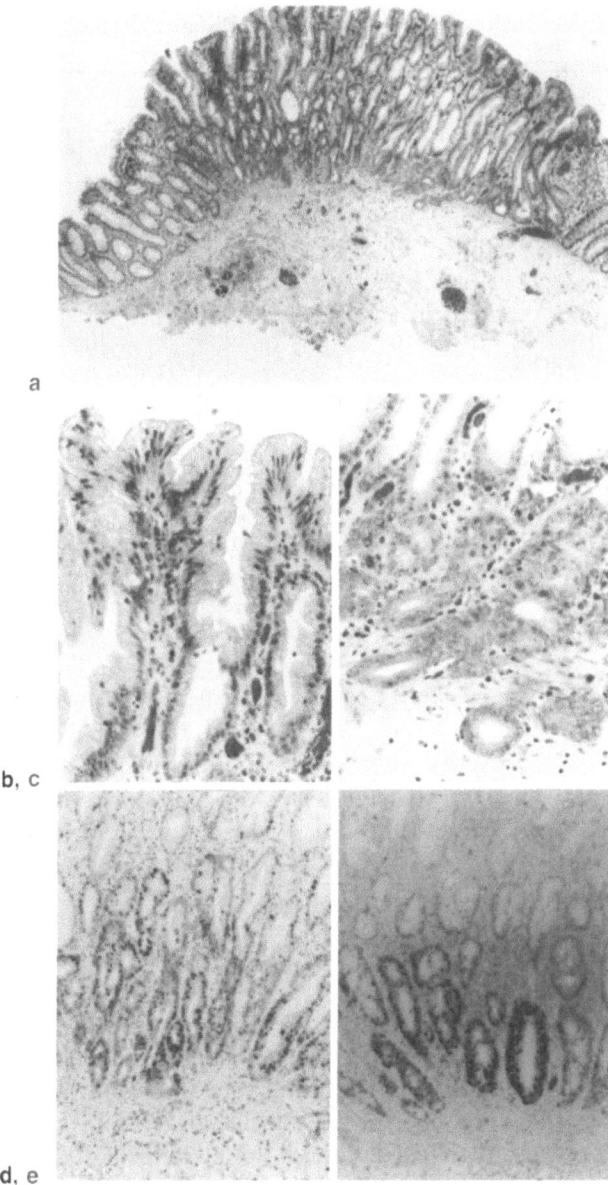

Fig. 3a–e. Superficial-type minute submucosal serrated adenocarcinoma in the transverse colon, 4mm in diameter. **a** This small polyp (endoscopically the subpedunculated type) spreads laterally with slight elevation, which is occupied by dysplastic glands. (H&E, ×40) **b** Note the serrated appearance with markedly decreased goblet cells and fewer dysplastic cells in the upper part of the crypts. (H&E, ×200) **c** Submucosal minute invasive carcinoma shows distinct nuclear atypia and complex glandular formation of the lower part of the crypt. (H&E, ×200) **d** Ki-67-positive cells with proliferation in the lower portion of the crypts. (×100) **e** Note P53 overexpression in the lower half of the crypts and submucosal invasive glands. (×100)

plays an important role in the development and progression of ordinary colorectal carcinomas [30–35]. Investigation of the accumulation of P53 protein would be also useful for histological diagnosis of colorectal tumors, as immunohistochemical expression of P53 protein increases according to the histological grade in ordinary adenomas.

Table 2 summarizes the relation between expression of P53 and the degree of atypia in serrated adenomas [18]. Of the 24 superficial-type serrated adenomas, 1 (14.2%) with moderate atypia, 3 (75.0%) with severe atypia, and 4 (66.7%) with focal carcinoma showed highly positive immunoreactivity (++ or +++) to P53 protein. Of the 27 polypoid-type adenomas, 4 (50.0%) with moderate atypia, 10 (83.3%) with severe atypia, and 4 (100%) with focal carcinoma showed highly positive immunoreactivity to P53. Both superficial- and polypoid-type serrated adenomas with severe atypia and focal carcinoma displayed a higher incidence of P53 expression than those with mild and moderate atypia; the difference was statistically significant ($P < 0.01$). Most of the P53-positive tumor cells could be identified in the proliferative area of the serrated adenoma. Therefore P53 overexpression of serrated adenomas may be useful for the diagnosis of serrated adenomas of the colorectum, as serrated adenomas are generally likely to be underdiagnosed as hyperplastic polyps [11, 17].

Hiyama et al. reported that mutation of the *p53* gene was found in 40% of serrated adenomas and all serrated adenocarcinomas in or with serrated adenoma; the *p53* gene mutations comprised missense and nonsense changes. Interestingly, identical *p53* gene mutations were detected in both serrated adenoma and invasive adenocarcinoma, suggesting a clonal origin for both lesions [36]. These observations indicate that serrated adenomas are truly neoplastic and that *p53* gene mutation is the most characteristic genetic alteration, appearing as a relatively early event in the multistep process of colorectal cancer, which may be distinct from the usual adenocarcinoma sequence of colorectal carcinogenesis.

Ki-67 Expression

Rubio and Rodensjoe first discovered the different patterns of cell proliferation of superficial-

Table 2. Relation between expression of P53 and Ki-67; and degree of atypia in 24 superficial-type and 27 polypoid-type serrated adenomas

Degree of atypia	No.	P53				Ki-67			
		−	+	++	+++	−	+	++	+++
Mild									
Type S	7 (29.2%)	2	5	0	0	0	0	7 (100%)	0
Type P	3 (11.1%)	1	2	0	0	0	2	1 (33.3%)	0
Moderate									
Type S	7 (29.2%)	0	6	1 (14.2%)	0	0	2	5 (71.4%)	0
Type P	8 (29.6%)	2	2	3 (50.0%)	1	0	1	6 (87.5%)	1
Severe									
Type S	4 (16.7%)	0	1	3 (75.0%)	0	0	0	3 (100%)	1
Type P	12 (44.4%)	0	2	4 (83.3%)	6	0	1	5 (91.7%)	6
Focal carcinoma									
Type S	6 (25%)	0	2	4 (66.7%)	0	0	0	4 (100%)	2
Type P	4 (14.8%)	0	0	0	4 (100%)	0	0	0	4 (100%)
Total	24 (100%)	2 (8.3%)	14 (58.3%)	8 (33.3%)	0	0	2 (8.3%)	19 (79.2%)	3 (12.5%)
	27 (100%)	3 (11.1%)	6 (22.2%)	7 (25.9%)	11 (40.7%)	0	4 (14.8%)	12 (44.4%)	11 (40.7%)

S, superficial-type serrated adenoma; P, polypoid-type serrated adenoma.

type serrated adenomas and flat tubular adenomas of the colorectum. They used the cell proliferation marker Ki-67 [20].

Ki-67-positive cells are found predominantly in the upper portion of the crypts in ordinary flat adenomas [20], whereas they are situated mainly in the lower one-third of the crypts in the superficial-type serrated adenoma (Fig. 2c). In polypoid-type serrated adenomas with a histologically flat and polypoid lesion, Ki-67 was not intensively positive in the lower portion of the crypts above the muscularis mucosa, whereas it was positive in the lower to middle portion of the crypts in the flat lesions and in the lower to upper portion of the crypts in the polypoid lesions (Fig. 1c,d). Interestingly, although cell proliferation of polypoid-type serrated adenomas has not been reported, the proliferative zone of flat lesions in the polypoid type, which might be histologically classified into the superficial type, is definitely different from that of the superficial type. This finding suggests that the difference in

growth patterns between the polypoid-type and superficial-type serrated adenomas may depend on the site of the proliferation zone in the crypts regardless of histological subclassification [23]. It would perhaps be useful to investigate the sites of Ki-67-positive cells in serrated adenomas to differentiate between the superficial and polypoid types (if the colonic polyps are small) and early polypoid-type serrated adenomas, which may arise from superficial-type serrated adenomas.

In the minute submucosal carcinoma arising in superficial-type serrated adenomas, P53-positive cells and Ki-67 proliferative cells are found in the lower portion of the crypt and in submucosal infiltrating tumor cells (Fig. 3d,e) [20, 22, 24]. Rubio and Rodensjoe suggested that the basal proliferative cells of the crypts in serrated adenomas aquire the capability of independent growth and concluded that flat serrated adenomas were a novel, independent phenotype of neoplastic lesions in the colorectum [20].

Hyperplastic Polyps and Hyperplastic Nodules

Clinical and Macroscopic Features

Hyperplastic polyps of the large intestine [37] are identical to metaplastic polyps [38]. Hyperplastic polyps show a striking predilection for the rectosigmoid [39] and are more common and more likely to be multiple in patients with colorectal adenomas and carcinomas [4, 40]. They have often been misdiagnosed in the past as either normal mucosa or adenomatous polyps [41]. No convincing examples of transition from hyperplastic polyp to traditional adenoma have been seen in large numbers of hyperplastic polyps of the colorectum [13, 14].

Hyperplastic polyps consist of serrated or sawtoothed crypts, and those without serrated features in the crypts are classified as hyperplastic nodules according to the histological criteria of the Japanese Research Society for Cancer of the Colon and Rectum.

Table 3 shows the clinicopathological features of 67 cases of hyperplastic nodule and 56 cases of hyperplastic polyp [42]. Among the patients with hyperplastic nodules, 50 were men and 17 women (M/F = 2.9:1). They ranged in age from 29 to 83 years (mean 58.3 years). Of those with hyperplastic polyps, 48 were men and 8 women (M/F = 6:1), with an age range of 41 to 81 years (mean 60.1 years). The major sites of hyperplastic nodules and hyperplastic polyps were the sigmoid colon and rectum, similar to the serrated adenomas. Macroscopically, the hyperplastic nodules and hyperplastic polyps were predominantly the sessile type (56.7% and 46.4%, respectively). The hyperplastic nodules ranged in size from 2 to 6mm diameter (mean 3.7mm) and were almost as large as the hyperplastic polyps, which ranged from 2 to 8mm (mean 4.0mm).

Histology

All hyperplastic nodules are characterized by nonserrated hyperplastic glands with mature goblet cells and no immature goblet cells; these cells were slightly dilated, distorted, and occasionally fused (Fig. 4a). The nuclei of the glands are round to ovoid and the nucleoli almost inconspicuous. Increased chronic inflammatory cell infiltration, sometimes with lymphoid follicles, is often found in the stroma of the lesions. Some hyperplastic nodules are transformed at an early stage to hyperplastic polyps, showing serrated patterns only in the surface epithelium of the upper crypts. A ordinary tubular adenoma is rarely found in hyperplastic nodules of the colorectum.

Table 3. Clinical and macroscopic features of hyperplastic nodules and hyperplastic polyps

Feature	Hyperplastic nodule	Hyperplastic polyp
No.	67	56
Sex (M:F)	2.9:1	6:1
Age (years)	29–83 (mean 58.3)	41–81 (mean 60.1)
Location		
Cecum	6 (8.9%)	1 (1.8%)
Ascending colon	6 (8.9%)	4 (7.1%)
Transverse colon	7 (10.4%)	2 (3.6%)
Descending colon	2 (3.0%)	1 (1.8%)
Sigmoid colon	24 (35.8%)	26 (46.4%)
Rectum	22 (32.8%)	22 (39.3%)
Macroscopic classification		
Ip	1 (1.5%)	1 (1.8%)
Isp	9 (13.4%)	8 (14.3%)
Is	38 (56.7%)	26 (46.4%)
IIa	5 (7.5%)	1 (1.8%)
Unknown	14 (20.9%)	20 (35.7%)
Size (mm)	2–6 (mean 3.7)	2–8 (mean 4.0)

Ip, pedunculated; Isp, subpedunculated; Is, sessile; IIa, flat and elevated.

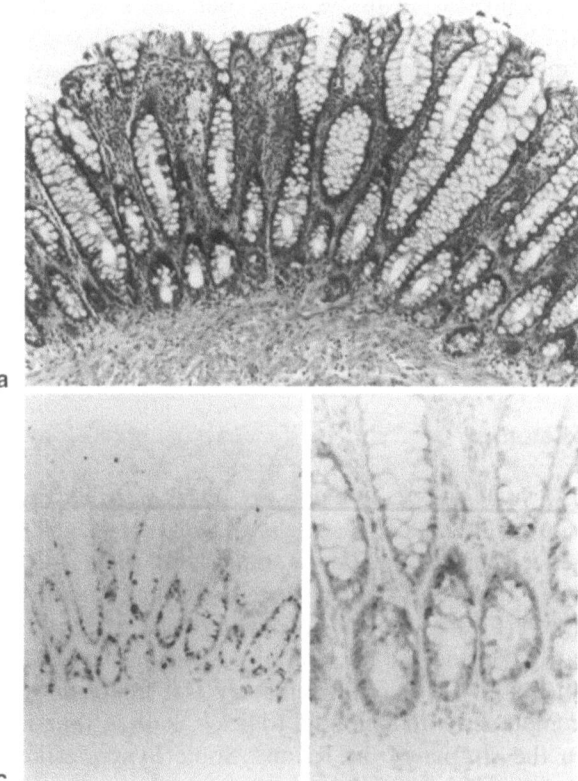

Fig. 4. Hyperplastic nodule in the rectum, 3mm in diameter. **a** Small polyp (endoscopically the subpedunculated type) is histologically considered to be a hyperplastic nodule because of the presence of nonserrated hyperplastic glands without dysplasia. (H&E, ×100) **b** Ki-67-positive cells in the lower portion of the crypt of this polyp are slightly increased over those of the adjacent normal mucosa. (×100) **c** P53-positive cells are sporadically detected in the lower portion of the crypts. (×100)

In contrast, in hyperplastic polyps, a serrated epithelial appearance is found only in the upper part of the crypts, composed of a varying degree of mixed mature and immature goblet cells and showing dilated, distorted, or sometimes fused glands with oval or round nuclei without prominent nucleoli or atypia (Fig. 5a).

Although most of the small pure hyperplastic polyps never exhibit dysplastic change, as the hyperplastic polyps increase in size mixed hyperplastic adenomatous polyps are occasionally encountered [2–8]. It is said that foci of dysplasia may be observed in hyperplastic polyps, but the incidence is low and dysplasia is probably overdiagnosed [12, 43]. Hyperplastic polyps showing pseudoinvasion across the muscularis

mucosa sometimes simulate adenocarinoma [44, 45].

If more than 10 hyperplastic polyps are present in the colon, the designation "hyperplastic polyposis" may be used. Some of these polyps are combined hyperplastic-adenomatous lesions [5, 6, 43] and are at low but definite risk of becoming malignant.

Oohara et al. [46] investigated the histogenesis of microscopic adenomas and hyperplastic (metaplastic) glands in nonpolyposis. They pointed out that when characteristic hyperplastic glands were followed up using complete serial sections, they were seen to connect with glands with reduced serrated patterns as did those in the above-described hyperplastic nodules. Moreover, with regard to the histogenesis of hyperplastic

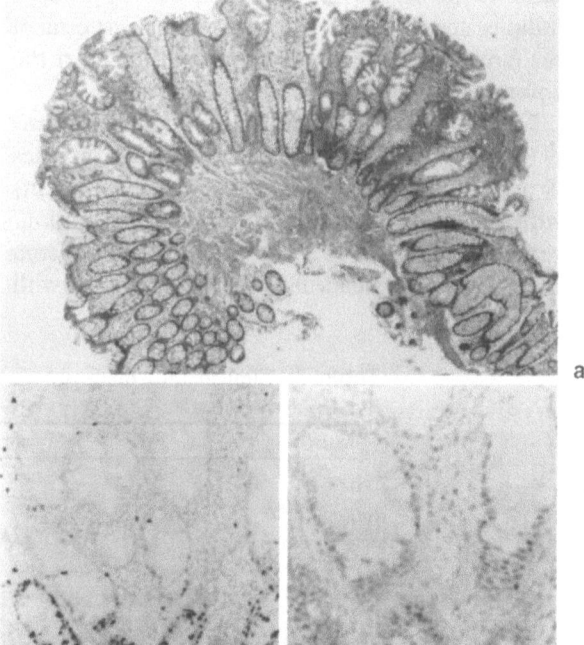

Fig. 5a–c. Hyperplastic polyp in the rectum, 5mm in diameter. **a** Small polyp (endoscopically the subpedunculated type) is composed of serrated and nonserrated glands. Note serrated epithelium only in the upper portion of the crypts and no dysplastic change of the glands. (H&E, ×40) **b** Ki-67-positive cells with nonserrated epithelium in the lower portion of the crypts. (×100) **c** P53-positive cells are sporadically found in the lower portion of the crypts. (×400)

polyps in the colorectum, Araki et al. first suggested that hyperplastic polyps originated by the apparent fusion of single abnormal crypts within a small region of mucosa and grew by fission of the crypt and fusion of the polycentrically arising polyp. They also noted that no serration of the epithelial lining could be seen during the early stages of hyperplastic polyps, as determined by advanced tissue digestive techniques and scanning electron microscopy [47].

p53 and Ki-67

Table 4 summarizes the relation between expression of P53 and Ki-67 and hyperplastic nodules and polyps. Of the 64 hyperplastic nodules, 30 (46.9%) showed weakly positive immunoreactivity (+) to P53 protein (Fig. 4c). In contrast, of the 55 hyperplastic polyps, 32 (58.2%) had weakly positive immunoreactivity to P53 (Fig. 5c); neither hyperplastic lesion (nodules or polyps) showed intense reactivity (++ to +++). The hyperplastic polyps display a slightly higher incidence of P53 expression than did the hyperplastic nodules. P53-positive cells were sporadically identified in the proliferative area, as in the serrated adenoma.

Rubio and Rodensjoe pointed out that weak P53 expression was unexpectedly demonstrated by nearly 12% of the flat hyperplastic polyps, in addition to a high incidence of P53 immunoreactivity in flat serrated adenomas, as shown in our study. The weak P53 immunoreactivity in flat hyperplastic polyps should be considered a false-positive reaction [22]. Extensive study of p53 gene alteration in hyperplastic lesions and serrated adenomas is necessary for understanding the carcinogenesis of the serrated adenoma. In fact, we have found p53 gene mutation in serrated adenomas and adenocarcinomas and suggested a multistep carcinogenesis pathway for serrated adenoma that is distinct from the usual adenoma-to-carcinoma sequence [29].

Ki-67-positive cells of hyperplastic nodules and polyps are situated mainly in the lower one-third of the crypts, and they appear in greater numbers than in normal glands (Figs. 4b, 5b). There was no statistical difference in the incidence of Ki-67-positive cells in regard to hyperplastic nodules and hyperplastic polyps.

Functional Alterations in Hyperplastic Polyps

There are functional alterations that overlap in hyperplastic polyps and severe adenomatous dysplasia and carcinomas of the colorectum [48]. Such changes include increased secretion of carcinoembryonic antigen (CEA) [49], reduced secretion of sialomucin [49], changes in blood group antigen expression [2], and an absence of cytoplasmic immunoglobulin A (IgA) secretory activity [48].

Ordinary Adenocarcinoma and Serrated Adenoma

For a long time normal-appearing hyperplastic mucosa adjacent to colorectal carcinoma was studied with particular attention to the morphological and histochemical changes [50, 51], colon carcinogenesis, ultrastructural findings [52], and karyotypic features [53]. Filipe et al., who first termed the adjacent mucosa as "transitional mucosa," suggested that the changes in transitional mucosa represented a specific premalignant alteration in the colon mucosa, represented by a consistent alteration of mucin histochemistry [50, 51]. Conversely, Isaacson and Attwood pointed out that mucosa adjacent to large bowel carcinoma was likely to represent a reactive phenomenon because the mucosal alteration described in the transitional mucosa could be demonstrated in mucosa from solitary ulcer syndrome and colostomies [54].

Table 4. Expression of P53 and Ki-67 in hyperplastic nodules and hyperplastic polyps

Lesion	No.	P53				Ki-67			
		−	+	++	+++	−	+	++	+++
HN	64	34 (53.1%)	30 (46.9%)	0	0	0	20 (31.3%)	39 (60.9%)	5 (7.8%)
HP	55	23 (41.8%)	32 (58.2%)	0	0	0	23 (41.8%)	32 (58.2%)	0

HN, hyperplastic nodule; HP, hyperplastic polyp.

Pandey et al. demonstrated that tissue adjacent (up to 3–4 cm) to a carcinoma has elevated levels of expression of cell cycle traverse-associated gene (c-Fos, c-Jun, and Cdc-2 protein) and down-regulation of non-proliferation-specific gene expression, such as statin. Consequently, they supported the concept that the transitional mucosa may represent a premalignant stage of tissue [55].

Table 5 summarizes the clinicopathlogical features of ordinary colorectal carcinomas with serrated lesions (hyperplastic polyps or serrated adenomas). In ordinary colorectal carcinomas, serrated lesions were observed in 37 (32.2%) of 115 submucosal early adenocarcinomas (Fig. 6) and 12 (24.5%) of 49 advanced adenocarcinomas. The serrated lesions are seen in the mucosa bordering the colorectal carcinoma and are histologically different from the transitional mucosa, which is thickened and composed of branched crypts lined by tall goblet cells [21]. Some ordinary colorectal carcinomas with serrated lesions had histological characteristics of complex pseudocribriform gland formation, sug-

gesting that they arose from hyperplastic polyps or serrated adenomas [17] (Fig. 6b). Among ordinary carcinomas the incidence of serrated lesions is higher in the flat-type traditional carcinomas (IIa, IIa + IIc, IIc + IIa) than in the polypoid-type ones (pedunculated, subpedunculated, sessile), and it is higher in the rectum and sigmoid colon than at other sites of the colon. The difference in these sites may be due to the incidence of hyperplastic polyps, most of which are located in the rectum and sigmoid colon. That the 37 (32.2%) and 12 (24.5%) serrated lesions were found in the mucosa immediately adjacent to early carcinoma and advanced carcinoma, respectively, histochemically and genetically suggests an early stage of carcinogenesis [51].

Histogenesis of Serrated Adenoma

Two hypotheses have been suggested to explain the histogenesis of serrated adenomas in the colorectum [8, 17, 20]. One hypothesis is that ser-

Table 5. Clinical and macroscopic features of early and advanced colorectal carcinomas with hyperplastic polyp or serrated adenoma

	Early (submucosal invasion)	Advanced
No.	37	12
Sex (M:F)	1.6:1	2:1
Age (years)	37–86 (mean 62.7)	55–76 (mean 59)
Location		
Cecum	0	0
Ascending colon	1 (2.7%)	0
Transverse colon	2 (5.4%)	1 (8.3%)
Descending colon	2 (5.4%)	0
Sigmoid colon	6 (16.2%)	2 (16.7%)
Rectum	26 (70.3%)	9 (75.0%)
Macroscopic classification		
Ip	4 (10.8%)	0
Isp	8 (21.6%)	0
Is	2 (5.4%)	0
IIa	9 (24.3%)	0
IIa + IIc	10 (27.0%)	0
IIc + IIa	1 (2.7%)	0
IIc	3 (8.1%)	0
II type	0	11 (91.7%)
III type	0	1 (8.3%)
Size (mm)	8–45 (mean 18.2)	22–80 (mean 43)

Ip, pedunculated; Ips, subpedunculated; Is, sessile; IIa, flat and elevated; IIc, depressed; II type, ulcerative and localized type; III type, ulcerative and infiltrative type.

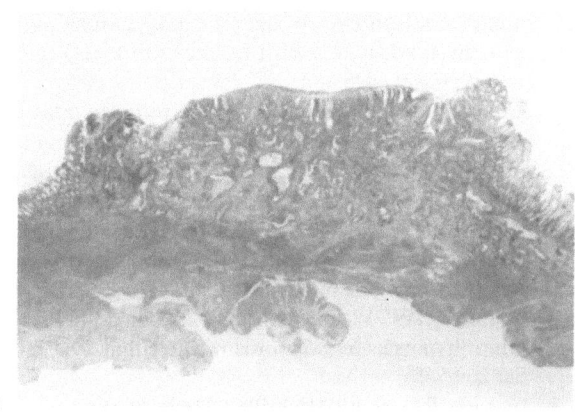

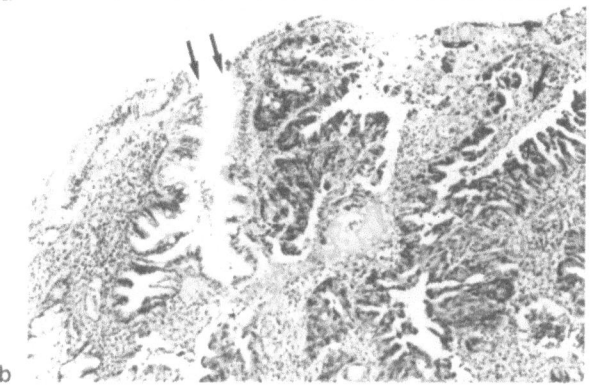

Fig. 6a,b. Traditional submucosal invasive carcinoma in the descending colon, 17 mm in diameter. **a** Flat carcinoma, macroscopically type IIa + IIc, massively invades the submucosa. (H&E, ×40) **b** Flat carcinoma surrounded by transitional mucosa of serrated adenomatous and hyperplastic epithelium with pseudocribriform formation (*single arrow*). Serrated adenomatous glands (*double arrows*) are composed of tumor cells with a pseudostratied elongated nucleus and immature goblet cells. (H&E, ×200)

rated adenomas arise from hyperplastic polyps [8, 20], and another is that they arise de novo, possibly owing to the neoplastic transformation of a more differentiated cell within the crypt than that which gives rise to the traditional adenoma, because a significant proportion of serrated adenomas are small (17.3% of serrated adenomas are less than 0.5 cm in diameter) [17].

Our study of the relations among hyperplastic nodules, hyperplastic polyps, and serrated adenomas reveals that some of the hyperplastic glands, which arise from some of the hyperplastic nodules or possibly directly from normal mucosa, may develop large polypoid-type serrated adenomas. In contrast, small superficial-type serrated adenomas may arise from small hyperplastic polyps or de novo without progression to a hyperplastic lesion.

The chronic inflammatory changes in the stroma of the hyperplastic polyp, which may be closely related to its histogenesis, is identified as often as the hyperplastic nodules. Chronic inflammation with lymphoid follicles drew attention, as human colonic adenomas and experimental rat carcinomas often developed in mucosal areas above lymphoid follicles [56, 57]. The following explanations have been proposed for the increased occurrence of tumors above colonic lymphoid follicles: (1) the more rapid turnover of epithelial cells may be responsible for the increased susceptibility to carcinogens inducing cancer above lymphoid follicles; (2) protrusion into the enteral lumen may cause nonspecific mucosal damage; (3) carcinogens or co-carcinogens may undergo increasing concentration here; and (4) immunologic control (surveillance) may be altered in the immediate perilymphatic surroundings [58]. These explanations suggest that the hyperplastic glands, from which colorectal serrated adenomas or carcinomas may develop, are particularly susceptible to carcinogenic or co-carcinogenic substances, such as bile or bile acids [59], and that they then support the histogenetically hyperplastic polyp–serrated adenoma–carcinoma sequence.

Hyperplastic polyps, which have been termed metaplastic polyps [39] and have been empirically noted to be histologically similar to intestinal metaplastic foveolar epithelium of the stomach, have been found to contain neutral/*MUC1* gene-related mucin. The latter is closely associated with the trefoil-peptide pS2, a major component of the ulcer-associated cell lineage (UACL) [60], which is expressed within the foveolar epithelium in the gastric antrum but not at as high a level as in normal small or large bowel. In additional, the pS2 peptide, epidermal growth factor/urogastrone (EGF/URO), EGF receptor, and *MUC1* gene immunoreactivity has been shown to be present throughout the hyperplastic polyps [61]. Hanby et al. suggested that hyperplastic polyps represent inappropriately activated UACL, switched on in the absence of ulceration, and that in this inappropriate, nonreparative setting EGF/URO-induced expansion of the proliferative compartment might lead to the mature and serrated appearances seen in hyperplastic polyps [61].

Finally, aberrant crypt foci (ACF), which were first identified in methylene blue-stained colonic mucosa from carcinogen-treated rodents, are now of interest in the carcinogenesis of human colorectal carcinoma [62, 63]. Otori et al. reported that their main histological finding was hyperplasia of glandular epithelium in human ACF and the high incidence of K-*ras* mutation in these ACF was a unique feature [64]. Histologically hyperplastic nodules, hyperplastic polyps, and serrated adenomas as described above may be partially included in the ACF lesions, which have been examined under a stereomicroscope after staining with methylene blue. The relations among ACF, hyperplastic lesions, serrated adenomas, and ordinary adenomas should be investigated in detail to further our knowledge of colorectal carcinogenesis.

Conclusion

One may hypothesize that serrated adenomas arise from hyperplastic nodules or hyperplastic polyps, which grow from polypoid-type or superficial-type adenomas, and are indicators of a high risk for colorectal carcinoma [1]. Some serrated adenomas show malignant transformation, similar to that seen in traditional adenomas, and may eventually develop into invasive, serrated colorectal adenocarcinomas. In particular, it should be clinically recognized that serrated adenocarcinomas arising from small superficial-type serrated adenomas have aggressive biological behavior and are difficult to detect endoscopically. They therefore may create considerable confusion during histological diagnosis [11, 17, 27]. Serrated adenomas should be regarded as a distinct form of colorectal neoplasia [17] and be correctly diagnosed, if necessary, using a marker of abnormal accumulation of P53 protein detected by immunohistochemistry. In the future, factors causing hyperplastic nodules or polyps should be thoroughly investigated to prevent ordinary carcinoma (or serrated adenocarcinoma) [48, 49].

References

1. Kearney J, Giovannucci E, Rimm EB, Stampfer MJ, Colditz GA, Ascherio A, Bleday R, Willett W (1995) Diet, alcohol, and smoking and the occurrence of hyperplastic polyps of the colon and rectum (United States). Cancer Causes Control 6:45–56
2. Cooper HS, Marshall C, Ruggerio F, Steplewski Z (1987) Hyperplastic polyps of the colon and rectum: an immunohistochemical study with monoclonal antibodies againt blood groups antigens (Sialosyl-Lea, Leb, Lex, Ley, A, B, H). Lab Invest 57:421–428
3. Gebbers JO, Laissue JA (1986) Mixed hyperplastic and neoplastic polyp of the colon: an immunohistological study. Virchows Arch [A] 410:189–194
4. Provenzale D, Martin ZZ, Holland KL, Sandler RS (1988) Colon adenomas in patient with hyperplastic polyps. J Clin Gastroenterol 10:46–49
5. Sumner HW, Wasserman NF, Mclain CJ (1981) Giant hyperplastic polyposis of the colon. Dig Dis Sci 26:85–89
6. Estrada RG, Spjut HJ (1980) Hyperplastic polyps of the large bowel. Am J Surg Pathol 4:127–133
7. Franzin G, Zamboni G, Scarpa A, Dina R, Iannucci A, Novelli P (1984) Hyperplastic (metaplastic) polyps of the colon: a histologic and histochemical study. Am J Surg Pathol 8:687–698
8. Goldman H, Ming S-C, Hickok DF (1970) Nature and significance of hyperplastic polyps of the human colon. Arch Pathol 89:349–354
9. Cooper HS, Patchefsky AS, Marks G (1979) Adenomatous and carcinomatous changes within hyperplastic colonic epithelium. Dis Colon Rectum 22:152–156
10. Franzin G, Novelli P (1982) Adenocarcinoma occurring in a hyperplastic (metaplastic) polyp of the colon. Endoscopy 14:28–30
11. Urbanski SJ, Marcon N, Kossakowska AE, Bruce WR (1984) Mixed hyperplastic adenomatous polyps—an underdiagnosed entity. Am J Surg Pathol 18:551–556
12. Morson BC, Dawson IMP, Day DW, Jass JR, Price AB, Williams GT (1990) Morson and Dawson's gastrointestinal pathology, 3rd edn. Blackwell, Oxford, pp 584–587
13. Arthur JF (1968) Structure and significance of metaplastic nodule in the rectal mucosa. J Clin Pathol 21:735–743
14. Wiebeck B, Brandts A, Eder M (1974) Epithelial proliferation and morphogenesis of hyperplastic adenomatous and villous polyps. Virchows Arch [A] 364:35–49
15. Kudo S (1993) Endoscopic mucosal resection of flat and depressed types of early colorectal cancer. Endoscopy 25:455–461
16. Muto T, Kamiya J, Sawada T, Konishi F, Sugihara K, Kubota Y, Adachi M, Agawa S, Saito Y, Morioka Y, Tanprayoon T (1985) Small "flat adenoma" of the large bowel with special reference to its clinicopathologic features. Dis Colon Rectum 28:847–846
17. Longacre TA, Fenoglio-Preiser CA (1990) Mixed hyperplastic adenomatous polyp/serrated adenoma: a distinct form of colorectal neoplasia. Am J Surg Pathol 14:524–537

18. Shimamoto F, Fujii M, Tanaka S, Haruma K, Tahara E (1994) Clinicopathological study of serrated adenomas in the colorectum. In: Proceedings of Japanese Cancer Association, 53rd Annual Meeting, p 542

19. Shimamoto F, Tanaka S, Haruma K, Tahara E (1995) Serrated epithelial lesion bordering traditional carcinoma of the colorectum. In: Transactiones societatis pathologicae japonicae, pp 84, 336

20. Rubio CA, Rodensjoe M (1995) Flat serrated adenomas and flat tubular adenomas of the colorectal mucosa: difference in the pattern of cell proliferation. Jpn J Cancer Res 86:756–760

21. Jass JR, Sobin LH (1989) Histological typing of intestinal tumours. In: WHO international histological classification of tumours. Springer, Berlin Heidelberg New York London Paris Tokyo Hong Kong, pp 29–40

22. Rubio CA, Rodensjoe M (1995) P53 overexpression in flat serrated adenomas and flat tubular adenomas of the colorectal mucosa. J Cancer Res Clin Oncol 121:571–576

23. Shimamoto F, Tanaka S, Hiraga Y, Hiyama T, Tahara E (1996) Cell proliferation in polypoid type and superficial type serrated adenomas of the colorectum. In: Recent advances in gastroenterological carcinogenesis, vol 1. Monduzzi Editore, Bologna, pp 773–778

24. Shimamoto F, Inai K, Kawamoto Y, Sasaki T, Ikeda T, Nishida T, Tanaka S, Hiraga Y, Tahara E (1995) A case of superficial minute submucosal carcinoma arising in colonic hyperplastic lesion (in Japanese). J Hiroshima Med Assoc 48:505–506

25. Wolber RA, Owen DA (1991) Flat adenomas of the colon. Hum Pathol 22:70–74

26. Teixeira CR, Tanaka S, Haruma K, Yoshihara M, Sumii K, Kajiyama G, Shimamoto F (1996) Flat-elevated colorectal neoplasms exhibit a high malignant potential. Oncology 53:89–93

27. Kasumi A, Kratzer GL, Takeda M (1995) Observation of aggressive, small, flat, and depressed colon cancer. Surg Endosc 9:690–694

28. Shimamoto F, Tanaka S, Hiraga Y, Haruma K, Tahara E (1995) Clinicopathological study of early colorectal carcinoma originating from minute superficial serrated adenomas. In: Proceedings of Japanese Cancer Association, 54th Annual Meeting, p 520

29. Shimamoto F, Tanaka S, Hiraga Y, Hiyama T, Tahara E (1996) Clinical significance of serrated adenomas in the colorectum. In: Proceedings of the Japanese Research Society for Cancer of the Colon and Rectum, 44th Meeting, p 31

30. Vogelstein B, Fearon ER, Hamilton SR, Kern SE, Preisinger AC, Leppert M, Nakamura Y, White R, Smits AMM, Bos JL (1988) Genetic alterations during colorectal-tumor development. N Engl J Med 319:525–532

31. Vogelstein B, Kinzler KW (1992) p53 Function and dysfunction. Cell 70:523–526

32. Greenblatt MS, Bennett WP, Hollstein M, Harris CC (1994) Mutations in the p53 tumor suppressor gene: clue to cancer etiology and molecular pathogenesis. Cancer Res 54:4855–4878

33. Ohue M, Tomita N, Monden T, Fujita M, Fukunaga M, Takami K, Yana I, Ohnishi T, Enomoto T, Inoue M, Shimano T, Mori T (1994) A frequent alteration of p53 gene in carcinoma in adenoma of colon. Cancer Res 54:4798–4804

34. Yukawa M, Fujimori T, Maeda S, Tabuchi M, Nagasako K (1994) Comparative clinicopathological and immunohistochemical study of ras and p53 in flat and polypoid type colorectal tumors. Gut 35:1258–1261

35. Yamamura-idei Y, Satonaka K, Fujimori T, Maeda S, Chiba T (1994) p53 Mutations in flat- and polypoid-type colorectal tumors detected by temperature-gradient gel electrophoresis. Dig Dis Sci 39:2043–2048

36. Hiyama T, Yokozaki H, Shimamoto F, Yasui W, Kajiyama G, Tahara E (1996) Frequent p53 gene mutations in serrated adenomas of the colorectum. In: The first international conference on gastroenterological carcinogenesis, Hiroshima, p 189

37. Schmieden V, Westhues H (1927) Zur klinik und pathologie der Dickdarmpolypen und deren klinischen und pathologisch-anatomischen Beziehungen zum Dickdarmkarzinom. Dtsch Z Chir 202:1–124

38. Morson BC (1962) Some peculiarities in the histology of intestinal polyps. Dis Colon Rectum 5:337–344

39. Stemmermann GN, Yanani R (1973) Diverticulosis and polyps of the large intestine: a necropsy study of Hawaii Japanese. Cancer 31:1260–1270

40. Eide TJ (1986) Prevalence and morphological features of adenomas of the large intestine in individuals with and without colorectal carcinoma. Histopathology 10:111–118

41. Lane N, Kaplan H, Pascal RR (1971) Minute adenomatous and hyperplastic polyps of the colon: divergent patterns of epithelial growth with special associated mesenchymal changes; contrasting roles in the pathogenesis of carcinoma. Gastroenterology 60:537–551

42. Shimamoto F, Tanaka S, Hiraga Y, Hiyama T, Nishida T, Tahara E (1996) Clinicopathological study of hyperplastic nodules and hyperplastic polyps in the colorectum. In: Transactiones societatis pathologicae japonicae, pp 85, 301

43. Williams GT, Arthur JF, Bussey HJR, Morson BC (1980) Metaplastic polyps and polyposis of the colorectum. Histopathology 4:155–170

44. Whittle TS, Varner W, Brown FM (1978) Giant hyperplastic polyps of the colon. Am J Surg Pathol 9:105–110

45. Sobin LH (1985) Inverted hyperplastic polyps of the colon. Am J Surg Pathol 9:265

46. Oohara T, Ogino A, Tohma H (1980) Histogenesis of microscopic adenoma and hyperplastic (metaplastic) gland in nonpolyposis coli. Dis Colon Rectum 24:375–384

47. Araki K, Ogata T, Kobayashi M, Yatani R (1995) A morphological study on the histogenesis of human of colorectal hyperplastic polyps. Gastroenterology 109:1468–1474

48. Jass JR (1983) Relation between metaplastic polyp and carcinoma of the colorectum. Lancet 1:28–30

49. Jass JR, Filipe MI, Abbas S, Falcon CAJ, Wilson Y, Lovell D (1984) A morphologic and histochemical study of metaplastic polyps of the colorectum. Cancer 53:510–515

50. Filipe MI (1969) Value of histochemical reactions for mucosubstances in the diagnosis of certain pathological conditions of the colon and rectum. Gut 10:577–586

51. Filipe MI, Branfoot AC (1974) Abnormal patterns of mucus secretion in apparently normal mucosa of large intestine with carcinoma. Cancer 34:282–290

52. Riddel RH, Levin B (1977) Ultrastructure of "transitional" mucosa adjacent to large bowel carcinoma. Cancer 40:2509–2522

53. Bibbo M, Michelassi F, Bartels PH, Dytch H, Bania C, Lerma E, Montag AG (1990) Karyometric marker features in normal appearing glands adjacent to human colonic adenocarcinoma. Cancer Res 50:147–151

54. Isaacson P, Attwood PRA (1979) Failure to demonstrate specificity of the morphological and histochemical changes in mucosa adjacent to colonic carcinoma (transitional mucosa). J Clin Pathol 32:214–218

55. Pandey S, Gordon PH, Wang E (1995) Expression of proliferative-specific genes in the mucosa adjacent to colon carcinoma. Dis Colon Rectum 38:462–467

56. Oohara T, Ogino A, Tohma H (1981) Microscopic adenoma in nonpolyposis coli: incidence and relation to basal cells and lymphoid follicles. Dis Colon Rectum 24:120–126

57. Shimamoto F, Vollmer E (1987) Change of intestinal mucosa above lymph follicles during carcinogenesis in rats. J Cancer Res Clin Oncol 113:41–50

58. Ross JS (1982) Experimental large intestinal adenocarcinoma induced by hydrazines, and human colorectal cancer: a comparative study. In: Malt RA, Williamson RCN (eds) Colonic carcinogenesis, Falk symposium. MTP Press, Lancaster, pp 31, 187–207

59. Narisawa T, Magadia NE, Weisburger JH, Wynder EL (1974) Promoting effect of bile acid on colon carcinogenesis after intrarectal instillation of MNNG in rats. J Natl Cancer Inst 53:1093–1098

60. Wright NA, Pike C, Elia G (1990) Induction of a novel epidermal growth factor secreting lineage by mucosal ulceration in human gastrointestinal stem cells. Nature 343:82–85

61. Hanby AM, Poulsonm R, Singh S, Jankowski J, Hopwood D, Elia G, Rogers L, Patel K, Wright NA (1993) Hyperplastic polyps: a cell lineage which both synthesizes and secretes trefoil-peptides and has phenotypic similarity with the ulcer-associated cell lineage. Am J Pathol 142:663–668

62. Roncucci L, Stamp D, Medline A, Cullen JB, Bruce R (1991) Identification and quantification of aberrant crypt foci and microadenomas in the human colon. Hum Pathol 22:287–294

63. Pretlow TP, Barrow BJ, Ashton S, O'Riordan A, Pretlow TG, Jurcisek JA, Stellato TA (1991) Aberrant crypts: putative preneoplastic foci in human colonic mucosa. Cancer Res 51:1564–1567

64. Otori K, Sugiyama K, Hasebe T, Fukushima S, Esumi H (1995) Emergence of adenomatous aberrant crypt foci (ACF) from hyperplastic ACF with concomitant increase in cell proliferation. Cancer Res 55:4743–4746

Carcinoma Cells at Deeply Infiltrated Sites: Role in Development of Metastases in Patients with Advanced Colorectal Adenocarcinomas

Kiyomi Taniyama[1], Naomi Sasaki[1], Hiroshi Maruyama[2], Hayao Nakai[2], Hirofumi Nakatsuka[3], Kazushige Toyama[4], and Eiichi Tahara[5]

Summary. Carcinoma cells that infiltrate beyond the muscularis propria ("ss" lesions) have a significant role in developing metastases in patients with advanced colorectal carcinoma. Examination of 363 resected colon carcinomas revealed a high frequency of metastasis when carcinoma cells invaded beyond the muscularis propria. The metastases found in 170 patients with advanced colorectal adenocarcinomas invading this tissue were divided into five groups according to the histology of the ss lesions and the overall predominant histology. Lymph node metastasis was significantly increased as the histologic grade of the ss lesion decreased. Poorly differentiated adenocarcinoma cells were rapidly infiltrative regardless of the proliferative state and were associated with peritoneal dissemination, distant metastasis, or local recurrence. In contrast, moderately differentiated adenocarcinoma cells were more proliferative with reduced expression of E-cadherin compared to well differentiated adenocarcinoma; they were closely associated with liver metastasis and overexpression of p53. In the DNA ploidy study, there was a relation between decreased histologic differentiation and an increased likelihood of changes of the DNA ploidy pattern. Overexpression of $\alpha2\beta1$- and $\alpha4\beta1$-integrins of carcinoma cells preceded disruption of the cadherin system, which was associated with the morphologic change, and were correlated with the high metastatic properties of the carcinoma cells. Tumor classification based on histology in the ss is a good indicator of metastasis or prognosis of advanced colorectal adenocarcinomas. Further study based on these findings will facilitate understanding of the metastasis.

Introduction

Modern molecular techniques have provided details on the development, invasion, and metastases of cancer. Gastrointestinal cancers involve genetic alterations in multiple oncogenes, multiple tumor suppressor genes, and multiple DNA repair genes. Alterations of these genes with malignancy include deletions, amplifications, and single-nucleotide mutations [1]. Several oncogenes function synergistically in the pathogenesis of colorectal cancer, and the same abnormalities are found with metastatic tumors [2]. Colorectal cancer remains one of the leading causes of neoplastic morbidity and mortality worldwide [3]. In Japan age-adjusted death rates for colorectal cancer per 100000 population were 22.0 for males and 13.9 for females in 1990. Mortality rates were 10.2% (males) and 12.9% (females) of deaths resulting from all malignancies. Moreover, the incidence of colorectal cancer is increasing [4].

About 30% to 50% of patients undergoing presumably curative resection have a recurrence within the first 2 years after surgery, with widespread metastases, particularly hepatic, in 45% of those patients; one-third develop local recurrence, which is particularly common after abdominoperineal resection [2]. One of the most im-

[1] Department of Clinical Pathology, Kure Kyosai Hospital, 2-3-28 Nishichuo, Kure, Hiroshima 737, Japan
[2] Department of Surgery, Kure Kyosai Hospital, 2-3-28 Nishichuo, Kure, Hiroshima 737, Japan
[3] Department of Surgery, Kure City Medical Association Hospital, 15-24 Asahi-cho, Kure, Hiroshima 737, Japan
[4] Department of Surgery, Shizuoka General Hospital, 4-27-1 Kitaando, Shizuoka 420, Japan
[5] First Department of Pathology, Hiroshima University School of Medicine, 1-2-3 Kasumi, Minami-ku, Hiroshima 734, Japan

portant and reliable predictors of local recurrence is the stage of the tumor at the time of surgery [2]. Although the stage is the final determinant of prognosis [5], several stages for colorectal carcinoma have been proposed, causing considerable confusion [6–9].

The classification for lymph node metastasis is also confusing [6–8, 10], although the number of lymph nodes with metastasis at the time of surgery has a great influence on the prognosis for colorectal adenocarcinoma [5]. Histologic classification of the tumors has been undertaken by many pathologists, but histologic grading is subjective and interobserver agreement poor [11]. Moreover, the histologic criteria for colorectal adenocarcinomas by Japanese pathologists are different from those used by pathologists in Western countries. With the classification of the Japanese Society for Cancer of the Colon and Rectum and the Histological Typing of Intestinal Tumors by the World Health Organization (WHO), malignant epithelial tumors are classified as adenocarcinoma, mucinous adenocarcinoma, signet-ring cell carcinoma, squamous cell carcinoma, adenosquamous carcinoma, undifferentiated carcinoma, small-cell carcinoma (oat cell carcinoma), and others. Small-cell carcinoma is included in the WHO classification but not in the Japanese classification. In the Japanese classification, small-cell carcinoma is classified as either undifferentiated carcinoma or "other." This difference is not an important matter because small-cell carcinoma is a rare tumor in the colorectum. An important difference is found, however, in the classification of adenocarcinoma. In Japan colorectal tumors are classified according to their predominant histology [9]. In contrast, with the WHO classification, well- and moderately differentiated adenocarcinomas are grouped together as low grade, and poorly differentiated adenocarcinoma and undifferentiated carcinoma are grouped as high grade. When a tumor shows different grades of differentiation, the higher grade should determine the final categorization [12]. Although some suggest that the disorganized glands commonly observed at the advancing edge of the cancer should not be considered a high-grade malignancy [12], this typing system pays little attention to the amount or localization of the higher-grade malignancy within a tumor. The various classifications for lymph node metastasis or histologic grading of the tumors have decreased the significance of tumor histology on the development of metastases.

In the present study, we clarify that carcinoma cells infiltrating lesions beyond the muscularis propria have a significant role in developing metastasis in patients with colorectal adenocarcinoma. Only advanced colorectal adenocarcinomas invading beyond the muscularis propria were selected for comparing the significance of histology at the deeply infiltrating sites and the potential to develop metastases. We also report the results concerning the DNA ploidy, cell kinetics, immunoreactivities for adhesion molecules or p53 suppressor gene, and serum levels of carcinoembryonic antigen (CEA) and CA19-9 of the carcinomas. Other suppressor genes that may relate to the metastases are also discussed. The histologic classification described in this study serves as a useful indicator of metastasis as well as for the prognosis of patients with advanced colorectal adenocarcinoma at the time of surgery.

Relations Among Tumor Histology, Depth of Invasion, and Metastases of Colorectal Carcinomas

In Japan most colorectal carcinomas are reported to be well-differentiated adenocarcinoma [13]. Poorly differentiated adenocarcinomas are rare [14]. In Western countries, however, approximately 20% are reported to be well-differentiated, 60% moderately differentiated and 20% poorly differentiated adenocarcinomas [5].

Altogether 363 colorectal malignant tumors were examined to determine the frequency of the tumors classified according to their predominant histology. The tumors were resected endoscopically or surgically in Kure Kyosai Hospital from 1993 to 1995 (Table 1). They consisted of 258 (71.1%) well-differentiated adenocarcinomas, 83 (22.9%) moderately differentiated adenocarcinomas, 6 (1.7%) poorly differentiated adenocarcinomas, 9 (2.5%) mucinous carcinomas, 4 (1.1%) carcinoids, 1 (0.3%) endocrine cell carcinoma, and 2 (0.6%) malignant lymphomas. The tumors were also classified according to their depth of invasion: 134 tumors were localized in the mucosa, 45 tumors invaded the submucosa, 19 tumors invaded the muscularis propria, and 165 tumors invaded beyond the muscularis propria. Of the 134 tumors localized to the mucosa, 132 (98.5%) were well-differentiated adenocarcinoma; the frequency of well-differenti-

Table 1. Depth of invasion and histology of 363 resected colorectal malignancies

Depth of invasion	Tumors (no.)	Adenocarcinoma, by differentiation (no.)			Mucinous (no.)	Carcinoid (no.)	ECC (no.)	ML (no.)
		Well	Moderately	Poorly				
M	134	132 (98.5%)	2 (1.5%)	0	0	0	0	0
SM	45	40 (88.9%)	1 (2.2%)	0	0	4 (8.9%)	0	0
PM	19	11 (57.9%)	8 (42.1%)	0	0	0	0	0
>PM	165	75 (45.5%)	72 (43.6%)	6 (3.6%)	9 (5.5%)	0	1 (0.6%)	2 (1.2%)
Total	363	258 (71.1%)	83 (22.9%)	6 (1.7%)	9 (2.5%)	4 (1.1%)	1 (0.3%)	2 (0.6%)

M, mucosa; SM, submucosa; PM, muscularis propria; >PM, beyond the muscularis propria; ECC, endocrine cell carcinoma; ML, malignant lymphoma.

ated adenocarcinoma decreased as the tumors invaded more deeply. In contrast, moderately differentiated adenocarcinoma was found in only 2 (1.5%) of the 134 tumors but increased in frequency as the tumors invaded more deeply. A total of 8 (42.1%) of 19 tumors that invaded the muscularis propria and 72 (43.6%) of 165 tumors that invaded beyond the muscularis propria were moderately differentiated adenocarcinoma. The latter frequency is almost equal to that of well-differentiated adenocarcinoma that invaded beyond the muscularis propria. Therefore almost all adenocarcinomas were considered well differentiated, and the predominant histology changed gradually as the tumors invaded more deeply. About half of the tumors were classified as moderately differentiated adenocarcinomas when they reached the level of the muscularis propria or invaded beyond.

Six poorly differentiated adenocarcinomas were observed to be invading beyond the muscularis propria. It has been reported that poorly differentiated cancers are, in any event, unlikely to present as an early growth [5]. In a previous study, 11 poorly differentiated adenocarcinomas of the colorectum were found to be invading beyond the muscularis propria. Four of the adenocarcinomas had minor foci of well- or moderately differentiated adenocarcinoma in the upper half of the tumors [14]. Therefore these poorly differentiated adenocarcinomas were considered to have changed their predominant histology from well or moderately-differentiated adenocarcinoma in the upper half (probably in the submucosa) of the colorectal wall.

Cancer metastasis is a critical point for treating patients with colorectal carcinoma. Almost one-third of the colon adenocarcinomas were reported to be localized at the time of diagnosis, with 20%

having distant metastases [15]. The risk of lymph node metastasis has been reported to be approximately 12% when the tumors extend into the muscularis propria and increases to 60% with spread beyond the muscularis propria into the pericolic or perirectal tissues [5]. To study the relation between the depth of invasion and metastases, 229 colorectal carcinomas surgically resected between 1993 and 1995 were analyzed (Table 2): We found that 1 (4.3%) of 23 tumors invading the submucosa, 4 (21.1%) of 19 tumors invading the muscularis propria, and 98 (60.1%) of the 163 tumors invading beyond the muscularis propria had metastases in lymph nodes, liver, peritoneum, or other organs at the time of surgery. The frequency of metastasis for the 163 tumors was significantly higher than that for other groups. These frequencies may be lower than the true frequencies of metastases found during the clinical course of the patients with these tumors or that found in all patients with the same tumors because the postoperative course of these patients was not considered; moreover, some inoperative cases were excluded from surgical treatment because of multiple metastases or complicating disease. These frequencies do suggest, however, that cancer metastasis requires a large number of carcinoma cells, and that carcinoma cells invading beyond the muscularis propria have a significant role in developing metastasis in patients with colorectal carcinoma.

The location of the tumors has been reported to have some significance for metastasis [16]. Rectal adenocarcinomas are reportedly associated with poorer survival than colon adenocarcinomas [15]. In the present study, carcinomas of the rectosigmoid were included with rectal tumors [8, 9]. Because metastases found in organs other than lymph nodes among the 163 patients with tumors

Table 2. Relation between depth of invasion and metastasis among 229 surgically resected colorectal carcinomas

Depth of invasion	Tumors (no.)	Tumors with metastasis (no.)				
		Lymph node	Liver	Peritoneum	Others	Total
M	24	0	0	0	0	0
SM	23	1 (4.3%)	0	0	0	1 (4.3%)*
PM	19	3 (15.8%)	1 (5.3%)	0	0	4 (21.1%)**
>PM	163	82 (50.3%)	8 (4.9%)	6 (3.7%)	2 (1.2%)	98 (60.1%)
Total	229	86 (37.6%)	9 (3.9%)	6 (2.6%)	2 (0.9%)	103 (45.0%)

See Table 1 for abbreviations.
$*P < 0.001$; $**P < 0.01$ versus >PM.

Table 3. Relation between predominant histology and metastasis among 163 advanced colorectal carcinomas

Predominant histology of tumor	Tumors (no.)	Tumors with metastasis (no.)				
		Lymph node	Liver	Peritoneum	Others	Total
Well	75	43 (57.3%)	4 (5.3%)	1 (1.3%)	1 (1.3%)	49 (65.3%)
Moderately	72	32 (44.4%)	4 (5.6%)	3 (4.2%)	1 (1.4%)	40 (55.6%)
Poorly	6	3 (50.0%)	0	0	0	3 (50.0%)
Mucinous	9	3 (33.3%)	0	2 (22.2%)	0	5 (55.6%)
ECC	1	1 (100%)	0	0	0	1 (100%)
Total	163	82 (50.3%)	8 (4.9%)	6 (3.7%)	2 (1.2%)	98 (60.1%)

Well, well-differentiated adenocarcinoma; Moderately, moderately differentiated adenocarcinoma; Poorly, poorly differentiated adenocarcinoma; Mucinous, mucinous adenocarcinoma; ECC, endocrine cell carcinoma.

invading beyond the muscularis propria were too small in number to examine, only the relation between the location of the tumors and lymph node metastasis found at the time of surgery was compared. The 82 tumors with lymph node metastasis were grouped according to their location: ascending colon, transverse colon, descending colon, sigmoid colon, and rectum; alternatively they were said to be in right half (including the ascending and transverse colon) or the left half (including the descending and sigmoid colon and rectum). There was no significant difference in the distribution between the tumors with lymph node metastasis and those without lymph node metastasis (data not shown).

Table 3 shows the relations between tumor histology and metastases found at the time of surgery in the 163 patients. Approximately 50% to 60% of patients with well-, moderately, or poorly differentiated adenocarcinomas and mucinous carcinomas had metastases elsewhere. There were no significant differences in the frequency of metastasis among these groups. In a previous study we also found no statistical difference in lymph node metastasis between the well-differentiated and the moderately differentiated adenocarcinomas of the colorectum, although the latter tended to have more widespread lymph node metastasis than the former [17]. Therefore classification of the tumors according to their predominant histology is considered to have little significance regarding the development of metastasis.

In Western countries, well- and moderately differentiated adenocarcinomas are grouped together as low-grade and poorly differentiated adenocarcinoma and undifferentiated carcinoma as high-grade [12]. Jass et al. reported that tumors were graded as either poorly differentiated or "other" [18]. These classifications are considered to be of practical importance concerning the prognosis, as the prognosis is known to be related to the absolute number of lymph nodes involved [19]; poorly differentiated tumors have been reported to be frequently associated with more than four lymph nodes being involved than other grades [20]. These classifications, however, do not consider other metastases.

Classification of Lymph Node Metastasis

In 1932 Dukes proposed a classification scheme for carcinoma of the rectum based on the depth of tumor penetration and the presence of regional node metastases as follows: A, tumor limited to the bowel wall; B, tumor extending into the perirectal adipose tissue; C, tumor with nodal metastasis, with no regard for tumor penetration [6]. Since the introduction of this classification scheme, there have been numerous efforts, particularly for patients with histologically positive nodes, to increase the predictive value of clinical pathologic staging [21]. In 1954 Astler and Coller introduced a modification of the Dukes scheme that consisted of subclassifying patients with histologically positive nodes on the basis of the depth of penetration of the primary tumor in the bowel wall. A C1 lesion referred to a tumor with positive nodes that had not penetrated the entire thickness of the bowel wall, whereas a C2 tumor manifested full-thickness penetration [7]. In 1958 Dukes and Bussey divided the C cases into C1, in which only the regional nodes contained metastases, and C2, in which there was more extensive lymphatic spread, including the nodes at the point of ligature of the blood vessels. In 1984 the Gastrointestinal Study Group subdivided patients with histologically involved nodes into those demonstrating one to four or more than four positive nodes. The two subsets were designated C1 and C2, respectively [10]. Needless to say, the classification of lymph node metastasis from colorectal carcinomas is confusing.

With the last TNM staging system (1992), nodal status was classified as follows: N0, no nodal metastasis; N1, one to three regional nodal metastases; N2, four or more regional nodal metastases; N3, nodal metastasis along the course of a named vascular trunk, metastasis to apical nodes, or both [8]. The Japanese Society for Cancer of the Colon and Rectum numbers and groups the lymph nodes according to their anatomical positions [9]. With this classification scheme, lymph node metastases confirmed by histologic examination were classified as follows: n0, negative lymph node metastasis; n1, metastasis in the pericolic or perirectal lymph nodes that are located mainly within 5 cm of the carcinoma along the colorectal wall; n2, metastasis in lymph nodes located 5 to 10 cm from the carcinoma along the colorectal wall or in the intermediate lymph nodes; n3, metastasis in lymph nodes located along the course of a named vascular trunk (almost the same as the N3 nodes in the TNM classification); and n4, metastasis in a more distant lymph node than n2 or in a more central lymph node than n3, without regard to the number of lymph nodes with metastasis. The n1 and n2

lymph nodes are the regional lymph nodes described in the TNM classification.

The degree of lymphatic invasion by carcinoma cells can be classified according to intensity as ly0, ly1, ly2, and ly3 [9]. We previously reported that the intensity values of ly2 and ly3 are found more frequently in moderately differentiated adenocarcinomas than in well differentiated adenocarcinomas [17]. Shirouzu et al. reported that the degree of lymphatic permeation is an important prognostic factor in patients with rectal carcinomas of stage IIIa of the TNM classification, with one to three nodes with metastasis. They differentiated lymphatic invasion from venous invasion or pseudolymphatic invasion due to tissue shrinkage by careful observation using hematoxylin-eosin and elastica van Gieson stains [22]. Therefore the degree of lymphatic permeation by carcinoma cells might be a useful tool for estimating lymphatic spread of carcinoma cells. This estimation, however, is subjective and not reliable because pseudolymphatic vessels are sometimes difficult to differentiate from true lymph vessels, even with careful observation using the hematoxylin-eosin and elastica van Gieson stains.

Lymph node metastasis is a result of carcinomatous lymphatic invasion. Classification of lymph node metastases theoretically reflects the likelihood that carcinoma cells will spread through the lymph vessels according to the anatomical course. Therefore in the present study lymph node metastases were grouped according to the classification of the Japanese Society for Cancer of the Colon and Rectum [9]. The degree of lymph node metastasis was estimated as being representative of carcinomatous lymphatic spread.

Histologic Grading at Deeply Infiltrated Sites

As mentioned previously, cancer cells that infiltrate beyond the muscularis propria have an important role in the development of metastasis in patients with advanced colorectal adenocarcinoma. We have already reported that low-grade differentiation of deeply infiltrating sites is significantly correlated with lymph node metastasis and that moderate differentiation is associated with hematogenous metastasis to the liver from advanced colorectal adenocarcinomas [16, 17]. These results were obtained with a small number of cases. In the present study, a large number of cases were examined to confirm these findings.

Lesions of adenocarcinoma invading beyond the muscularis propria of the colorectum were described as ss lesions and were classified as 1, 2, or 3 depending on the number of cancer cells. According to the histologic criteria described in previous studies [16, 17], adenocarcinoma cells in the ss lesions were subclassified based on the degree of their glandular differentiation, including

the following levels of differentiation: well, well to moderate, moderate, and poor. The well differentiated (Wel) type showed small or large acinar arrangements, with or without papillary structures (Fig. 1a). The well-to-moderately differentiated (W/M) type (Fig. 1b) was intermediate between the Wel and the moderately differentiated (Mod) types. The Mod type showed cribriform-like arrangements or fused glands (Fig. 1c). The Wel, W/M, and Mod types closely corresponded to the grade 1, 2, and 3 tumors, respectively, re-

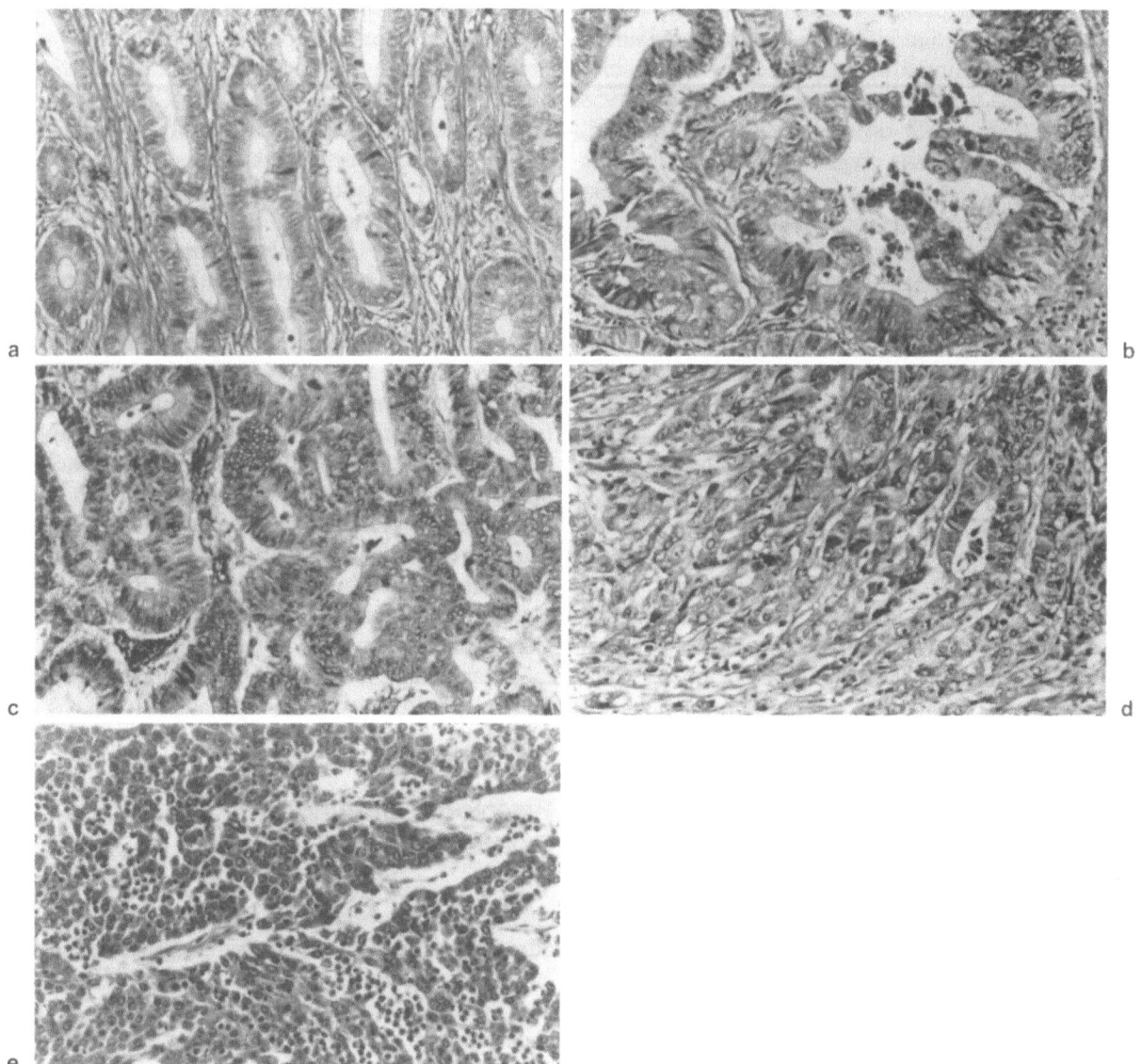

Fig. 1a–e. Histologic grading of adenocarcinoma. **a** Well-differentiated type showing acinar arrangements. **b** Well-to-moderately differentiated (W/M) type. **c** Moderately differentiated (Mod) type showing fused glands. **d** Poorly differentiated adenocarcinoma cells intermingled with Wel-type cells. **e** Predominantly poorly differentiated (poor) adenocarcinoma. (**a–e**: H&E, ×175)

ported by Dukes [23]. Poorly differentiated adenocarcinoma cells showed a trabecular arrangement or individual infiltration of cancer cells. When poorly differentiated adenocarcinoma cells intermingled with Wel-, W/M-, or Mod-type cells in the ss lesions of the predominantly well- or moderately differentiated adenocarcinomas, they were subclassified as Por subtype (Fig. 1d). Poorly differentiated adenocarcinoma cells in ss lesions were found exclusively with the predominantly poorly differentiated (poor) adenocarcinomas (Fig. 1e), which corresponded with Dukes' histologic grade 4.

In 1937 Dukes reported that the most common form of rectal carcinoma is adenocarcinoma grade 2, which accounts for approximately 50% of the tumors. Next in order of frequency were grade 3 (26%), colloid growths (12%), grade 1 (6%), and grade 4 (2%) [23]. Mucinous adenocarcinoma has been reported to be involved in 10% of colon carcinomas and approximately 6% of rectal carcinomas [15]. As mucinous or colloid colorectal carcinomas are biologically different from other adenocarcinomas [15], they were excluded from the present study.

Comparison of Tumor Grading at Deeply Infiltrated Sites and Metastases

To clarify the significance of histologic typing of tumors in relation to metastases, 170 colorectal adenocarcinomas were examined. All adenocarcinomas invaded beyond the muscularis propria and were surgically resected at the departments of surgery of the Shizuoka General Hospital, Kure City Medical Association Hospital, or Kure Kyosai Hospital between 1983 and 1994. Some of these cases were included in previously reported studies [14, 16, 17]. None of the patients received any treatment before surgery. Surgical specimens were fixed in formalin and examined microscopically by preparing tissue strips (5–10mm). The tumor tissue was embedded in paraffin wax for light microscopic examination. The adenocarcinomas consisted of 71 well differentiated, 86 moderately differentiated, and 13 poorly differentiated types. The 71 well differentiated adenocarcinomas were subclassified into 16 (22.5%) Wel, 42 (59.2%) W/M, 4 (5.6%) Mod, and 9 (12.7%) Por subtypes. The 86 moderately

differentiated adenocarcinomas were also subclassified into 12 (14.0%) W/M, 36 (41.9%) Mod, and 38 (44.2%) Por subtypes. Although the moderately differentiated adenocarcinomas were more likely than the well-differentiated adenocarcinomas to be subclassified as Por subtype, it was difficult to predict the histology of ss lesions from the predominant histology of the tumor.

Table 4 summarizes the clinicopathologic findings. Among the five groups there were no significant differences in the mean age of the patients. The male/female ratios of the Wel-subtype tumors and the poor tumors were 0.8 and 0.9, respectively, whereas those of the other three groups ranged form 1.4 to 2.2. Male predominance was not seen in the former two groups. The poor tumors tended to be found in the right half of the colorectum, although there were no significant differences in the colon/rectum ratio or the right/left ratio among the five groups. Mean tumor diameter of the Por-subtype tumors was 45.1mm—significantly smaller than those of the other four groups. The mean size of the ss lesion, however, tended to increase as the degree of histologic differentiation of carcinoma cells in the ss lesion decreased in the well- or moderately differentiated adenocarcinomas. The mean size of the ss lesion of the Por-subtype tumors was 2.3 and was not significantly different from the mean size of the ss lesion (2.1) among the poor tumors, although the latter tumors had the largest diameter. From these results, the Por-subtype tumors were considered to be the most rapidly infiltrative into the deep tissue, forming small tumors; and the poor tumors were rapidly infiltrative in all directions, forming larger tumors. This difference may be due to the difference in the amount of poorly differentiated adenocarcinoma cells.

Por-subtype tumors were differentiated from W/M- and Mod-subtype tumors by the minor components of poorly differentiated adenocarcinoma cells, not by the predominant histology; and poorly differentiated adenocarcinoma cells related to the rapidly infiltrative growth of the Por-subtype tumors. Therefore they should be more rapidly infiltrating than well or moderately differentiated adenocarcinoma cells. This finding may relate to the tumor size or size of the ss lesion. Por-subtype tumors may have had poorly differentiated adenocarcinoma cells in the deep tissue, which formed a minor but deeply infiltrating component in the tumor. In contrast, the poor tumors

Table 4. Relation between tumor histology and clinicopathologic data for 170 patients with advanced colorectal adenocarcinoma

Predominant histology of tumor (differentiation) and subtype	Tumors (no.)	Patients		Tumor				Survival rate (%)
		Age (years)	M/F ratio	Diameter (mm)	ss	Colon/ rectum ratio	Right/ left ratio	
Well (Wel)	16	67.9	0.8	55.8*	1.8	3.0	0.5	91.7
Well or moderate								
W/M	54	66.1	2.2	54.5*	2.0	1.7	0.7	84.1
Mod	40	67.9	1.4	59.3**	2.2***	1.5	0.3	74.1[‡]·****
Por	47	66.3	1.8	45.1	2.3****	1.8	0.7	53.9[§]·***
Poor	13	63.4	0.9	64.6*	2.1	1.6	1.2	44.9[†,††]·****

Data for age, M/F (male/female) ratio, tumor diameter, and ss lesion of tumor are mean values.

Wel, well-differentiated type; W/M, well-to-moderately differentiated type; Mod, moderately differentiated type; Por, admixture of poorly differentiated adenocarcinoma cells with other type cells; ss, amount of cancer cells invading beyond the muscularis propria of the colorectum; Survival rate, cumulative survival rates 3 years after surgery.

* $P < 0.05$; ** $P < 0.01$ versus Por. *** $P < 0.01$; **** $P < 0.05$ versus Wel. [†]$P < 0.001$; [§]$P < 0.001$, [‡]$P < 0.05$ versus W/M. [††]$P < 0.05$ versus Mod.

Table 5. Relation of lymph node metastasis and clinicopathologic data for 169 patients with advanced colorectal adenocarcinoma

Grade of lymph node metastasis	Tumors (no.)	Lymph nodes with metastasis (no.)	Patients		Tumor		Right/left ratio
			Age (years)	M/F ratio	Size (mm)	ss (mm)	
n0	88	0	67.7***	1.9	57.1*****	2.0***	0.5
n1	34	1.8	66.9****	1.1	51.0	2.2	0.4
n2	33	5.1*	66.3****	0.9	49.2	2.2	0.5
n3,n4	14	6.6**	58.6	2.5	51.4	2.5	1.0

Data for lymph node number, patient age, tumor size, and ss lesion of tumor are mean values.

n0, no lymph node metastasis; n1, metastasis in the regional pericolic or perirectal node only; n2, metastasis in the intermediate lymph node; n3, metastasis in the main lymph node; n4, metastasis in a more distant lymph node than those in n3.

* $P < 0.001$; ** $P < 0.05$ versus n1. *** $P < 0.01$; **** $P < 0.05$ versus n3,n4; ***** $P < 0.05$ versus n2.

were considered to have had the poorly differentiated adenocarcinoma cells in the submucosa, where they formed large tumors.

Metastases at the time of or after surgery were compared among the five groups. Of the 170 patients, 19 died of carcinoma and 5 were excluded from the follow-up study because of non-cancer-related death within 1 year after surgery. Other patients were followed more than 1 year (up to 10 years). As most recurrences of the colorectal adenocarcinomas are reported to be found within 2 years of surgery [24], the follow-up data in the present study should be sufficient. If different metastases are observed among the five groups, they could be attributable, at least in part, to the different histology or number of carcinoma cells in the ss lesion.

Lymph Node Metastasis

Table 5 shows lymph node metastases found at the time of surgery. In 1 of 54 patients with W/M-subtype tumors, lymph node resection was not performed because of the presence of multiple liver metastases. Therefore lymph node metastasis was compared among 169 patients.

Lymph node metastasis was found in 81 (47.9%) of 169 patients. Of the 81 patients, 34 had n1, 33 n2, and 14 n3 or n4 lymph node metastasis. The mean numbers of lymph nodes with metastasis found were 1.8 in n1, 5.1 in n2, and 6.6 in n3 or n4. There was a statistically significant difference between n1 and n2, n3, or n4 in the number of lymph nodes with metastasis. The patient's age with n3 or n4 was younger than that with n0, n1, or n2. The mean diameters of the tumors were

Table 6. Relation between tumor histology and lymph node metastasis among 169 advanced colorectal adenocarcinomas

Predominant histology of tumor and subtype	Tumors (no.)	Tumors with lymph node metastasis at the time of surgery (no.)		
		n1 or more*	n2*	n3 or n4
Well (Wel)	16	3 (18.8%)	1 (5.6%)	0
Well or moderate				
W/M	53	19 (35.8%)	5 (9.4%)	1 (1.9%)
Mod	40	17 (42.5%)	8 (20.0%)	0
Por	47	32 (68.1%)	13 (27.7%)	9 (19.1%)
Poor	13	10 (76.9%)	6 (46.2%)	4 (30.8%)

See Table 4 for abbreviations.
*$P < 0.01$.

57.1 mm for n0, 51.0 mm for n1, 49.2 mm for n2, and 51.4 mm for n3 or n4. In contrast, the mean sizes of the ss lesions in these tumors were 2.0 (n0), 2.2 (n1), 2.2 (n2) and 2.5 (n3 or n4). There was a significant difference in the tumor diameter between n0 and n2 and in the size of the ss lesion between n0 and n3 or n4. These results indicate that lymph node metastases are likely to be found in tumors with a small diameter but large ss lesion. Therefore adenocarcinoma cells infiltrating rapidly into the deep tissue have a high probability for developing lymph node metastasis. Although tumors with n3 or n4 metastasis tended to be found in the right half of the colorectum, the development of lymph node metastasis did not depend on the location of the tumor.

Table 6 shows the relation between the histologic grade of the tumors in the ss lesion and the degree of lymph node metastasis. The frequency of n1 or more or n2 was significantly increased as the histologic differentiation of the tumors decreased ($P < 0.01$). In particular, 13 of 14 tumors with n3 or n4 metastasis were either Por-subtype tumors or poor tumors. These results indicate that adenocarcinoma cells with different histologic differentiation in the ss lesion have different potentials for lymph node metastasis, and that poor differentiation, primarily loss of tubular differentiation, may have a critical role in forming lymph node metastases. This finding is consistent with the finding that rapidly infiltrating adenocarcinoma cells in the deep tissue have a high probability of developing lymph node metastases, as described above.

Chung et al. examined 246 patients with colorectal adenocarcinoma and reported that, irrespective of the size of the primary tumor, site of the tumor, or depth of invasion, patients with grade 3 lesions (poorly differentiated adenocarcinoma) had an increased likelihood of nodal metastasis compared to those with grade 1 lesions (well differentiated adenocarcinoma) or grade 2 lesions (moderately differentiated adenocarcinoma) [24]. According to their histologic criteria for tumors, both the Por-subtype tumor and the poor tumor in the present study might belong to the grade 3 tumor group. Chung et al. also found distant metastases during a follow-up study of 34 patients. Of these 34 patients, 15 had metastasis in the liver, 6 in the lung, 5 in the bone, 4 in the supraclavicular area, 3 in the brain, and 1 in the spinal cord. They reported that patients with grade 3 lesions had more local recurrences, distant metastasis, or both than those with grade 1 or 2 lesions. They did not find any difference for grade 3 tumors, however, between patients with liver metastasis and those with other metastases.

Liver Metastasis

Liver metastases are reportedly found in as many as one-fifth to one-fourth of patients operated on for colorectal carcinoma and are an important contributory cause of death [25]. Kelvin and Maglinte reported that with approximately 45% of colorectal adenocarcinoma distant metastases were found predominantly in the liver [26]. In the present study, liver metastasis was found in 22 patients (12.9%) at the time of surgery and in another 22 patients after surgery, accounting for approximately one-fourth of the 170 patients examined. Their clinicopathologic findings are sum-

Table 7. Relation between liver metastasis and clinicopathologic data for 170 patients with advanced colorectal adenocarcinoma

Liver metastasis		Tumors (no.)	Patients		Tumors			
At surgery	After surgery		Age (years)	M/F ratio	Size (mm)	ss	Colon/rectum ratio	Right/left ratio
Positive		22	62.5	1.4	51.7	2.6	2.1	0.5
Negative	Positive	22	66.5	2.7	50.5	2.3	1.4	0.3
Negative	Negative	126	67.3*	1.4	54.9	2.0**	1.7	0.4

M/F, male/female.

Data for patient age, tumor size, and ss lesion of tumor are mean values.

* $P < 0.05$ versus positive. ** $P < 0.05$ versus positive.

Table 8. Relation between tumor histology and several metastases for 170 patients with advanced colorectal adenocarcinoma

Predominant histology of tumor and subtype	Tumors (no.)	Tumors with metastasis (no.)						Local rec
		Liver		Peritoneum		Others		
		At	All	At	All*	At	All	
Well (Wel)	16	1 (6.3%)	1 (6.3%)	0	1 (6.3%)	0	0	0
Well or moderate								
W/M	54	5 (9.3%)	13 (24.1%)	2 (3.7%)	4 (7.4%)	1 (1.9%)	4 (7.4%)	3 (5.6%)
Mod	40	9 (22.5%)	14 (35.0%)	4 (10.0%)	4 (10.0%)	0	2 (5.0%)	1 (2.5%)
Por	47	6 (12.8%)	17 (36.2%)	6 (12.8%)	10 (21.3%)	2 (4.3%)	7 (14.9%)	6 (12.8%)
Poor	13	1 (7.7%)	1 (7.7%)	3 (23.1%)	3 (23.1%)	1 (7.7%)	3 (23.1%)	2 (15.4%)

At, at the time of surgery; All, all metastases found during the clinical course; Local rec, retroperitoneal recurrence after surgery. See Table 4 for other abbreviations.

* $P < 0.05$.

marized in Table 7. The mean age of patients with liver metastasis at the time of surgery was 62.5 years, which was approximately 5 years younger than that of patients having no liver metastasis during the clinical course ($P < 0.05$). The mean size of the ss lesion in the tumors with liver metastasis at the time of surgery was significantly greater than that of tumors without liver metastasis during the clinical course. Moreover, the mean size of the ss lesion in the former tumors tended to be larger than that of tumors having liver metastasis after surgery, although this difference was not statistically significant. Therefore liver metastasis tended to be found in younger patients and with tumors having larger ss lesions.

There was no significant difference in the male/female ratio of the patients, tumor diameter, colon/rectum ratio, or right/left ratio of the tumors for patients with or without liver metastasis. In a postmortem study, Schulz et al. examined 26 livers containing metastases from colon carcinoma and reported an approximately homogeneous distri-bution of metastases from colon carcinoma in the hepatic parenchyma, irrespective of the location of the primary tumor [27]. Although the highest frequency of blood-borne metastasis was found in the middle third of the rectum for rectal carcinomas [28], the rectum was not divided into smaller portions in the present study.

Table 8 shows the relations between the histologic grades of the tumors and liver metastasis. At the time of surgery, 1 (6.3%) of 16 Wel-, 5 (9.3%) of 54 W/M-, 9 (22.5%) of 40 Mod-, 6 (12.8%) of 47 Por-subtype tumors, and 1 (7.7%) of 13 poor tumors had liver metastasis. These frequencies were different from those observed for lymph node metastasis. After surgery, 8 W/M-, 5 Mod-, and 11 Por-subtype tumors were also found to have liver metastasis. No additional liver metastasis was found in any of the Wel-subtype tumors or the poor tumors. Overall frequencies of liver metastasis among these five groups were 6.3%, 24.1%, 35.0%, 36.2% and 7.7%, respectively. From the findings that greater ss lesion size is significantly correlated to liver metastasis, the smaller ss lesion size of the Wel-subtype tumors might correlate to the lower frequency of liver metastasis than in W/M-, Mod-, or Por-subtype tumors. The ss lesion size of poor tumors, however, was not different from that of the W/M-, Mod-, or Por-subtype tumors. Por-subtype tumors frequently presented with liver metastasis as well as lymph node metastasis. Differences in liver metastasis between the Por-subtype tumors and the poor tumors might be partially attributable to the difference in the predominant histology of these tumors. Therefore moderate differentiation of carcinoma cells may be associated with liver metastasis.

Peritoneal Dissemination, Metastases to Other Organs, and Local Recurrence in the Retroperitoneum

Peritoneal dissemination can occur when carcinoma cells are exposed to the peritoneal surface at either the primary or the metastatic site. Therefore organs covered by the peritoneum are the sites in which peritoneal dissemination occurs.

Twenty-one tumors were found to be associated with peritoneal dissemination. Of these 21 tumors, 15 were found at the time of surgery and 6 were found after surgery. The mean size of the ss lesion of these tumors was 2.6, and 18 were found in colon tumors. Thirteen were associated with liver metastasis, and six of eight tumors without liver metastasis were associated with lymph node metastasis of n2 or more. Therefore peritoneal dissemination of carcinoma cells was likely to be found with colon tumors that had large ss lesions and liver or widespread lymph node metastasis (data not shown). According to the histologic grade of the tumors with ss lesions less differentiated tumors were associated with a higher frequency of peritoneal dissemination ($P < 0.05$) (Table 8).

Distant metatases were found in other organs in 16 patients: lung (10), brain (3), spleen (1), skin (1), and bone (1). Of these 16 patients, 9 had liver metastasis. Six of the other seven patients had lymph node metastasis of n2 or more (data not shown). The distant metastases tended to be found in the patients with Por-subtype tumors or poor tumors (Table 8).

Local recurrence in the retroperitoneum was found in 12 patients. The mean diameter of the tumors was 50.1mm and the mean size of the ss lesions of their tumors 2.3. Ten had rectal tumors, and the other two had colon tumors 80 and 75mm diameter, respectively. Therefore local recurrence is related to the rectal tumor or to a large tumor of the colon (data not shown). Moreover, 8 of the 12 tumors were either Por-subtype tumors or poor tumors (Table 8). These results indicate that, in addition to the location and size of the tumors, poorly differentiated adenocarcinoma cells may have a role in the development of peritoneal dissemination, distant metastases, and local recurrence.

Relations Between Lymph Node Metastasis and Other Metastases

Newland et al. reported that the survival of 910 patients with no known residual tumor and no lymph node metastasis after resection of colorectal carcinoma was equivalent to that of the general population with the exception of male patients with stage B tumors (tumors that invade beyond the muscularis propria with no lymph node metastasis). They reported that the reduced survival of the male patients with stage B tumors was largely due to clinical factors, such as postoperative complications, and suggested that the risk of occult metastasis is low for patients with no lymph node metastasis at the time of surgery [29]. In the present study, metastasis after surgery in patients without lymph node metastasis was found in 16 (18.2%) of 88 patients (Table 9). Therefore even for patients without lymph node metastasis at the time of surgery careful follow-up should be undertaken.

Table 9 shows the relations between the degree of lymph node metastasis and other metastases found during the clinical course of 169 patients. Patients with lymph node metastasis had more metastases than those with no lymph node metastasis. Peritoneal dissemination significantly correlated with the degree of lymph node metastasis. The highest frequency of liver metastasis, distant metastasis, or local recurrence in the retroperitoneum, however, was found in patients with n2 lymph node metastasis and not in those with n3 or n4 metastasis. Moreover, liver metastasis was found in 12 (13.6%) of 88 patients with no lymph node metastasis. As mentioned previously, distant metastasis tended to be found in patients

Table 9. Relation between lymph node metastasis and other metastases for 169 patients with advanced colorectal adenocarcinoma

Grade of lymph node metastasis	Patients (no.)	Patients with metastasis (no.)				
		Liver	Peritoneum	Others	Local	Total
n0	88	12 (13.6%)	7 (8.0%)	4 (4.5%)	3 (3.4%)	16 (18.2%)
n1	34	13 (38.2%)*	3 (8.8%)	2 (5.9%)	2 (5.9%)	16 (47.1%)**
n2	33	14 (42.4%)**	7 (21.2%)***	7 (21.2%)**	5 (15.2%)***	22 (66.7%)*
n3,n4	14	4 (28.6%)	4 (28.6%)***	2 (14.3%)	1 (7.1%)	9 (64.3%)*

*$P < 0.001$; **$P < 0.01$; ***$P < 0.05$ versus n0.

with liver or lymph node metastasis of n2 or more; and local recurrence relates to the rectal tumor or large tumor of the colon, although both were related to poorly differentiated adenocarcinoma cells. These results indicate that the mechanism of liver metastasis may be different from that of lymph node metastasis.

It is well known that cancer metastasis is not formed by chance according to the anatomic position of organs involved [30]. As indicated in the present study, moderately differentiated adenocarcinoma cells are closely associated with liver metastasis, and poorly differentiated adenocarcinoma cells are closely associated with other metastases or local recurrence. Analysis of the carcinoma cells in the ss lesion might elucidate the metastatic mechanisms.

Prognosis

Cumulative survival rates of 170 patients were calculated using the Kaplan-Meier method and were analyzed using the generalized Wilcoxon test. Differences were assumed significant when the P value was less than 0.05. Cumulative survival rates after 3 years were 91.7% in 16 patients with Wel-subtype tumors, 84.1% in 54 patients with W/M-subtype tumors, 74.1% in 40 patients with Mod-subtype tumors, 53.9% in 47 patients with Por-subtype tumors, and 44.9% in 13 patients with poor tumors (Table 4). As the 2-year survival rate is reported to be reliable for the purpose of comparing various treatment results [24] the 3-year survival rates are also reliable for comparing the biologic behavior of the tumors classified according to the histology of the ss lesion. These results indicate that the histologic grades of carcinoma cells in the ss lesion closely relate to the

prognosis of the patients, which reflects the different metastases.

In Japan W/M-subtype tumors are classified as well differentiated tumors and Por-subtype tumors as well- or moderately differentiated adenocarcinomas according to their predominant histology [9]. In contrast, in Western countries, W/M-subtype tumors may be classified as moderately differentiated tumors and Por-subtype tumors as poorly differentiated adenocarcinomas [5]. These differences in histologic classifications may have failed to provide important data on the metastasis or prognosis of advanced colorectal adenocarcinomas.

Factors Relating to Metastasis or Prognosis

DNA Ploidy

The DNA ploidy pattern is reported to be a useful prognostic factor for colorectal carcinomas [14, 31]. Intratumoral differences in DNA ploidy were reported in 7.4% of colorectal carcinomas [32] and in 71 colorectal carcinomas [14, 17]. All were adenocarcinomas invading beyond the muscularis propria and were classified histologically according to their predominant histology. Altogether 24 were well differentiated, 36 moderately differentiated, and 11 poorly differentiated. A total of 12 (50%) of the well-differentiated, 20 (55.6%) of the moderately differentiated, and 8 (72.7%) of the poorly differentiated tumors were associated with lymph node metastasis.

The DNA ploidy patterns were analyzed by flow cytometry (Coulter, EPICS-Profile or Elite, Hialeah, FL, USA) in paraffin-embedded tissue using the method of Hedley et al. [33] with some modification [14, 17]. The representative paraffin block of the primary tumor was divided horizontally into two portions, and the superficial and deep halves were defined as Sup and Deep, respectively. Aneuploid tumors were found in 14 (58.3%) of 24 well differentiated, 22 (61.1%) of 36 moderately differentiated, and 6 (54.5%) of 11 poorly differentiated adenocarcinomas. The DNA ploidy pattern of Deep differed from that of Sup in 2 (28.6%) of 14 aneuploid tumors of well differentiated, 11 (50.0%) of 22 aneuploid tumors of moderately differentiated, and 4 (66.7%) of 6 aneuploid tumors of poorly differentiated adenocarcinomas. The aneuploid stem line was more frequently found in the Deep than in the Sup in well or moderately differentiated adenocarcinomas; however, in poorly differentiated adenocarcinomas the aneuploid stem line was more frequently found in the Sup than in the Deep. These results may indicate a relation between decreased histologic differentiation and a greater liability in changing the DNA ploidy pattern of the tumor [17].

Scott et al. reported the DNA histograms of rectal carcinomas from 121 patients along with a detailed clinicopathologic assessment of the same tumors; they also reported the incidence of postresection tumor recurrence and patient survival over an extended period of 15 years. They found that DNA nondiploid rectal carcinomas had a statistically significant increase in the incidence of vascular invasion, tumor fibrosis, and high Dukes' stage and concluded that the most important independent prognostic variables for rectal carcinomas were DNA ploidy pattern and the operative assessment of tumor spread [31].

Goh et al. reported an independent contribution of DNA content to survival after an analysis of 203 cases of rectal cancer with a follow-up of at least 15 years. They reported that the contribution of DNA content was small [34]. Rowley et al. reported that the significant effect of ploidy was restricted to patients with Dukes' A and C tumors, representing 51 (28%) of the 179 patients with colorectal carcinoma, followed for up to 9 years. There was some doubt as to its clinical value as a prognostic indicator, and the authors reported that the Dukes' classification remains superior to the ploidy status for prognostication [35].

Cumulative survival rates of the 29 patients with diploid tumors and the 42 patients with aneuploid tumors were calculated in the present study as being 52.5% and 65.1%, respectively, 5 years after surgery. There was no statistical difference in cumulative survival rates between these two groups. This result may be attributable to the small number of patients examined or the short duration of the follow-up. On the other hand, we previously reported that the DNA ploidy pattern of a primary tumor is correlated with the degree of metastasis or prognosis in the poor tumors [14] but also that the histology of Deep should have a greater significance than DNA content on lymph node metastasis in well- or moderately differentiated adenocarcinomas of the colorectum [17]. Therefore heterogeneous histology in the deeply infiltrating sites of the 71 tumors may result in no significant differences in the cumulative survival rates between patients with diploid and aneuploid tumors in the present study. Practically, it is important to examine the DNA content of Deep to determine if there is aneuploidy in well- or moderately differentiated adenocarcinoma of the colorectum [17].

Cell Kinetics

Proliferative activity has been reported to be a more significant predictor of survival than the tumor DNA ploidy pattern [36]. Proliferative activity has been estimated by use of nonradioactive reagents, such as the monoclonal antibody to bromodeoxyuridine (BrdU), [17] proliferating cell nuclear antigen (PCNA) [37], and Ki-67 [38]. The number of argyrophilic nuclear organizer regions (AgNOR) has also been reported as a tool to assess the malignant potential of the tumor [39]. Previously, we compared the proliferative activities of different histologic areas in colorectal adenocarcinomas by means of PCNA and Ki-67 labeling and by AgNOR impregnation [16, 17]. Twenty-three colorectal adenocarcinomas for BrdU analysis and 28 colorectal adenocarcinomas for PCNA labeling and AgNOR impregnation were examined. Of the latter 28 tumors, 9 were also used for Ki-67 labeling. All of these adenocarcinomas had invaded beyond the muscularis propria.

For in vitro BrdU labeling, tumor tissues were obtained separately from the superficial peripheral and deeply invading central lesions of the tumors immediately after tumor excision. The tissues were treated according to the method of

Sasaki et al. [40] with some modification [17]. BrdU labeling indices (LIs) of superficial peripheral lesions of the well- and moderately differentiated adenocarcinomas were 15.2% and 15.6%, and those of deeply infiltrating lesions were 6.9% and 11.8%, respectively. After dividing the deeply infiltrating regions into well-, well-to-moderately, moderately, and moderately-to-poorly differentiated areas, their BrdU LIs were 5.5%, 12.1%, 11.0%, and 10.6%, respectively. These areas corresponded with the Wel, W/M, Mod, and Por subtypes in the present study. There was no significant difference in BrdU LIs among W/M-, Mod-, and Por-subtype tumor cells, although all three subtypes had higher BrdU LIs than did the Wel-subtype tumor cells.

The PCNA and Ki-67 LIs were reported to be larger than the BrdU LI in lung tumors [38]. The PCNA and Ki-67 LIs being higher than the BrdU LI might make it possible to distinguish between the proliferative activity of Mod areas in Mod-subtype tumors and Por areas in Por-subtype tumors. Hence the PCNA LI and Ki-67 LI for various histologic areas in the moderately differentiated adenocarcinomas of the colorectum were determined even when BrdU LI values were similar [17]. Such analysis revealed that the PCNA LI, Ki-67 LI, and AgNOR values determined for the poorly differentiated adenocarcinoma cells in the Por-subtype tumors were significantly lower than those of moderately differentiated adenocarcinoma cells in the Mod-subtype tumors. In cells from tumors classified as Por subtype, poor differentiation was associated with a decreased PCNA LI but an unchanged Ki-67 LI and AgNOR values [16]. Therefore adenocarcinoma cells with high proliferative activity may proliferate more rapidly in the tubular gland, resulting in formation of tubulopapillary or fused glands; and loss of glandular formation (i.e., poor differentiation) is possibly unrelated to the proliferative activity of adenocarcinoma cells.

The mechanisms for a decrease in the PCNA LI and unchanged BrdU LI, Ki-67 LI, or AgNOR value for poor differentiation is not clear. The BrdU LI reportedly corresponds with the S phase of the cell cycle [17]. Ki-67 antigen is present at all stages of the cell cycle except G0 [41]. The Ki-67 LI has been reported to correlate best with the BrdU LI when compared with the PCNA LI and DNA polymerase alpha LI [38]. PCNA is an auxiliary protein of DNA polymerase delta and is expressed in normal and neoplastic cells during the proliferation cycle, particularly during the late G1 and S phases of the cell cycle [42]. PCNA LI does not necessarily express the reproduction rate, however (unpublished work). The decreased PCNA LI may reflect a shorter late G1 phase of the poorly differentiated adenocarcinoma cells [16].

Cadherin and Integrin

It is reported that varying genetic abnormalities of cell adhesion molecules may participate in the processes of invasion and metastasis of carcinoma cells [43]. For formation of a metastatic nodule, carcinoma cells must leave the primary tumors, invade the surrounding host tissue, enter the circulation, lodge in the distant vascular bed, extravasate into the target organ, and proliferate, resulting in formation of a metastatic nodule [44]. The most crucial step is the dissociation of carcinoma cells from the tumor [43].

Cadherins are reported to be a family of cell adhesion receptors crucial for the mutual association of vertebrate cells. The regulated expression of cadherins also controls cell polarity and tissue morphology [45]. Basal lamina formation is not necessary for glandular structure formation in colon cancer cells [46]. In humans the gene for epithelial (E)-cadherin is located on chromosome 16q22.1 [47, 48]. Its expression is reportedly strong in well-differentiated carcinomas, whereas it is generally reduced in undifferentiated carcinomas having a strong invasive property [43]. It has been reported that E-cadherin expression in colorectal carcinomas is related inversely to tumor differentiation. Down-regulation of E-cadherin levels was associated with cellular dissociation, progression, invasion, and metastasis [49–51].

Adhesion of cells to basement membranes and extracellular matrices is mediated by members of the integrin family of cell surface receptors [52]. Integrins are heterodimeric cell surface glycoproteins comprised of noncovalently linked α and β chains [53]. $\alpha2\beta1$-Integrin is a receptor for collagen and laminin [54], and $\alpha4\beta1$-integrin is a receptor for fibronectin and vascular endothelial cells [48]. Both are reported to relate to the metastasis [55]. Immunoreactivity for the $\alpha2$-subunit, but not for $\alpha4\beta1$-integrin, is found in normal colonic epithelium [56].

In a previous study, the expressions of E-cadherin and integrins ($\alpha2\beta1$ and $\alpha4\beta1$) in the predominant histology of the tumors were examined in 61 acetone-methanol-fixed colorectal adenocarcinomas [57] which were included in the 170 tumors. They consisted of 30 well-differentiated and 31 moderately differentiated adenocarcinomas, divided into 26 W/M-, 17 Mod-, and 18 Por-subtype tumors. Reduced expression of E-cadherin (Fig. 2a) was observed in 11.5% of W/M-, 35.3% of Mod-, and 27.8% of Por-subtype tumors. There was no difference in frequency of reduced expression of E-cadherin between the latter two groups. Predominant histology revealed that W/M- and Mod-subtype tumors were composed mainly of well- and moderately differentiated adenocarcinomas, respectively. The predominant histology of the Por-subtype tumors, however, was a mixture of well-

or moderately differentiated adenocarcinoma. Moderately differentiated adenocarcinoma cells had a more reduced expression of E-cadherin than did well differentiated adenocarcinoma cells, indicating that E-cadherin expression was closely associated with the morphology. Its reduction, however, cannot precede the morphologic change from well- or moderately differentiated to poorly differentiated [57].

Cadherins form a complex with the actin-based cytoskeleton via catenins [58]. It is reported that cells in epithelial proliferative breast lesions proliferate within the basement membrane-bound spaces, losing their evenly spaced arrangement, and form secondary lumens. In these lesions the actin-binding, cytoskeletal protein fodrin (part of the cadherin cascade) is abnormally distributed

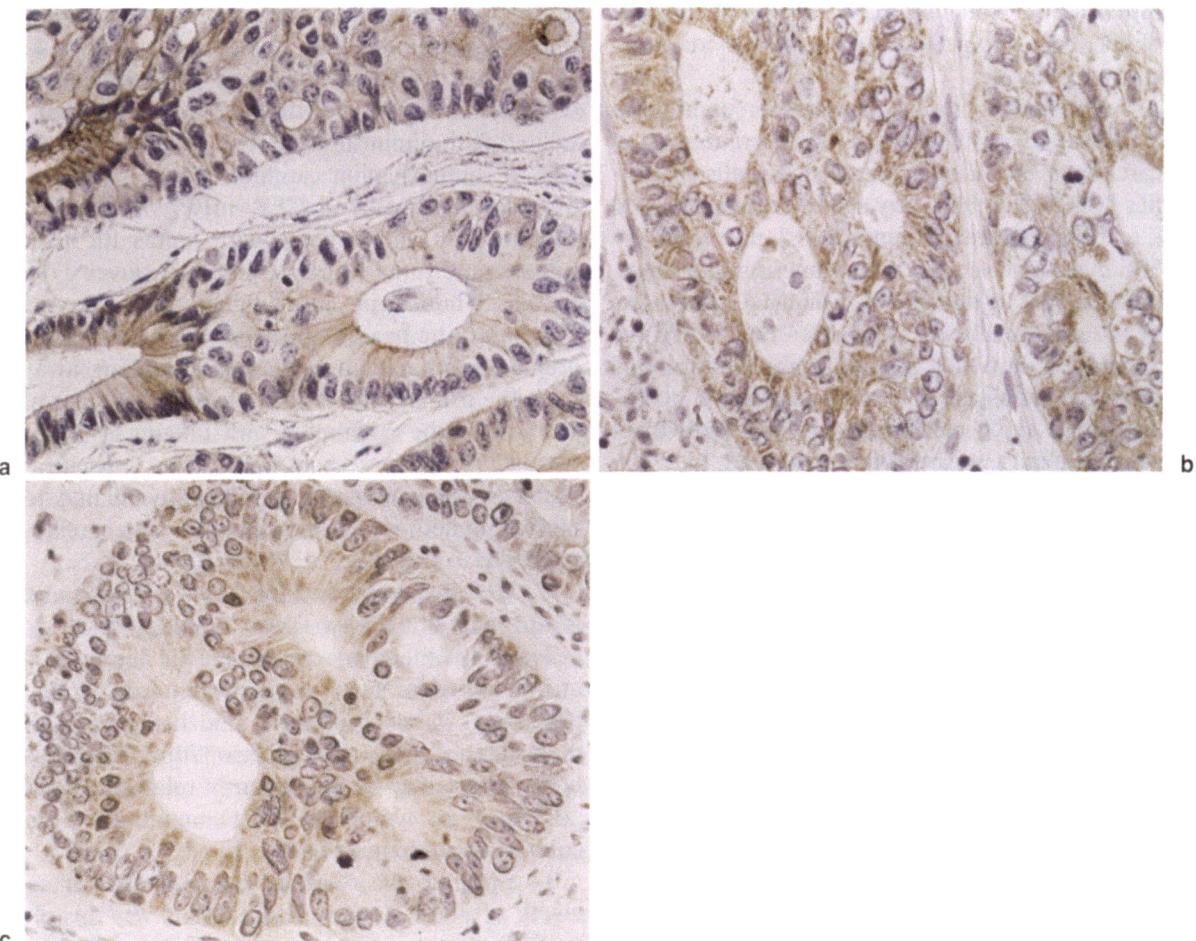

Fig. 2a–c. Immunohistochemical expressions of E-cadherin and integrins (α2β1 and α4β1) in acetone-methanol-fixed adenocarcinomas. **a** Expression of E-cadherin on the cell membrane is reduced in W/M-type cells. **b,c** Overexpression of α2β1-integrin (**b**) and α4β1-integrin (**c**) is observed in Mod-type cells of Por-subtype tumors. (*a–c*: labeled with avidin-biotin, ×400)

[59]. As W/M- or Mod-subtype carcinoma cells are more proliferative with higher BrdU LIs than Wel-subtype carcinoma cells, they are considered to form papillary, cribriform-like, or fused glands associated with reduced expression of E-cadherin.

On the other hand, expressions of $\alpha2\beta1$-integrin (Fig. 2b) in the predominant histology were found in 76.9%, 76.5%, and 94.4%; and those of $\alpha4\beta1$-integrin (Fig. 2c) were in 7.7%, 5.9%, and 27.8% of W/M-, Mod-, and Por-subtype tumors, respectively. Although these differences were not statistically significant, stronger expression of $\alpha2\beta1$- and $\alpha4\beta1$-integrins in the predominant histology of the Por-subtype tumors than in the W/M- or Mod-subtype tumors suggest that overexpression of $\alpha2\beta1$- and $\alpha4\beta1$-integrins in the predominant histology relates to the poor differentiation at the deeply infiltrating sites from well- or moderately differentiated carcinoma cells or more metastases of the Por-subtype tumors than W/M- or Mod-subtype tumors.

Overexpression or underexpression of integrins is reportedly correlated with dedifferentiation of carcinoma and acquisition of metastatic properties [13]. During the early stages of tumor growth (i.e., release from the tumor mass), decreased adhesion to the basement membranes or matrix proteins may be advantageous. Enhanced expression of integrins on tumor cells after they reach the circulation, however, might aid implantation and promote metastasis [55]. Overexpression of $\beta1$-integrin is implicated in the invasive growth of gastric scirrhous carcinomas [60] and the liver metastasis of human gastric carcinoma cells [61]. Overexpression of $\alpha4\beta1$-integrin relates to the invasive ability by an enhanced interaction with fibronectin, increased mRNA for type IV collagenase, and pulmonary metastasis of osteogenic or fibrosarcoma cells [62]. To form metastatic foci in the lungs, however, laminin receptors such as $\alpha2\beta1$-integrin on tumor cells might be necessary to bind to subendothelial basement membranes because $\alpha4\beta1$-integrin on tumor cells is reported only to initiate adhesion to lung endothelial cells [62].

Sakamoto et al. [13] examined alterations of cell morphology and adhesion molecules in response to phorbol ester treatment of a human colon cancer cell line, which forms a well-differentiated tubular structure even under standard culture conditions. They suggested that activation of the integrin system in association with tyrosine phosphorylation of paxillin, which is a focal adhesion protein [63], secondarily promotes disruption of the cadherin system [13]. Taken together, those results indicate that overexpression of $\alpha2\beta1$- and $\alpha4\beta1$-integrins precedes disruption of the cadherin system in well- or moderately differentiated adenocarcinoma cells to change their morphology to poorly differentiated cells; and it relates to the high probability of metastases of the Por-subtype tumors.

Serum Levels of CEA and CA19-9

Serum levels of CEA and CA19-9 are well-known serologic markers for colorectal carcinoma [64]. CEA is a heavily glycosylated 180-kDa protein that was described not only as an oncofetal tumor marker of colorectal carcinoma [65] but also as a homotypic intercellular adhesion molecule [66, 67] of the immunogloblin supergene family [68]. A CEA level elevation of more than 5 ng/ml is observed with advanced disease and has been correlated with diminished survival [2]. Liver metastasis of human colon carcinomas is reported to produce high levels of CEA mRNA, and CEA protein [69]; and patients with metastatic liver tumors tend to have high serum CEA levels [70]. Increased homotypic intercellular adhesion favors the metastatic process, probably because cell aggregates, rather than single cells breaking away from the primary tumor, have a greater chance of survival in the circulation and lodging in other organs [71]. A decreasing CEA tissue concentration was reported to be significantly related to increasing dedifferentiation of colorectal carcinomas [64].

CA19-9 is defined as sialyl-Lewis-a (SLA) and is a product of the Lewis gene [72]. SLA serves as a ligand for members of the selectin family [73] and is noted to have an important role in the process of vascular invasion and hematogenous metastasis of carcinomas in vitro [74]. CA19-9 has been reported to be significantly related to liver [25], lung, or lymph node [75] metastasis from colorectal carcinoma [76].

To evaluate the relations between the serum levels of these tumor markers and the histologic grade of the colorectal adenocarcinoma, preoperative serum levels of CEA (normal < 2.5 ng/ml) were measured in 85 patients and CA19-9 (normal < 37 U/ml) in 53 patients (Table 10). All of the tumors, resected at Kure Kyosai

Table 10. Relation between preoperative serum CEA and CA19-9 and lymph node metastasis, liver metastasis, and tumor histology

Factor	Tumors (no.)	Serum CEA (ng/ml)	Serum CA19-9 (U/ml)
Lymph node metastasis			
n0	44	4.9	33.4 ($n = 28$)
n1	18	6.5	36.0 ($n = 10$)
n2	14	8.4	31.3 ($n = 11$)
n3	9	8.3	44.3 ($n = 4$)
Liver metastasis			
Present			
All	18	11.3	25.9 ($n = 10$)
At surgery	6	13.2	27.3 ($n = 3$)
After surgery	12	10.3	25.3 ($n = 7$)
Absent (other metastases present)	29	6.2	35.4 ($n = 20$)
Absent (no metastasis)	38	3.7**	37.0 ($n = 23$)
Tumor histology and subtype			
Well (Wel)	5	5.5	13.5 ($n = 2$)
Well or moderately			
W/M	31	3.8	36.6 ($n = 18$)
Mod	16	4.8	18.4 ($n = 12$)
Por	29	9.9*	47.0 ($n = 19$)
Poorly	4	4.2	9.0 ($n = 2$)

All data are mean values.
CEA, carcinoembryonic antigen. See Table 4 for other abbreviations.
* $P < 0.05$ versus W/M. ** $P < 0.05$ versus All.

Hospital between July 1992 and September 1995, had invaded beyond the muscularis propria of the colorectum. Sixty-two of the patients were included among the 170 patients of our study, and all patients were followed for more than 5 months after surgery. Lymph node metastasis at the time of surgery was found in 41 patients, of which 18 had n1, 14 had n2, and 9 had n3 grade lymph node metastasis. Preoperative serum levels of CEA and CA19-9 in patients with lymph node metastasis of n3 grade were 8.3 ng/ml and 44.3 U/ml, and those in patients with no lymph node metastasis were 4.9 ng/ml and 33.4 U/ml, respectively. Serum CEA levels in patients with lymph node metastasis of n1 and n2 were 6.5 ng/ml and 8.4 ng/ml, respectively. Elevated serum CEA or CA19-9 levels tended to related to the lymph node metastasis, although there was no statistical difference.

Of the 85 patients, liver metastasis was found in 6 patients at the time of surgery and in 12 after surgery. Twenty-nine patients had no liver metastasis but had other metastases during their clinical courses. Thirty-eight patients had no metastases during their clinical courses. Serum CEA levels of these patients were 13.2, 10.3, 6.2, and 3.7 ng/ml, respectively. The serum CEA level of 18 patients with liver metastasis during their clinical courses was 11.3 ng/ml, which was significantly higher than the 3.7 ng/ml in the 38 patients without metastases. No significant difference was found in serum CA19-9 levels among those patients. Hence the serum CEA level relates more significantly to liver metastasis than to lymph node metastasis. The serum CA19-9 level does not relate to liver metastasis, although it has some relation to lymph node metastasis.

The 85 tumors were classified as 5 Wel, 31 W/M, 16 Mod, and 29 Por subtypes and 4 poor tumors. Serum CEA levels were 3.8 ng/ml for the 31 patients with W/M-subtype tumors, 4.8 ng/ml for the 16 patients with Mod-subtype tumors, and 9.9 ng/ml for the 29 patients with Por-subtype tumors. Serum CA19-9 levels of these patients were 36.6, 18.4, and 47.0 U/ml, respectively. Hence serum CEA and CA19-9 levels were expressing well the high malignant potential of Por-subtype tumors.

p53 and Other Suppressor Genes

The *p53* tumor suppressor gene is involved in the pathogenesis of a large number of human neoplasms as a major biochemical regulator of growth control [77]. *p53* mutant tumor cells have been reported to have a survival advantage over cells with intact *p53* [78]. Starzynska et al. reported that immunohistochemical detection of p53 protein is correlated with a poor prognosis [79], although literature on the prognostic value of p53 immunoreactivity is controversial [77]. Ayhan et al. discussed the diversity of *p53* alterations in the development and progression of colon carcinoma and found no relation between p53 immunoreactivity and histologically defined tumor subtype [80]. We previously reported that p53 immunoreactivity tended to be correlated with liver metastasis, and the Mod-subtype tumors had a stronger immunoreactivity for p53 than did the Por-subtype tumors. However, p53 overexpression was not well correlated with the histologic change at the deeply infiltrating sites [16].

With colorectal carcinoma, loss of heterozygosity (LOH) on chromosome 17p is reported to be correlated with vascular invasion, whereas 18q LOH is correlated with lymphatic invasion and hepatic metastasis, and 22q LOH correlates with lymph node metastasis [81]. The *p53* gene mapped on chromosome 17p13 [82] and the *DCC* gene on 18q [81]. *Nm23-h1* has been located on 17q21.3-22. Deletions of *Nm23-h1* are reported to be relatively more frequent in poorly differentiated adenocarcinomas and to be associated with shorter patient survival [82]. The close relation between tumor histology at deeply infiltrated sites of advanced colorectal adenocarcinomas and metastasis and the genetic alterations of those carcinoma cells, with special attention to the LOH of suppressor genes, must be further elucidated.

References

1. Tahara E (1995) Genetic alterations in human gastrointestinal cancers. Cancer 75:1410–1417
2. Levin B, Raijman I (1995) Malignant tumors of the colon and rectum. In: Haubrich WS, Schaffner F, Berk JE (eds) Gastroenterology. Saunders, Philadelphia, pp 1744–1772
3. Borring CC, Squires TS, Tong T, Montgomery S (1994) Cancer statistics, 1994. CA Cancer J Clin 44:7–26
4. Kuroishi T, Hirose K, Tajima K, Tominaga S (1994) Cancer mortality in Japan (1950–1990). In: Tominaga S, Aoki K, Fujimoto I, Kurihara M (eds) Gann Monograph on Cancer Research No. 41. Cancer mortality and morbidity statistics. Japan and the world—1994. Japan Scientific Societies Press, Tokyo, pp 1–105
5. Morson BC, Dawson IMP, Day DW, Jass JR, Price AB, Williams GT (1990) Morson & Dawson's gastrointestinal pathology, 3d edn. Blackwell Scientific, Oxford, pp 597–629
6. Dukes CE (1932) The classification of cancer of the rectum. J Pathol Bacteriol 35:323–332
7. Astler VB, Coller FA (1954) The prognostic significance of direct extension of carcinoma of the colon and rectum. Ann Surg 139:846–852
8. Spiessl B, Beahrs OH, Hermanek P, Hutter RVP, Scheibe O, Sobin LH, Wagner G (1992) TNM Atlas, 3d edn, 2nd revision. Springer, Berlin, pp 87–95
9. Japanese Research Society for Cancer of Colon and Rectum (1994) General rules for clinical and pathological studies on cancer of the colon, rectum and anus, 5th edn. Kanehara, Tokyo (in Japanese)
10. Group GS (1984) Adjuvant therapy of colon cancer: results of a prospectively randomized trial. N Engl J Med 310:737–743
11. Jass JR, Morson BC (1987) Reporting colorectal cancer. J Clin Pathol 40:1016–1023
12. Jass JR, Sobin LH (1989) Histological typing of intestinal tumours, 2nd edn. Springer, Berlin
13. Sakamoto M, Ino Y, Ochiai A, Kanai Y, Akimoto S, Hirohashi S (1996) Formation of focal adhesion and spreading of polarized human colon cancer cells in association with tyrosine phosphorylation of paxillin in response to phorbol ester. Lab Invest 74:199–208
14. Taniyama K, Suzuki H, Matsumoto M, Hakamada K, Toyama K, Tahara E (1991) Flow cytometric DNA analysis of poorly differentiated adenocarcinoma of the colorectum. Jpn J Clin Oncol 21:406–411
15. Thomas RM, Sobin LH (1995) Gastrointestinal cancer. Cancer 75:154–170
16. Taniyama K, Sasaki N, Wada S, Sasaki M, Miyoshi N, Nakai H, Kodama S, Nakatsuka H, Tahara E (1996) Comparison of proliferative activities and metastases between two subtypes classified at the deeply infiltrating sites of colorectal moderately differentiated adenocarcinomas. Pathol Int 46:195–203
17. Taniyama K, Suzuki H, Matsumoto M, Hakamada K, Toyama K, Tahara E (1993) Relationships between nodal status and cell kinetics, DNA ploidy pattern and histopathology of the deeply infiltrating sites in colorectal adenocarcinoma. Acta Pathol Jpn 43:590–596

18. Jass JR, Love SB, Northover JMA (1987) A new prognostic classification of rectal cancer. Lancet 1:1303–1306

19. Association of Directors of Anatomic and Surgical Pathology (1996) Recommendations for the reporting of resected large intestinal carcinomas. Hum Pathol 27:5–8

20. Phillips RKS, Hittinger R, Blesovsky L, Fry JS, Fielding LP (1984) Large bowel cancer: surgical pathology and its relationship to survival. Br J Surg 71:604–610

21. Wolmark N, Fisher B, Wieand HS (1986) The prognostic value of the modifications of the Dukes' C class of colorectal cancer. Ann Surg 203:115–122

22. Shirouzu K, Isomoto H, Morodomi T, Kakegawa T (1995) Carcinomatous lymphatic permeation: prognostic significance in patients with rectal carcinoma—a long term prospective study. Cancer 75:4–10

23. Dukes CE (1937) Histological grading of rectal cancer. Proc R Soc Med 30:371–376

24. Chung CK, Aaino RJ, Stryker JA (1982) Colorectal carcinoma: evaluation of histologic grade and factors influencing prognosis. J Surg Oncol 21:143–148

25. Nagai E, Yao T, Sakamoto M, Akazawa K, Utsunomiya T, Tsuneyoshi M (1994) Risk factors related to liver metastasis in colorectal carcinoma: a multivariate analysis of clinicopathologic and immunohistochemical variables. Jpn J Cancer Res 85:1280–1287

26. Kelvin FM, Maglinte DT (1987) Colorectal carcinoma: a radiologic and clinical review. Radiology 164:1–8

27. Schulz W, Hagen C, Hort W (1985) The distribution of liver metastases from colonic cancer. Virchows Arch Pathol Anat 406:279–284

28. Dionne L (1965) The pattern of blood-bone metastasis from carcinoma of rectum. Cancer 18:775–781

29. Newland RC, Dent OF, Chapuis PH, Leslie B (1995) Survival after curative resection of lymph node negative colorectal carcinoma. Cancer 76:564–571

30. Paget S (1889) Distribution of secondary growths in cancer of the breast. Lancet 1:571–573

31. Scott NA, Rainwatter LM, Wieand HS, Weiland LH, Pemberton JH, Beart RW, Lieber MM (1987) The relative prognostic value of flow cytometric DNA analysis and conventional clinicopathologic criteria in patients with operable rectal carcinoma. Dis Colon Rectum 30:513–520

32. Sasaki K, Hashimoto T, Kawachino K, Takahashi M (1988) Intramural regional differences in DNA ploidy of gastrointestinal carcinomas. Cancer 62:2569–2575

33. Hedley DW, Friedlander ML, Taylor IW, Rugg CA, Musgrove EA (1983) Method for analysis of cellular DNA content of paraffin-embedded pathological material using flow cytometry. J Histochem Cytochem 31:1333–1335

34. Goh HS, Jass JR, Atkin WS, Cuzick J, Northover JMA (1987) Value of flow cytometric determination of ploidy as a guide to prognosis in operable rectal cancer: a multivariate analysis. Int J Colorectal Dis 2:17–21

35. Rowley S, Newbold KM, Gearty J, Keighley MRB, Donovan JA, Neoptolemos JP (1990) Comparison of deoxyribonucleic acid ploidy and nuclear expressed p62 c-myc oncogene in the prognosis of colorectal cancer. World J Surg 14:545–551

36. Bauer KD, Lincoln ST, Vera-Roman JM, Wallemark CB, Chmiel JS, Madurski ML, Murad T, Scarpelli DG (1987) Prognostic implications of proliferative antivity and DNA aneuploidy in colonic adenocarcinomas. Lab Invest 57:329–335

37. Suzuki T, Takano Y (1993) Comparative immunohistochemical studies of p53 and proliferating cell nuclear antigen expression and argyrophilic nucleolar organizer regions in pancreatic duct cell carcinoma. Jpn J Cancer Res 84:1072–7077

38. Hayashi Y, Fukayama M, Koike M, Kaseda S, Ikeda T, Yokoyama T (1993) Cell-cycle analysis detecting endogenous nuclear antigens: comparison with BrdU-in vivo labeling and application to lung tumors. Acta Pathol Jap 43:313–319

39. Aoki K, Sakamoto M, Hirohashi S (1994) Nucleolar organizer regions in small nodular lesions representing early stages of human hepatocarcinogenesis. Cancer 73:289–293

40. Sasaki K, Matsumura K, Tsuji T, Shinozaki F, Takahashi M (1988) Relationship between labeling indices of Ki-67 and BrdUrd in human malignant tumors. Cancer 62:989–993

41. Weidner N, Moore II DH, Vartanian R (1994) Correlation of Ki-67 antigen expression with mitotic figure index and tumor grade in breast carcinomas using the novel "paraffin"-reactive MIB1 antibody. Hum Pathol 25:337–342

42. Kawai K, Serizawa A, Hamana T, Tsutumi Y (1994) Heat-induced antigen retrieval of proliferating cell nuclear antigen and p53 protein in formalin-fixed, paraffin-embedded sections. Pathol Int 44:759–764

43. Kanai Y, Shimoyama Y, Oda T, Hirohashi S (1994) Abnormalities of cell adhesion molecules in multistage carciniogenesis. Gann Monogr Cancer Res 42:127–137

44. Liotta LA, Steeg PS, Stetler-Stevenson WG (1991) Cancer metastasis and angiogenesis: an imbalance of positive and negative regulation. Cell 64:327–336

45. Takeichi M (1991) Cadherin cell adhesion receptors as a morphogenetic regulator. Science 251:1451–1455

46. Fukamachi H, Kim YS (1989) Glandular structure formation of LS174T human colon cancer cells cul-

126   K. Taniyama et al.

tured with collagen gels. Dev Growth Differ 31:
107–112

47. Mansouri A, Spurr N, Goodfellow PN, Kemler R
(1988) Characterization and chromosomal localization of the gene encoding the human cell adhesion
molecule uvomorulin. Differentiation 38:67–71

48. Pignatelli M, Vessey CJ (1995) Adhesion molecules: novel molecular tools in tumor pathology.
Hum Pathol 25:849–856

49. Dorudi S, Sheffield JP, Poulsom R, Northover
JMA, Hart IR (1993) E-cadherin expression in
colorectal cancer. Am J Pathol 142:981–986

50. Kinsella AR, Lepts GC, Hill CL, Jones M (1994)
Reduced E-cadherin expression correlates with increased invasiveness in colorectal carcinoma cell
lines. Clin Exp Metast 12:335–342

51. Frixen UH, Behrens J, Sachs M, Eberle G, Voss B,
Warda A, Lochner D, Birchmeier W (1991) E-
cadherin-mediated cell–cell adhesion prevents invasiveness of human carcinoma cells. J Cell Biol
113:173–185

52. Hynes RO (1987) Integrin: a family of cell surface
receptors. Cell 48:549–554

53. Hynes RO (1992) Integrins: versatility, modulation
and signaling in cell adhesion. Cell 69:11–25

54. Dedhar S (1990) Integrins and tumor invasion.
Bioassays 12:583–590

55. Alberda SM (1993) Biology of disease: role of
integrins and other cell adhesion molecules in
tumor progression and metastasis. Lab Invest
68:4–17

56. Koukoulis GK, Virtanen I, Moll R, Quaranta V,
Gould VE (1993) Immunolocalization of integrins
in the normal and neoplastic colonic epithelium.
Virchows Arch Cell Pathol [B] 63:373–383

57. Taniyama K, Sasaki N, Tahara E (1996) Expres-
sions of CEA, E-cadherin, integrin ($\alpha2\beta1$, $\alpha4\beta1$)
and bcl-2 in the predominant histology of advanced
colorectal adenocarcinomas. In: Proceedings, Japanese Society of Tumor Marker Research, vol 11, pp
67–69 (in Japanese)

58. Yasui W, Kuniyasu H, Akama Y, Kitahara K,
Nagafuchi A, Ishihara S, Tsukita S, Tahara E
(1994) Expression of E-cadherin, α- and β-catenins
in human gastric carcinomas: correlation with histology and tumor progression. Oncol Rep 2:111–
117

59. Page DL, Simpson JF (1995) Are catenins and
cadherins relevant to tumor biology? Good fences
make good neighbors. Lab Invest 72:491–493

60. Kozako Y, Yasui W, Tahara E (1994) Expression of
$\beta1$ integrin in human gastric carcinomas: correlation with histological type and tumor progression.
Int J Oncol 5:225–230

61. Yasoshima T, Denno R, Kawaguchi S, Sato N,
Okada Y, Ura H, Kikuchi K, Hirata K (1996) Establishment and characterization of human gastric
carcinoma lines with high metastatic potential in

the liver: changes in integrin expression associated
with the ability to metastasize in the liver of nude
mice. Jpn J Cancer Res 87:153–160

62. Kawaguchi S, Kikuchi K, Ishii S, Takada Y,
Kobayashi S, Uede T (1992) VLA-4 molecules on
tumor cells initiate an adhesive interaction with
VCAM-1 molecules on endothelial cell surface. Jpn
J Cancer Res 83:1304–1316

63. Turner CE, Glenney JR, Burridge K (1990)
Paxillin: a new vinculin-binding protein present in
focal adhesions. J Cell Biol 111:1059–1068

64. Quentmeier A, Moller P, Schwarz V, Abel U,
Schlag P (1987) Carcinoembryonic antigen, CA19-
9, and CA125 in normal and carcinomatous human
colorectal tissue. Cancer 60:2261–2266

65. Jothy S, Yuan SY, Shirota K (1993) Transcription
of carcinoembryonic antigen in normal colon and
colon carcinoma: in situ hybridization study and
implication for a new in vivo functional model. Am
J Pathol 143:250–257

66. Benchimol S, Fuks A, Jothy S, Beauchemin N,
Shirota K, Stanners CP (1989) Carcinoembryonic
antigen, a human tumor marker, functions as an
intercellular adhesion molecule. Cell 57:327–334

67. Levin LV, Griffin TW (1991) Specific adhesion of
carcinoembryonic antigen-bearing colorectal cancer cells to immobilized carcinoembryonic antigen.
Cancer Lett 60:143–152

68. Hostetter RB, Augustus LB, Mankarious R, Chi K,
Fan D, Toth C, Thomas P, Jessup JM (1990)
Carcinoembryonic antigen as a selective enhancer
of colorectal cancer metastasis. J Natl Cancer Inst
82:380–385

69. Boucher D, Cournoyer D, Stanners CP, Fuks A
(1989) Studies on control of expression the carcinoembryonic antigen family in human tissue.
Cancer Res 49:847–852

70. Shuster J, Thomson DMP, Fuks A, Gold P (1980)
Immunologic approaches to the diagnosis of malignancy. Prog Exp Tumor Res 25:89–139

71. Updyke TV, Nicholson GL (1986) Malignant
melanoma cell lines selected in vitro for increased
homotypic adhesion properties have increased experimental metastatic potential. Clin Exp Methods
4:273–284

72. Narimatsu H, Iwasaki H, Nishihara S, Kimura H,
Kudo T, Yamauchi Y, Hirohashi S (1996) Genetic
evidence for the Lewis enzyme, which synthesizes
type-1 Lewis antigens in colon tissue, and intracellular localization of the enzyme. Cancer Res 56:
330–338

73. Berg EL, Magnani J, Warnock RA, Robinson MK,
Butcher EC (1992) Comparison of L-selectin and
E-selectin ligand specificities: the L-selectin can
bind the E-selectin ligands sialyl Le^x and sialyl Le^a.
Biochem Biophys Res Commun 184:1048–1055

74. Takada A, Ohmori K, Yoneda T, Tsuyuoka K,
Hasegawa A, Kiso M, Kannagi R (1993) Contribu-

tion of carbohydrate antigen sialyl Lewis a and sialyl Lewis x to adhesion of human cancer cells to vascular endothelium. Cancer Res 53:354–361

75. Nakayama T, Watanabe M, Katsumata T, Teramoto T, Kitajima M (1995) Expression of sialyl Lewis[a] as a new prognostic factor for patients with advanced colorectal carcinoma. Cancer 75:2051–2056

76. Shimono R, Mori M, Akazawa K, Adachi Y, Sugimachi K (1994) Immunohistochemical expression of carbohydrate antigen 19-9 in colorectal carcinoma. Am J Gastroenterol 89:101–105

77. Battifora H (1994) p53 immunohistochemistry; a word of caution. Hum Pathol 25:435–437

78. Graber TG, Osmanian C, Jacks T, Housman DE, Koch CJ, Lowe SW, Giaccia AJ (1996) Hypoxia-mediated selection of cells with diminished apoptotic potential in solid tumours. Nature 379:88–91

79. Starzynska T, Bromley M, Ghosh A, Stern SL (1992) Prognostic significance of p53 over-expression in gastric and colorectal carcinoma. Br J Cancer 66:558–562

80. Ayhan A, Yasui W, Yokozaki H, Ito H, Tahara E (1992) Genetic abnormalities and expression of *p53* in human colon carcinomas. Int J Oncol 1:431–437

81. Iino H, Fukayama M, Maeda Y, Koike M, Mori T, Takahashi T, Kikuchi-Yanoshita R, Miyaki M, Mizuno S, Watanabe S (1994) Molecular genetics for clinical management of colorectal carcinoma. Cancer 73:1324–1331

82. Campo E, Miquel R, Jares P, Bosch F, Juan M, Leone A, Vives J, Cardesa A, Yague J (1994) Prognostic significance of the loss of heterozygosity of *nm23-h1* and *p53* genes in human colorectal carcinomas. Cancer 73:2913–2921

Glycoprotein Histochemistry and the Histogenesis of Colorectal Cancer

Jeremy R. Jass

Summary. The nature and synthesis of the carbohydrate and protein components of colorectal mucin are discussed before drawing together particular carbohydrate structures, types of apomucin, and associated cell lineages. In normal goblet cells MUC2 is co-expressed with type 1 carbohydrate chains and sialylated structures including SLe^a, SLe^x, and STn. MUC1 is expressed normally by immature crypt base cells and shows co-localization with type 2 carbohydrate chains (Le^x and Le^y). Colorectal cancers may secrete mucin-like material that is mainly MUC2 and non-mucin-like material that is mainly up-regulated MUC1. These secretions are characterized by distinct patterns of morphologic distribution, MUC2 being within goblet cells and extracellular pools, MUC1 being glycocalyceal, luminal, and within intracytoplasmic lumens. It appears that cancer "mucin" is derived from different lineages and needs to be characterized accordingly. The distribution of mucins in normal tissue, precancerous and cancer-associated lesions, and cancer is considered in light of the lineage-based model. The essential molecular processes involved in carcinogenesis must be largely independent of the genetic control of mucin synthesis. By relating the characterization of mucin to cell lineage, it may be possible to derive classifications that are biololgically meaningful and relevant to the pathogenesis and behavior of colorectal cancer.

Introduction

It is accepted that structural differences exist between mucins expressed by normal colorectal epithelium and those expressed by adenocarcinoma, but there is little appreciation of the pathogenesis

Department of Pathology, University of Queensland, Queensland, Australia

of these differences or of their biologic or clinical significance. Colorectal mucins have been studied by various technologies including histochemistry, biochemistry, and molecular biology. These techniques have their own limitations and pitfalls, and the findings associated with each must be integrated to provide a comprehensive overview. This presentation focuses on the histochemical approach but begins with an account of the chemical structure of epithelial mucin.

Mucins are glycoproteins containing up to 85% carbohydrate, and it is necessary to consider the carbohydrate and protein components separately. The carbohydrate component is best approached from the standpoint of blood group biochemistry, as the peripheral region consists of blood groups, substances that provide the main structural (antigenic) variability. The protein component (apomucin) includes several distinct species coded for by different genes. Many of these genes have been cloned, and monoclonal antibodies have been raised to the specific repetitive amino acid sequences. It is then necessary to combine the carbohydrate and protein components and relate the unified molecule to particular regions and cell lineages within the gastrointestinal tract. This exercise provides a firm basis for studying the changes that occur during the course of neoplastic evolution.

Carbohydrate Component

The carbohydrate component is arranged in oligosaccharide chains of varying length and degree of branching, and the chains are attached to the protein backbone by covalent linkage. Oligosaccharide chains containing 2 to 12 monosaccharides have been demonstrated in colonic mucin [1–3]. During the course of biosynthesis, monosaccharides are added in stepwise fashion by specific glycosyl transferases. Compositional analysis has demonstrated the presence of five saccharides: the hexosamines *N*-acetyl-D-galactosamine (GalNAc) and *N*-acetyl-D-glucosamine (GlcNAc); the hexose D-galactose (Gal); smaller amounts of 6-deoxyhexose L-fucose (Fuc); and a variety of neuraminic (sialic) acid derivatives. Sulfation of certain sugars contributes further to the acidity [4]. Examples of long and short oligosaccharide chains are shown in Fig. 1.

The oligosaccharide chains can be considered to have three structurally distinct domains: a core region incorporating the linkage to the protein, a backbone, and a peripheral region [5, 6]. Among the four best-established core structures, core 3 structure is the best represented within colorectal mucin: GlcNAcβ1→3GalNAc-O-serine/threonine [1, 2]. The precursor of core structure 3 is the Tn antigen (GalNAc-O-R). The presence of core 1 structure (Galβ1→3GalNAc-O-R) (T antigen) within either normal or cancerous mucin is generally accepted [7] but may be an erroneous view. The abnormal expression of T antigen within colorectal cancer was apparently demonstrated by means of the lectin peanut agglutinin (PNA) [8–10] and by immunohistochemistry [11]. However, apart from the fact that core 3 structure predominates in structural analyses of human colonic mucin [1, 2], PNA is not in fact specific for T antigen, binding also to the backbone disaccharide sequence (Galβ1→3/4GlcNAc-R) [5,

6]. Furthermore, highly specific monoclonal antibodies to the T antigen fail to localize this structure in either normal or malignant tissues of the colorectum [12].

The backbone of the oligosaccharide chain is made up of one or more disaccharide repeats (Galβ1→3/4GlcNAc–). There are two types of backbone depending on whether the linkage is 1→3 (type 1) or 1→4 (type 2). This variable also determines the type of peripheral blood group substance (see below). The mucins of normal colorectal goblet cells are constituted predominantly but not exclusively of type 1 oligosaccharide chains (hence type 1 blood group substances). Increased amounts of type 2 chain are found in colorectal cancer mucin [13, 14].

As noted above, the terminal component of the oligosaccharide chain is a blood group substance, the type (1 or 2) being determined by the underlying backbone. The terminal component is the most variable part of the molecule, and the variability is genetically determined. There are several models to explain the genetic basis of blood group substance expression, and they center on the Lewis (Le) system and the secretor (Se) gene. The simplest, most recently formulated model is probably the correct one [15]. The synthesis of blood group substances begins with the precursor structure Le^c, which is the most peripheral backbone disaccharide (Galβ1→3GlcNAc-R). Fucose

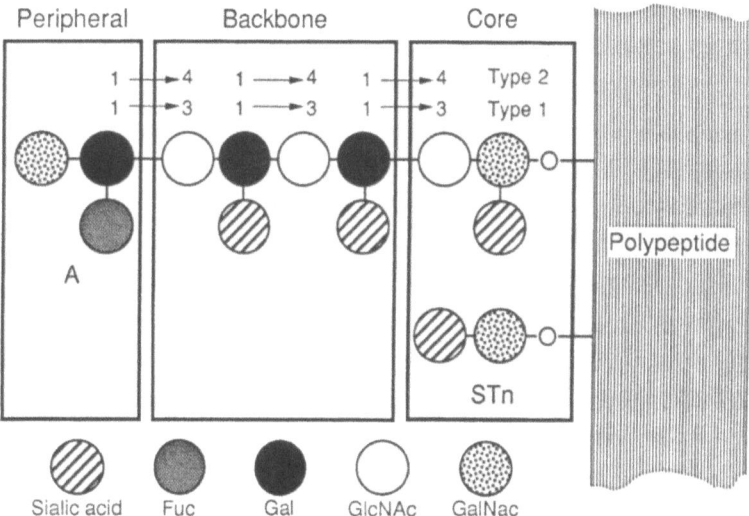

Fig. 1. The shortest carbohydrate chain is formed through α2,6-sialylation of Tn, the precursor of core structure 3. Sialosyl Tn (STn) is expressed within normal goblet cell mucin, but *O*-acetylation of sialic acid renders the structure cryptic without prior alkaki saponification. The long chain is made up of core structure 3, a repetitive backbone, and peripheral blood group A. Sialylation is shown at several sites

is linked to galactose to give substance H. However, there are two α-2-fucosyltransferase genes, one for type 1 chains (Se) and one for type 2 chains (H). About 75% of caucasians [5] carry the Se gene (which is expressed in endoderm), and these individuals therefore secrete gastrointestinal mucins that carry blood group structures. The Se gene converts Le^c to Le^d (H type 1) substance. The Le gene converts Le^c to Le^a and Le^d (H Type 1) to Le^b. The Le and Se genes compete with each other and with other transferases involved with chain elongation or branching, as well as with sialyltransferases (giving sialosyl-Le^a). Additionally, substances A or B may be produced according to blood group status. The structures and synthetic pathways are illustrated in Fig. 2. The type 2 chain homologs of Le^a, Le^b, and sialosyl-Le^a are Le^x, Le^y, and sialosyl-Le^x, respectively. The latter show limited expression in normal mucosa and increased expression in colorectal cancer mucin. Le^x is synonymous with Hapten X, CD15, and stage-specific embryonic antigen (SSEA) and is recognized by a variety of monoclonal antibodies [16] including Leu-M1.

Protein Component

Seven mucin genes (MUC1–MUC7) have been cloned, and three of them are expressed by normal colorectal goblet cells: MUC2 [17–20], MUC3 [19, 21, 22], and MUC4 [21, 23, 24]. MUC2 is regarded as the predominant goblet cell mucin [17]. MUC3 is secreted within small vesicles by both columnar cells and goblet cells [19]. One study indicated that MUC2 is expressed by columnar cells as well as goblet cells [18], but MUC2 is otherwise held to be goblet cell-specific [19] (Fig. 3). Immunolocalization studies have revealed MUC2 to be in a characteristic perinuclear distribution [19] (Fig. 3), a finding confirmed by in situ hybridization of MUC2 mRNA [19]. The repetitive amino acid sequences characteristic of human mucins MUC1 to MUC4 are shown in Table 1.

The MUC1 gene differs from the other mucin genes in that it codes for the protein backbone of membrane-bound, nonsecretory glycoproteins. The latter, distributed along the apical membrane (glycocalyx) of columnar cells of glandular tissues such as breast and pancreas, are characterized as

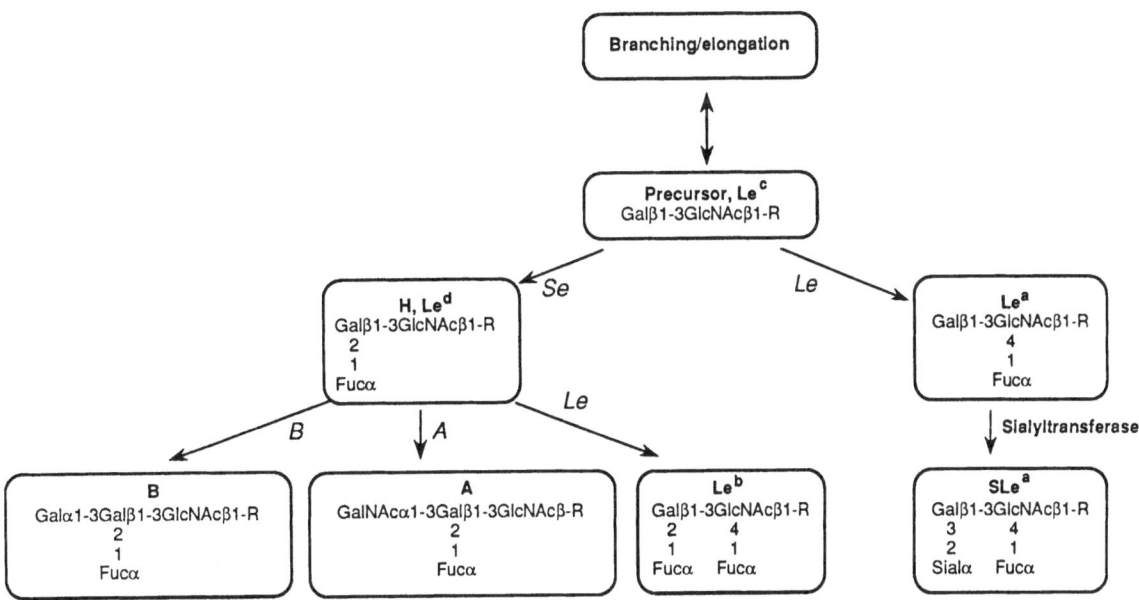

Fig. 2. Synthetic pathways for the formation of type 1 Lewis structures within goblet cell mucin. All subjects express Le^a and sialosyl Le^a within goblet cell mucus with a pancolonic distribution. H and Le^b are found only in secretors (Se⁺) and are expressed in the proximal but not distal colon. A and B are expressed in the proximal colon according to blood group status. The type 2 equivalents of Le^a, Le^b, and SLe^a are Le^x, Le^y, and SLe^x, respectively. Of the latter, only SLe^x is demonstrable within goblet cell mucin. Although both SLe^a and SLe^x are components of goblet cell mucin, sialic acid is heavily O-acetylated, rendering these structures nonantigenic with respect to available monoclonal antibodies. Antigenicity can be unmasked by saponification

EMA and are structures recognized by the monoclonal antibodies HMFG-1 and HMFG-2 [25, 26, 31]. Increased expression of MUC1 is a feature of a variety of adenocarcinomas (Fig. 4). MUC1 is acknowledged to be minimally expressed in normal colorectum [26], though immunoreactivity is influenced by the choice of monoclonal antibody and use of pretreatments. When periodate oxidation precedes immunostaining with MUSE11 [32], a distinctive pattern of immunolocalization is observed, highlighting the apical membranes of immature columnar cells within the crypt base (Fig. 5). Colorectal adenocarcinomas may show marked upregulation of MUC1 [26].

The protein backbone of the mucin molecule is termed an apomucin. It comprises a central do-

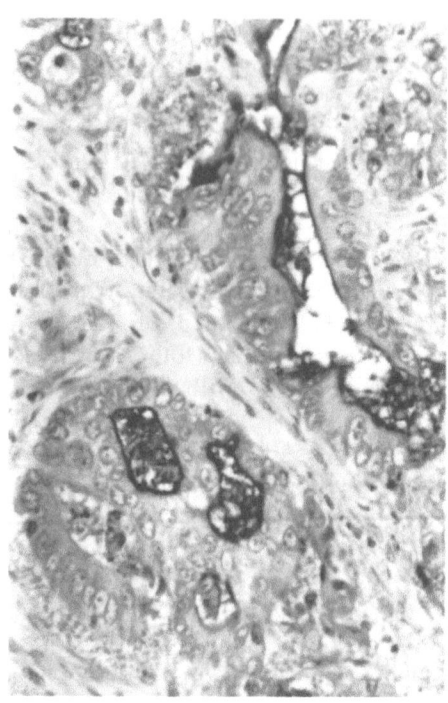

Fig. 4. MUC1 expression within a moderately differentiated adenocarcinoma showing typical glycocalyceal and intraluminal distribution. The intraluminal material was "non-mucin-like," being dense, eosinophilic, and weakly positive with mild PAS (specific for non-*O*-acetyl sialic acid). The material is assumed to be derived from cells of columnar lineage. (Immunoperoxidase reaction with MUSE11 [32])

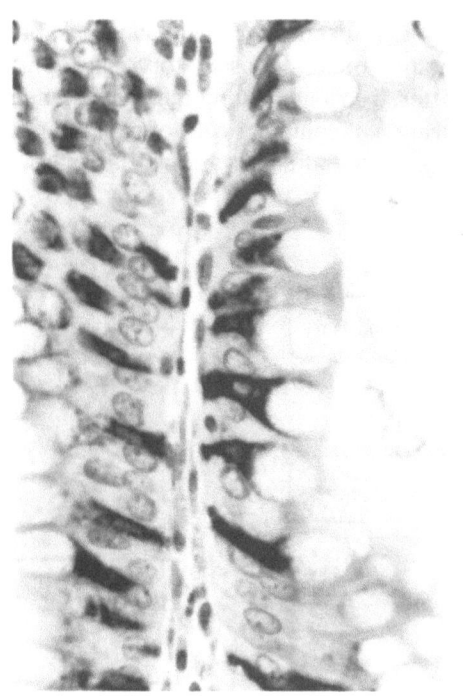

Fig. 3. MUC2 showing restricted immunolocalization to the perinuclear cytoplasm of normal goblet cells. (Immunoperoxidase reaction with CCP58 [18])

main bearing the carbohydrate chains and peripheral domains [31]. Apomucins are linked together, forming a polymeric macromolecule through disulfide bonds within the peripheral domains. The central domains include multiple tandem repeating amino acid sequences. In MUC2, for example, the length of each repeat is 23 amino acids, which is repeated 51 to 115 times [20]. Fourteen of the amino acids are threonine (Table 1), and it is to this hydroxy amino acid that the oligosaccharide chain is attached covalently. Monoclonal antibodies have been developed that

Table 1. Mucin genes expressed in large intestine

Mucin	Amino acid sequence	Chromosome	Tissue expression	References
MUC1	PGSTAPPAHGVTSAPDTRPA	1q21–24	Multiple epithelia	25–29
MUC2	PTTTPITTTTTVTPTPTPTGTQT	11p15	Intestine, lung, cervix	17–20
MUC3	HSTPSFTSSITTTETTS	7q22	Small and large intestine	19, 21, 22, 30
MUC4	TSSASTGHATPLPVTD	3q29	Large intestine, trachea	21, 23, 24

structures show a similar apical or glycocalyceal distribution within colorectal cancers. On the basis of these observations, it is clear that the expression of particular carbohydrate structures may be determined by the underlying apomucin, which in turn is influenced by lineage differentiation. For example, if a colorectal cancer shows loss of the goblet cell lineage (expressing MUC2), the secretory material described loosely as "mucin" may be up-regulated MUC1, MUC3, or both, expressed by cells of columnar lineage. It would then be unnecessary to invoke the induction of altered pathways of oligosaccharide synthesis to explain mucin changes. The "changes" would, rather, reflect the substitution of one secretory lineage by another owing to an altered program of differentiation.

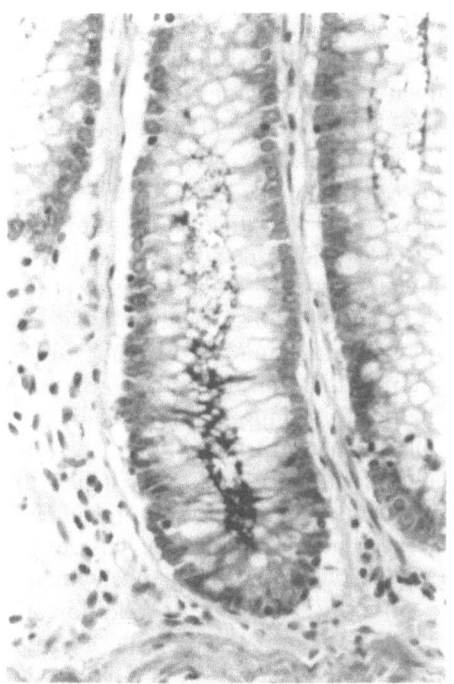

Fig. 5. MUC1 expression along the apical membrane of immature crypt base columnar cells within normal large bowel mucosa. MUC1 reactivity was evident only after periodate oxidation. (Immunoperoxidase reaction with MUSE11 [32])

recognize the amino acid sequences forming the repeats [33]. Antibodies to MUC2 do not recognize the glycosylated apomucin but may do so following neuraminidase digestion and periodate oxidation (Fig. 6).

Relation Between Classes of Apomucin and Carbohydrate Chain

It is likely that different classes of apomucin are associated with particular oligosaccharide structures. It is known, for example, that MUC2 predominates in normal colorectal goblet cell mucin, which is constituted mainly of type 1 oligosaccharide chains. Conversely, cancer secretions may show up-regulation of MUC1 and type 2 carbohydrate chains with associated blood group structures (Le^x, Le^y, SLe^x). Interestingly, in normal colon MUC1 and type 2 oligosaccharide chains (Le^x and Le^y) are co-expressed within crypt base columnar cells (Fig. 7). Up-regulated MUC1 and type 2 blood group

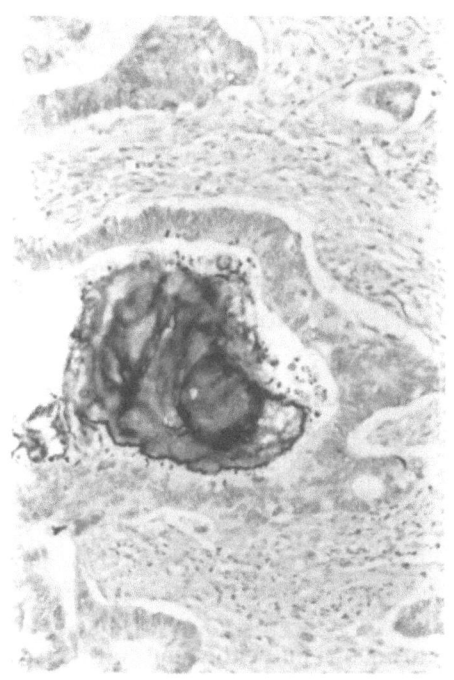

Fig. 6. Demonstration of MUC2 within mucin-like secretory material of colorectal cancer following sialic acid removal (saponification followed by neuraminidase digestion and periodate oxidation. Saponification presumably denatures the nonglycosylated apomucin that would normally be present within the cytoplasm of subjacent goblet cells. The unmasking effect is not seen in the normal goblet cell theca, perhaps because of the presence of longer oligosaccharide chains that would conceal MUC2 apomucin despite pretreatment. (Immunoperoxidase staining with CCP58 [18] preceded by KOH-neuraminidase-periodate)

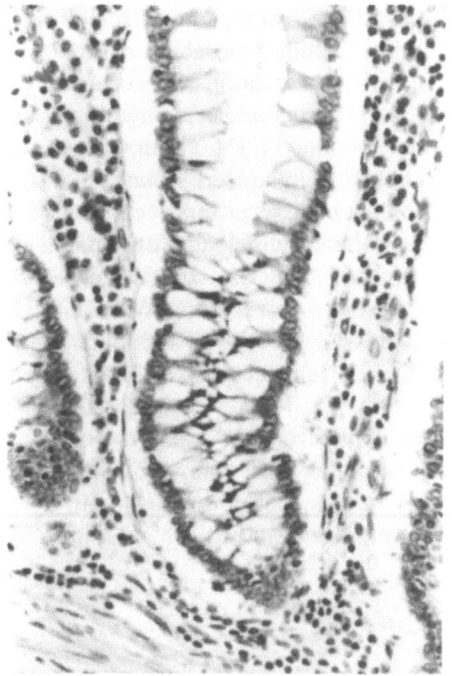

Fig. 7. Expression of Le^x within the normal crypt base. Note the granular staining within the apical cytoplasm of crypt base columnar cells. (Immunoperoxidase reaction with monoclonal antibody CMRF7 [16])

Characterization of Colorectal Cancer Secretions

A fundamental characteristic of all adenocarcinomas is the production of diastase-periodic acid Schiff (dPAS)-positive mucin. In some cancers this material is clearly a product of cells belonging to the goblet cell lineage, most obvious in mucinous adenocarcinomas. The secretory material appears foamy or wispy and is basophilic; goblet cells may be identified in the adjacent malignant epithelium. In other cancers, secretions are more eosinophilic, homogeneous, and admixed with necrotic debris. Such non-mucin-like material may be seen within lumens lined by columnar epithelium lacking goblet cells. Similar material occurs in intracytoplasmic lumens (ICLs), which are intracytoplasmic invaginations of the apical membrane of columnar cells. Mucin stains identify a ring representing the glycocalyceal covering of microvilli projecting into the ICLs together with a central secretory droplet (Fig. 8). The mucin-like and non-mucin-like secretions have been classed type I and type II and differ in their histochemical profiles [34].

Type I secretions are strongly mild periodic acid Schiff (mPAS)-positive and stain with antibodies to sialylated carbohydrate structures (STn, SLe^a, SLe^x) [35, 36]. When treated with neuraminidase and periodate oxidation, MUC2 apomucin may be demonstrated (Fig. 6). Type II secretions are less obviously mPAS-positive and stain with antibodies or lectins specific for sialylated and nonsialylated type 2 blood group substances (Le^x, Le^y, SLe^x) and the core structure Tn [35]. Type II secretions include the MUC1 apomucin (Fig. 4).

In the past there has been little attempt to link histochemical staining patterns with secretory material originating from different cell lineages. Although the attempt to do so is logical, it is not simple to achieve in practice. Malignant cells may show either lineage infidelity or failure of differentiation (expressing simultaneously the products of two different lineages). In addition, there is mixing of intraluminal secretions derived from different cell types. Furthermore, some carbohy-

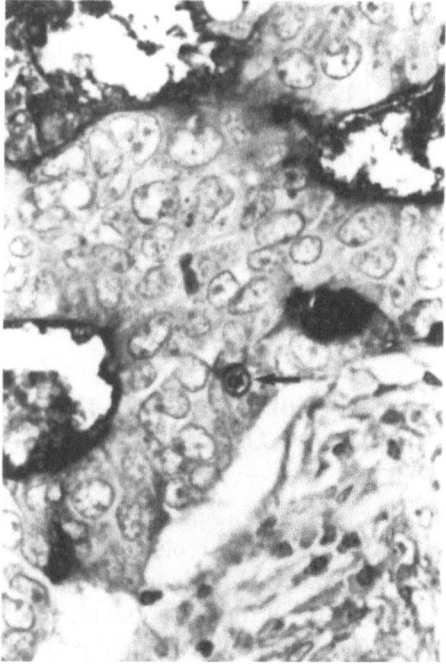

Fig. 8. Intracytoplasmic lumens (ICLs) within a moderately differentiated adenocarcinoma (*arrow*). The outer ring, equivalent to glycocalyx coating microvilli, surrounds a secretory droplet, and both express MUC1. The ICL is a marker of the columnar cell lineage, being a cytoplasmic invagination of the columnar cell apical membrane. ICLs co-express Le^y (identified with UEA-1), Le^x, and SLe^x. (Immunoperoxidase with monoclonal antibody MUSE11 [32])

drate structures, such as sialosyl-Le^x, may be common to different classes of mucin (MUC1 and MUC2) [27, 36, 37]. Nevertheless, recognition of the fact that dPAS-positive secretions are not necessarily derived from cells of goblet cell lineage is of fundamental importance for the proper characterization of colorectal cancer mucin. It is likely that the type I, or mucin-like, secretions are indeed of goblet cell origin, whereas type II, or non-mucin-like, secretions are the up-regulated products of columnar cells [35]. Although data are far from complete, it appears that cancer mucin derived from cells of the goblet lineage differs only in subtle ways from normal colorectal goblet cell mucin. Central to this difference is an alteration in the structure of sialic acid.

Sialic Acid and Goblet Cell Mucin

Sialic acid differs from the other four sugars making up the carbohydrate chain in goblet cell mucus in having an acidic carboxy group, a three-carbon side chain ($C_{7,8,9}$) and existing in a number of variant forms [38–42]. Sialic acid is added at a relatively late stage during chain synthesis, either to the backbone or to terminal blood group structures (Fig. 1). The sialic acid variants are of two major types, with or without O-acetyl substituents. The O-acetyl groups are substituted within the three-carbon side chain ($C_{7,8,9}$) or at C_4. O-Acetyl substitution renders sialic acid resistant to neuraminidase digestion. O-Acetyl sialic acid is found in the large intestine, whereas small intestinal goblet cell mucin is largely non-O-acetylated. These main structural forms confer different antigenicities. Structures incorporating non-O-acetyl sialic acid are recognized by the monoclonal antibodies AM-3 [43] and TKH2 [35] and a panel of antibodies to small intestinal mucin antigen (SIMA) [44]. Structures incorporating O-acetyl sialic acid are recognized by the monoclonal antibodies PR3A5 [45], 3NM [46, 47], and MMM-17 [48].

In colorectal cancer mucin secreted by cells of goblet cell lineage, sialic acid is consistently altered from the usual colonic O-acetylated type to the small intestinal non-O-acetylated type [34]. The increased or neoexpression of sialylated blood groups substances (SLe^a, SLe^x, STn) within colorectal cancer mucin is more apparent than real, being due merely to the alteration in sialic acid structure. Appreciation of the cryptic presence of SLe^a, SLe^x, and STn within normal colorectal goblet cells renders invalid many of the conclusions promulgated in prestigious journals over the last decade. The cryptic presence of SLe^a, SLe^x, and STn within normal colorectal mucosa can be appreciated following alkali saponification to remove O-acetyl groups. STn is then revealed within goblet cells of the lower crypt, whereas SLe^a and SLe^x (representing the peripheral blood group structures characterizing longer chains) are expressed by more mature goblet cells of the upper crypt and surface epithelium [35, 36, 49] (Fig. 9). The short-chain STn is presumably included within mature goblet cell mucin but is obscured by the presence of surrounding long-chain oligosaccharides. Type 1 blood group substances (A, B, H, Le^a, Le^b) and the sugar GalNAc (identified with the lectin DBA) are also (when present) displayed within goblet cells of the upper crypt and surface epithelium [50–52].

The simplest technique for demonstrating small intestinal-type non-O-acetyl sialic acid is mPAS staining. Interestingly, the normal

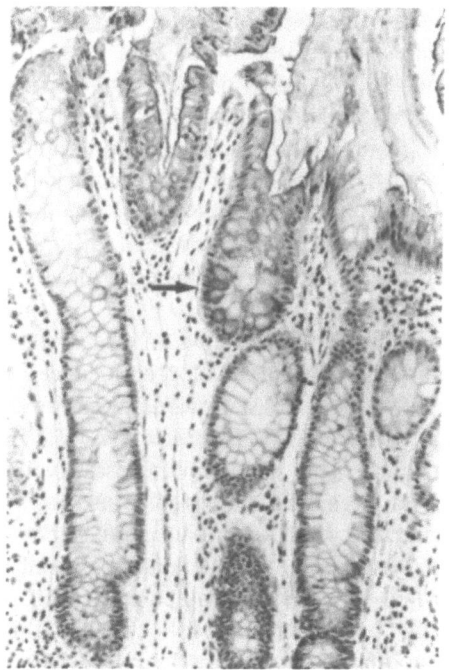

Fig. 9. Presence of sialosyl-Le^x within normal goblet cells of the upper crypt and surface epithelium of the large bowel mucosa (*arrow*). Normally cryptic due to O-acetylation of sialic acid, SLe^x can be demonstrated following alkali saponification. (KOH-immunoperoxidase reaction using monoclonal antibody Km-93: Serotec)

colorectal goblet cells in about 9% of caucasians [53] and a higher proportion of Asians [54] are stained with mPAS. This secretion of non-O-acetyl sialic acid is explained by genetic variability in the expression of the enzyme O-acetyl transferase (OAT). Nine percent of the caucasian population is homozygous for inactive OAT genes (OAT$^-$/OAT$^-$). This subgroup shows no increased susceptibility to cancer or any other colorectal disease. From the Hardy-Weinburg equilibrium, approximately 42% of the population would be predicted to be heterozygous (OAT$^+$/OAT$^-$). The presence of one active OAT gene allows O-acetylation to proceed because the inactive gene has a recessive effect. However, inactivation of the OAT$^+$ gene (through mutation or mitotic loss) would canvert the stem cell and its clonal progeny to the genotype OAT$^-$/OAT$^-$. This situation is visualized as a single mPAS-positive crypt, thereby proving that the crypt is a clonal unit [55]. The same crypt can be shown to express sialylated blood group structures (STn) without requiring the saponification step [49, 56].

The switch to the small intestinal phenotype by colorectal cancer is not limited to sialic acid but implicates the expression of type 1 blood group substances (in cancers of the distal large bowel) [14, 52, 57] and small intestinal brush border enzymes [58–61]. The concerted expression within colorectal cancer of type 1 blood group substances (SLe^a, SLe^x) and STn is likely to be due to a single underlying switch in direction of differentiation toward the small intestinal phenotype (as occurs in gastric cancer) [4, 62].

Sialic acid generally shows an $\alpha2,3$ linkage with the underlying sugar. Colorectal cancer mucin shows increased $\alpha2,6$ sialic acid linkage as demonstrated with the lectin *Sambucus nigra* agglutinin (SNA) [63]. This need not necessarily indicate induction of a new sialyltransferase, as STn is characterized by $\alpha2,6$ linkage and is present in cryptic form (due to O-acetylation of sialic acid) in normal large bowel goblet cells. This lectin-detected change may merely be "seeing" the sialic acid modification described above. The lectin *Trichosanthes japonica* has a high affinity to sialic acid in $\alpha2,6$ linkage with type 2 blood group structures, although the expression of such a structure [64] could be a component of concerted up-regulation of MUC1 in association with type 2 blood group substances.

Regional Variation Within Normal Colorectum and Intracryptal Variability

In the fetus, blood group substances are expressed throughout the gastrointestinal tract (as determined by Se and blood group genes—see above) but disappear from the distal large bowel during postnatal life [52, 65–67]. The sugar that is central to the Lewis blood group system is fucose. *Ulex europaeus* agglutinin-1 (UEA-1) binds to fucose, but its greatest affinity is for fucose in the configurations found in the type 2 chains H type 2 and Le^y [68]. UEA-1 binds to goblet cells in the proximal bowel (presumably H type 2 substance) and the columnar cell glycocalyx throughout the colorectum. In the distal bowel, UEA-1 binding is restricted to the apical membrane of crypt base columnar cells. Unlike goblet cell binding, the glycocalyceal pattern is independent of secretor status and presumably reflects the expression of Le^y. In cancers UEA-1 binding is enhanced, and its distribution follows non-mucin-like luminal material, MUC1, and sites that would indicate up-regulation of columnar cell secretory activity (glycocalyx and intracytoplasmic lumens) [69–73].

The binding pattern with the lectin *Dolichos biflorus* agglutinin (DBA) shows a pancolonic distribution [51, 69–71, 74, 75]. Binding is most marked within goblet cells of the upper crypt and surface epithelium (as with blood group substances) (Fig. 10). In the proximal colon it is restricted mainly to goblet cells within the surface epithelium, whereas in the distal bowel goblet cells are stained within the upper two-thirds of the crypt. DBA binds to GalNAc in terminal locations. GalNAc is also the first sugar to be added to the apoprotein (Fig. 1). STn is generated by $\alpha2,6$ sialylation of core GalNAc, which acts to stop further chain elongation [76, 77]. STn can be demonstrated indirectly within normal colorectal goblet cells by removing the sialic acid through the step of saponification-neuraminidase digestion [35]. DBA then binds to core GalNAc (Tn antigen) within goblet cells of the lower crypt. These observations indicate that mucins within goblet cells of the lower crypt contain a relatively high proportion of short carbohydrate chains, whereas long chains with a terminal GalNAc are more numerous in the goblet cells of the upper crypt. The

explained by the same mechanism, whether it occurs in normal goblet cells of the crypt base, goblet cells throughout transitional mucosa, or colorectal cancer mucin. Thus increased α2,6 sialyltransferase activity stops chain elongation through generation of the disaccharide sialosyl-Tn.

Columnar Cells as Sources of Secretory Material in Colorectal Cancer

Columnar cells are generally regarded as nonsecretory and absorptive in function. Yet it has been known for years that immature columnar cells within the normal crypt base region are secretory, with glycoprotein-containing vacuoles in the apical cytoplasm. These cells have been termed differentiating cells [80], intermediate cells [81], and, in species other than humans, vacuolated columnar cells [82]. Within this immature cell population evidence of glycoprotein production can be demonstrated with lectins (UEA-1) and monoclonal antibodies to Le^y [83], monoclonal antibodies to Le^x [16, 84, 85], PNA (probably recognizing the carbohydrate backbone structure Gal→GlcNAc) [86], and MUC1 probes (following periodate oxidation) (Figs. 5, 7). Sialosyl-Le^x is not normally seen in this location except focally in the hyperplastic (transitional) mucosa bordering colorectal cancer [84]. The lack of co-expression of SLe^x and MUC1 in normal mucosa has been demonstrated biochemically [27].

It is likely that colorectal cancer columnar cells are closely related to the immature columnar cell population within normal crypts. It would explain the co-localized expression of MUC1, Le^x, and Le^y within cancer secretions, albeit upregulated in comparison with normal. Expression of SLe^x, given the presence of Le^x, would be explained most simply by increased sialyltransferase activity.

In summary, cancer mucin production can be linked to two major lineages: goblet cells and columnar cells. The normal counterparts are immature crypt base goblet cells with their relative preponderance of short-chain oligosaccharides and, similarly, immature crypt base columnar cells.

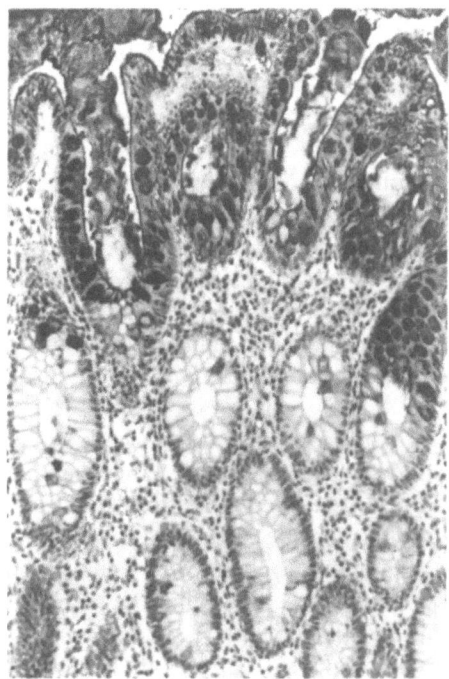

Fig. 10. Binding by lectin *Dolichos biflorus* agglutinin to goblet cells of the upper crypt and surface epithelium of normal proximal colon, indicating peripheral GalNAc. Goblet cells in the lower crypt are reactive after removal of sialic acid by the sequence KOH-neuraminidase (revealing structure Tn). (Direct lectin-peroxidase: Sigma)

short-chain mucins would be less viscous, thereby facilitating the upward extrusion of the crypt contents into the bowel lumen. The saponification-neuraminidase-DBA effect is particularly marked within the transitional mucosa (thickened and hyperplastic) bordering colorectal cancers [35, 69]. This finding indicates an excess of short chains (sialosyl-Tn) and would account for the lack of sulfation [78], reduced binding with DBA (without neuraminidase pretreatment) [35, 69], and increased binding with particular monoclonal antibodies to small intestinal mucin antigens [79]. Precisely the same observations apply to colorectal cancer mucin, indicating a relative preponderance of short-chain carbohydrates (sialosyl-Tn). This reaction would explain why cancer mucin can be more readily stripped of carbohydrate to reveal immunoreactive MUC2 than normal goblet cell mucin (through the sequence of saponification-neuraminidase-periodate oxidation) (Fig. 6). Short-chain preponderance can be

Biologic and Clinical Significance of Mucin Changes

Traditional models to explain the mucin changes in colorectal cancer have ignored the fundamental issues relating to lineage and lineage-specific function and have introduced convoluted biochemical explanations to account for the differences between normal tissue and cancer. There has been an uncritical tendency to regard particular biomarkers as cancer-specific and a general failure to integrate information gathered through different but complementary approaches. Not surprisingly, therefore, the traditional models have added little to our understanding of the pathogenesis, classification, or behavior of colorectal cancer. Furthermore, several decades of research have failed to enlighten or change the reporting practices of diagnostic pathologists. In the following section the lineage-based model is applied to precancerous and cancer-associated lesions and to cancer diagnosis, classification, and prognosis.

Precancerous and Cancer-Associated Lesions

Colorectal cancer mucus derived from cells of the goblet cell lineage can be distinguished from that of normal goblet cells by a variety of methods. However, many of these methods are based on the fact that sialic acid has switched from the colonic type (O-acetylated) to the small intestinal type (non-O-acetylated). This switch can be shown by means of mucin histochemistry and by numerous monoclonal antibodies to sialylated blood group structures (whose reactivities are influenced by the sialic acid change). This mucin change is seen with modifications of the PAS technique such as mPAS [87] in precancerous adenomas, where it is associated particularly with the grade of dysplasia, rather than size or villosity [62, 88]. The same change occurs in a high proportion of hyperplastic polyps [89] but is not especially evident in the transitional mucosa bordering colorectal cancer [90].

Distal bowel cancers show reappearance of type 1 blood group substances [52, 65–67]. This change also occurs in distal adenomas but is not related to adenoma size or villosity [91]. Hyperplastic polyps do not show this phenomenon but do reveal (like adenomas) deletion of Le^a [91].

The type 2 blood group structure Le^y is expressed within the normal crypt base [83, 92], but extended forms of Le^y are more cancer-specific and show correlations with increasing adenoma size, villosity, and dysplasia [92]. MUC1 (expressed only minimally within normal mucosa) does not show significant up-regulation in adenomas, except within areas of severe dysplasia amounting to carcinoma in situ [26]. Expression of SLe^x also correlates with increasing dysplasia [43], but this epitope co-localizes with both goblet cell- and columnar cell-derived secretions [27, 36, 37].

Hyperplastic polyps do not show cancer-associated change relevant to the columnar cell lineage, such as up-regulation of MUC1 or type 2 blood group substances (Le^x and Le^y) [85, 92]. The most fundamental change is one of lineage. The "columnar" cell population secretes large amounts of mucin, and the same cells express MUC2 (Fig. 1.11). It appears that the immature crypt base cells have switched their program of differentiation to produce a population of small goblet cells compressed between the larger, more conventional goblet cells. These smaller goblet cells may express SLe^x [85] (rendered noncryptic

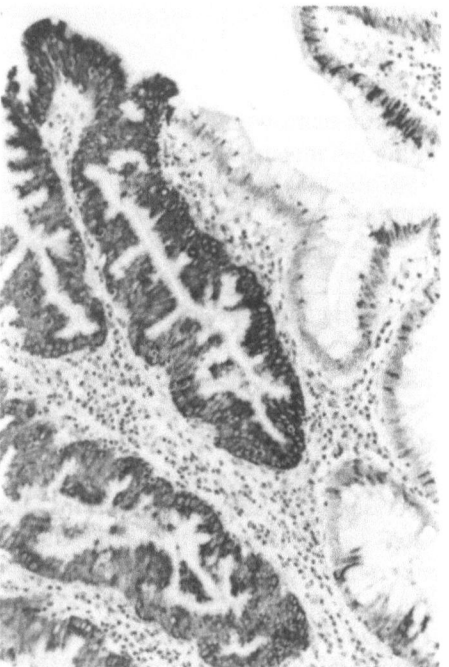

Fig. 11. Hyperplastic polyp showing enhanced MUC2 expression within large and small goblet cell populations. (Immunoperoxidase with monoclonal antibody CCP58 [18])

by the sialic acid modification) (Fig. 12). Focal STn expression may also occur in hyperplastic polyps [93]. The switch from columnar to goblet cell lineage explains the loss of secretory component production and immunoglobulin A (IgA) translocation [94], which is a normal function of both enterocytes and colonocytes. The hyperplastic polyp combines epithelial hyperplasia with altered differentiation (goblet cell metaplasia) and is probably a focal, reactive growth disorder secondary to ischemia, ulceration, or inflammation. Hyperplastic type change is common in the solitary rectal ulcer/mucosal prolapse syndrome and in ulcerative colitis [86], conditions associated with inflammation and ulceration.

The preceding observations are consistent with the widely accepted view of adenoma, rather than a hyperplastic polyp, being the important precursor of colorectal cancer. Cancer-associated changes occur in both but more consistently in adenomas. Although none of the changes is cancer-specific, it is their association with increasing grades of dysplasia in adenomas that provides powerful circumstantial evidence in favor of the adenoma–carcinoma sequence. Nevertheless, the hyperplastic polyp may be associated with a

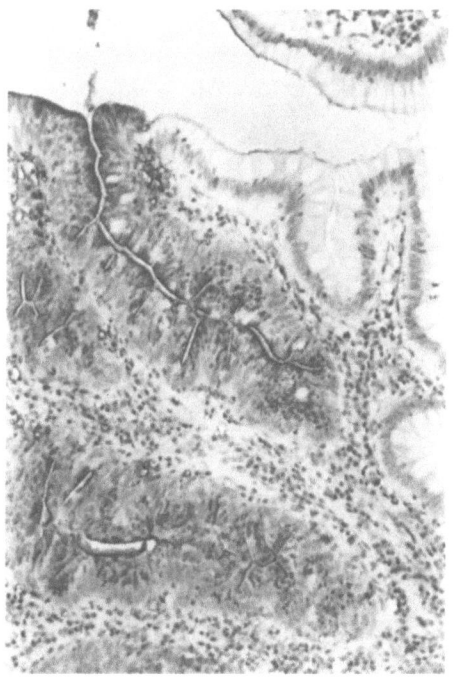

Fig. 12. Hyperplastic polyp showing enhanced expression of SLe^x, particularly in the population of small goblet cells. (Immunoperoxidase with monoclonal antibody Km-93)

separate histogenetic pathway involving the mixed polyp or serrated adenoma. This hypothesis is supported by recognition of the precancerous and familial nature of hyperplastic polyposis [95].

The concept of a precancerous field continues to retain some popularity, despite a number of conceptual difficulties. Such a field could not be neoplastic (clonal with cancer gene mutations), as crypts are clonal units and show little tendency to divide in the normal adult colon. With ulcerative colitis, however, regeneration following ulceration could lead to formation of a clonal patch, which could explain the demonstration of nondysplastic patches showing aneuploidy or *p53* mutation [96]. The hyperplastic mucosa (transitional mucosa) bordering colorectal cancer has been considered to represent a precancerous field change, but the change must be reactive rather than neoplastic for the reason given above. Transitional mucosa is characterized by a number of mucin changes, most obviously the switch from brown to blue with high iron diamine-alcian blue staining, indicating a relative increase in sialic acid over sulfate [78]. Although cancer mucin may show a similar change, it is not cancer-specific. Transitional mucosa has been shown to occur in a variety of settings, notably in all situations causing colorectal mucosal prolapse [97, 98]. It may be seen in the vicinity of various tumor types, epithelial and nonepithelial, primary and secondary [99]. Clearly, it is a secondary, reactive change and not a precancerous field change.

Nevertheless, there is evidence to suggest that a subset of colorectal cancers does not arise within adenoma but originates de novo. It has been suggested that positive immunostaining for MUC2 identifies cancers that arise from adenomas, whereas MUC2-negative cancers arise de novo [18]. This point is considered in more detail in the following section.

Attempts have been made to identify mucin changes in nondysplastic mucosa from subjects with ulcerative colitis, which might indicate an increased risk of developing cancer. Although no mucin changes are cancer-specific, alterations within nonneoplastic mucosa could be a marker of severe, long-standing injury and therefore serve as a cancer risk factor. The switch from *O*-acetyl to non-*O*-acetyl sialic acid has been demonstrated with mPAS [86] and by antibodies to STn [100] and has been shown to be associated with cancer risk in colitis. This sialic acid change coincides with morphologic evidence of hyperplasia [86], indicating that it is likely to be injury-related and not a marker of neoplastic progression per se. The difficult distinction between reactive and dysplastic change in ulcerative colitis is not facilitated by mucin histochemistry because of the lack of markers with a high degree of specificity and sensitivity for neoplastic change.

Diagnosis and Classification of Colorectal Cancer

Differences in the secretions of cancer versus normal mucosa have rarely been exploited for diagnostic purposes in clinical practice. Particular situations in which markers of altered goblet cell sialic acid could be usefully employed are the distinction between genuine and pseudoinvasion (particularly when epithelium is relatively well differentiated) and the diagnosis of well-differentiated mucinous adenocarcinoma. The change in sialic acid structure (O-acetyl to non-O-acetyl) is the basis for this distinction and can be demonstrated by mucin histochemistry (mPAS) or antibodies to sialosyl-Tn or sialosyl-Le^x. Upregulation of columnar cell secretory activity has a distinct morphologic counterpart: the presence of luminal (including intracytoplasmic luminal) secretions with an apparent absence of epithelial cells containing mucus. PAS staining of this material is intense and highlights an abnormally prominent glycocalyx. A similar pattern is seen with markers of columnar cell secretory activity: MUC1, Le^x (Fig. 13), Le^y, and sialosyl-Le^x. Sialosyl-Le^x would be a useful broad-spectrum marker of colorectal cancer, as it detects malignant goblet cell mucin without prior saponification as well as up-regulated columnar cell secretory material. Pathologists differ in their criteria for distinguishing dysplasia and carcinoma, and the preceding techniques could play a role in this debate.

It is in the classification of colorectal cancer that lineage-specific markers (or sets of markers) could be especially useful. The information derived from this approach may provide new insight into the etiology, pathogenesis, and behavior of cancer. If MUC2 and MUC1 are specific for goblet cells and columnar cells, respectively, the pattern closest to normal is MUC2$^+$/MUC1$^-$. This pattern is seen also in adenomas of all types. The pheno-

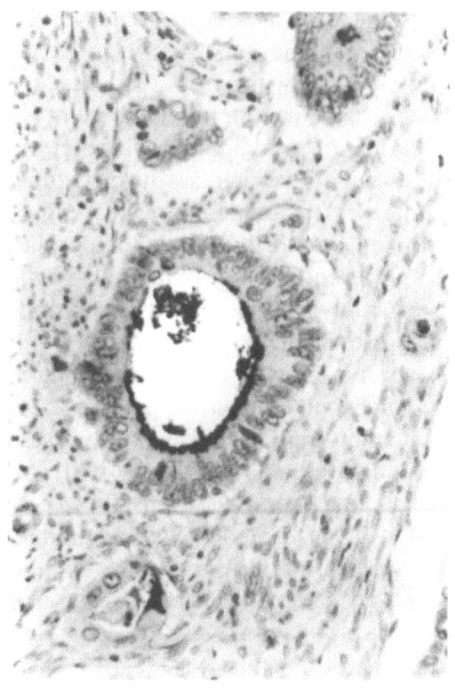

Fig. 13. Expression of Le^x within apical cytoplasm and glycocalyx of moderately differentiated adenocarcinoma. (Immunoperoxidase with monoclonal antibody CMRF7 [16])

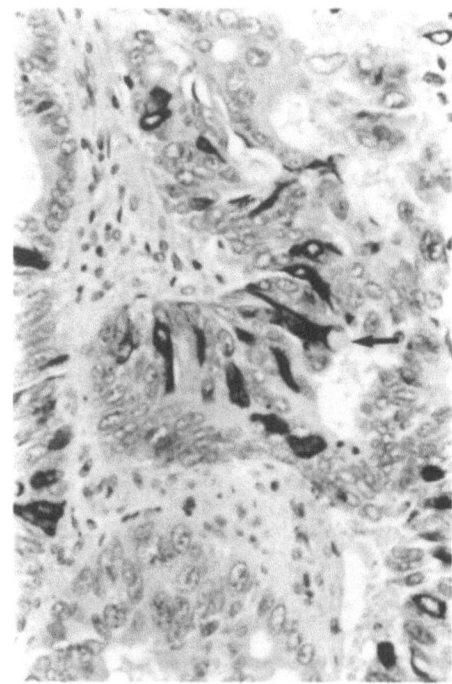

Fig. 14. Presence of MUC2$^+$ cells within a moderately differentiated adenocarcinoma. Note the obvious goblet cell theca in one cell (*arrow*). (Immunoperoxidase staining with monoclonal antibody CCP58 [18])

Table 2. MUC1/MUC2 phenotypes in relation to grade of differentiation of colorectal cancer

Differentiation	MUC2$^+$/MUC1$^-$	MUC2$^+$/MUC1$^+$	MUC2$^-$/MUC1$^+$	MUC2$^-$/MUC1$^-$
Good	0	1 (6.7%)	4 (17.4%)	0
Moderate	9 (100%)	11 (73.3%)	12 (52.2%)	3 (75.0%)
Poor	0	3 (20.0%)	7 (30.4%)	1 (25.0%)

The distribution does not differ significantly from the expected, though 8 of 11 poorly differentiated cancers were MUC2$^-$.

type MUC2$^+$/MUC1$^-$, was seen in 9 of 51 cancers (17.6%) (Fig. 14) (unpublished observations). Of these lesions, only one (11.1%) was associated with lymph node metastases. Conversely, MUC1 expression is known to be associated with a poor prognosis [101]. The phenotype MUC2$^+$/MUC1$^+$ included four of the five cancers within the series considered to be mucinous, the fifth being MUC2$^+$/MUC1$^-$. Mucinous cancers are associated with villous adenomas [102]. The mucinous phenotype probably results from a generalized secretory up-regulation of MUC1, MUC2, and presumably MUC3 and MUC4.

Phenotypes MUC2$^-$/MUC1$^+$ and MUC2$^-$/MUC1$^-$ would differ most from normal, but the MUC2 negativity could arise through either the absence of goblet cells or the cessation of mucin production by a population of nonfunctioning goblet cells. Interestingly, no cancers considered to arise de novo expressed MUC2 [18]. Further research is required to confirm the suggestion that MUC2$^-$ cancers arise de novo (from transformed undifferentiated cells within the normal crypt base). It is notable that the MUC2/MUC1 phenotype showed no significant correlation with grade of differentiation (Table 2), despite the relation with pathogenesis, mucinous type cancer, and lymph node spread.

The production of abundant mucin affects prognosis adversely, but the mechanism for this effect is unclear [103]. Physical dissection of the normal layers of the bowel wall could be one factor. A lymphocyte reaction is a good prognostic feature but is rarely evident in mucinous carcinomas. Mucin could act as an immunosuppressant. Particular carbohydrate structures, such as SLe^x, may serve as ligands to receptors expressed by endothelial cells (E-selectin), permitting cell–cell attachment, which would be a critical step in the process of metastasis [104, 105]. Because SLe^x is expressed constitutively by normal colorectal goblet cells [36], it may be loss of secretory polarity

(expression by lateral and basal membranes) that is more important in influencing cell–cell adhesion than the mere presence of particular carbohydrate structures.

Conclusion

The production of mucin is a process of considerable complexity requiring the synthesis of multiple gene products and subsequent coordinated bioassembly of one of the largest molecules in nature. Nevertheless, this highly energy-dependent activity may proceed within malignant cells in a manner essentially unchanged from that of their normal counterparts (just as keratin production may occur in squamous cell carcinomas). The distribution of mucin types within cancers may even recapitulate the normal crypt pattern [50], which suggests that the genetic control of mucin synthesis is largely independent of the essential molecular processes involved in carcinogenesis. Whether mucin production is increased or decreased depends on master genes involved in lineage differentiation and maturation. When relating function to lineage, one's ability to define differentiation and maturation in objective terms is greatly enhanced, but alterations in glycoprotein biochemistry must be regarded as epiphenomenal to the more fundamental changes within the malignant cell.

References

1. Podolsky DK (1985) Oligosaccharide structures of human colonic mucin. J Biol Chem 260:8262–8271
2. Podolsky DK (1985) Oligosaccharide structures of isolated human colonic mucin species. J Biol Chem 260:15510–15515
3. Slomiany BL, Murty VLN, Slomiany A (1980) Isolation and characterization of oligosaccharides from rat colonic mucus glycoprotein. J Biol Chem 255:9719–9723

4. Jass JR, Roberton AM (1994) Colorectal mucin histochemistry in health and disease: a critical review. Pathol Int 44:487–504

5. Feizi T, Gooi HC, Childs RA, Picard JK, Uemura K, Loomes LM, Thorpe SJ, Hounsell EF (1984) Tumour-associated and differentiation antigens on the carbohydrate moieties of mucin-type glycoproteins. Biochem Soc Trans 12:591–596

6. Picard JK, Feizi T (1983) Peanut lectin and anti-li antibodies reveal structural differences among human gastrointestinal glycoproteins. Mol Immunol 20:1215–1220

7. Campbell BJ, Finnie IA, Hounsell EF, Rhodes JM (1995) Direct demonstration of increased expression of Thomsen-Friedenreich (TF) antigen in colonic adenocarcinoma and ulcerative colitis mucin and its concealment in normal mucin. J Clin Invest 95:571–576

8. Ørntoft TF, Langkilde NC, Wiener H, Ottosen PD (1991) Cellular localization of PNA binding in colorectal adenomas: comparison with differentiation, nuclear:cell height ratio and effect of desialylation. APMIS 99:275–281

9. Boland CR, Montgomery CK, Kim YS (1982) Alterations in human colonic mucin occurring with cellular differentiation and malignant transformation. Proc Natl Acad Sci USA 79:2051–2055

10. Boland CR, Montgomery CK, Kim YS (1982) A cancer-associated mucin alteration in benign colonic polyps. Gastroenterology 82:664–672

11. Ørntoft TF, Mors NPO, Eriksen G, Jacobsen NO, Poulsen HS (1985) Comparative immunoperoxidase demonstration of T-antigens in human colorectal carcinoma and morphologically abnormal mucosa. Cancer Res 45:447–452

12. Ørntoft TF, Harving N, Langkilde NC (1990) O-linked mucin-type glycoproteins in normal and malignant colon mucosa: lack of T-antigen expression and accumulation of Tn and sialosyl-Tn antigens in carcinomas. Int J Cancer 45:666–672

13. Hanski C, Hanisch FG, Riecken EO (1992) Alteration of mucin-bound carbohydrate moieties in malignant transformation of colonic mucosa. Cancer J 5:332–342

14. Dabelsteen E, Graem N, Clausen H, Hakomori S-I (1988) Structural variations of blood group A antigens in human normal colon and carcinomas. Cancer Res 48:181–187

15. Henry S, Oriol F, Samuelson B (1995) Lewis histo-blood group system and associated secretory phenotypes. Vox Sang 69:166–182

16. Davidson SE, McKenzie JL, Beard MEJ, Hart DNJ (1988) The tissue distribution of the 3α-fucosyl-N-acetyl lactosamine determinant recognized by the CD15 monoclonal antibodies CMRF-7 and 27. Pathology 20:24–31

17. Tytgat KMAJ, Büller HA, Opdam FJM, Kim YS, Einerhand AWC, Dekker J (1994) Biosynthesis of human colonic mucin: MUC2 is the prominent secretory mucin. Gastroenterology 107:1352–1363

18. Blank M, Klussmann E, Kruger-Krasagakes S, Schmitt-Graff A, Stolte M, Bornhoeft G, Stein H, Xing P-X, McKenzie IFC, Verstijnen CPHJ, Riecken EO, Hanski C (1994) Expression of MUC2-mucin in colorectal adenomas and carcinomas of different histological types. Int J Cancer 59:301–306

19. Chang S-K, Dohrman AF, Basbaum CB, Ho SB, Tsuda T, Toribara NW, Gum JR, Kim YS (1994) Localization of mucin (MUC2 and MUC3) messenger RNA and peptide expression in human normal intestine and colon cancer. Gastroenterology 107:28–36

20. Toribara NW, Gum JR, Culhane PJ, Lagace RE, Hicks JW, Petersen GM, Kim YS (1991) MUC-2 Human small intestinal mucin gene structure: repeated arrays and polymorphism. J Clin Invest 88:1005–1013

21. Audie JP, Janin A, Porchet N, Copin MC, Gosselin B, Aubert JP (1993) Expression of human mucin genes in respiratory, digestive and reproductive tracts ascertained by in situ hybridisation. J Histochem Cytochem 41:1479–1485

22. Ho SB, Niehans GA, Lyftogt C, Yan PS, Cherwitz DL, Gum ET, Dahiya R, Kim YS (1993) Heterogeneity of mucin gene expression in normal and neoplastic tissues. Cancer Res 53:641–651

23. Porchet N, van Chong N, Dufosse J, Audie JP, Guyonnet-Duperat V, Gross MS, Denis C, Degand P, Bernheim A, Aubert JP (1991) Molecular cloning and chromosomal localisation of a novel human tracheo-bronchial mucin cDNA containing tandemly repeated sequences of 48 base pairs. Biochem Biophys Res Commun 175:414–422

24. Ogata S, Uehara H, Chen A, Itzkowitz SH (1992) Mucin gene expression in colonic tissues and cell lines. Cancer Res 52:5971–5978

25. Burchell J, Gendler S, Taylor-Papadimitriou J, Girling A, Lewis A, Millis R, Lamport D (1987) Development and characterization of breast cancer reactive monoclonal antibodies directed to the core protein of the human milk mucin. Gancer Res 47:5476–5482

26. Zotter S, Lossnitzer A, Hageman PC, Delemarre JFM, Hilkens J, Hilgers J (1987) Immunohistochemical localization of the epithelial marker MAM-6 in invasive malignancies and highly dysplastic adenomas of the large intestine. Lab Invest 57:193–199

27. Hanski C, Drechsler K, Hanisch FG, Sheehan J, Manske M, Okorek D, Klussmann E, Hanski M, Blank M, Xing P-X, McKenzie IFC, Devine PL,

Riecken EO (1993) Altered glycosylation of the MUC-1 protein core contributes to the colon carcinoma-associated increase of mucin-bound sialyl-Lewis[x] expression. Cancer Res 53:4082–4088

28. Gendler SJ, Lancaster CA, Taylor-Papadimitriou J, Duhig T, Peat N, Burchell J, Pemberton L, Lallani E-N, Wilson D (1990) Molecular cloning and expression of human tumour associated polymorphic epithelial mucin. J Biol Chem 265:15286–15293

29. Strous GJ, Dekker J (1992) Mucin-type glycoproteins. Crit Rev Biochem Mol Biol 27:57–92

30. Gum JR, Byrd JC, Hicks JW, Toribara NW, Lamport DTA, Kim YS (1989) Molecular cloning of human intestinal mucin cDNAs: sequence analysis and evidence for genetic polymorphism. J Biol Chem 264:6480–6487

31. Gum JR (1992) Mucin genes and the proteins they encode: structure, diversity, and regulation. Am J Respir Cell Mol Biol 7:557–564

32. Ohe Y, Hinoda Y, Irimura T, Imai K, Yachi A (1994) Expression of sulfated carbohydrate chains detected by monoclonal antibody 91.9H in human gastric cancer tissues. Jpn J Cancer Res 85:400–408

33. Carrato C, Balague C, De Bolos C, Gonzalex E, Gambus G, Planas J, Perini JM, Andreu D, Real FX (1994) Differential apomucin expression in normal and neoplastic human gastrointestinal tissues. Gastroenterology 107:160–172

34. Jass JR, Smith M (1992) Sialic acid and epithelial differentiation in colorectal polyps and cancer—a morphological, mucin and lectin histochemical study. Pathology 24:233–242

35. Jass JR, Allison LJ, Edgar SG (1995) Distribution of sialosyl Tn and Tn antigens within normal and malignant colorectal epithelium. J Pathol 176:143–149

36. Ogata S, Ho I, Chen A, Dubois D, Maklansky J, Singhal A, Hakomori S, Itzkowitz SH (1995) Tumor-associated sialylated antigens are constitutively expressed in normal human colonic mucosa. Cancer Res 55:1869–1874

37. Hanski C, Hanski ML, Zimmer T, Ogorek D, Devine P, Riecken EO (1995) Characterization of the major sialyl-Le(X)-positive mucins present in colon, colon carcinoma, and sera of patients with colorectal cancer. Cancer Res 55:928–933

38. Culling CFA, Reid PE, Clay MG, Dunn WL (1974) The histochemical demonstration of O-acylated sialic acid in gastrointestinal mucins: their association with the potassium hydroxide-periodic acid-Schiff effect. J Histochem Cytochem 22:826–831

39. Culling CFA, Reid PE, Worth AJ, Dunn WL (1977) A new histochemical technique of use in the interpretation and diagnosis of adenocarcinoma and villous lesions in the large intestine. J Clin Pathol 30:1056–1062

40. Reid PE, Culling CFA, Dunn WL, Ramey CW, Magil AB, Clay MG (1980) Differences between the O-acetylated sialic acids of the epithelial mucins of human colonic tumours and normal controls: a correlative chemical and histochemical study. J Histochem Cytochem 28:217–222

41. Reid PE, Dunn WL, Ramey CW, Coret E, Trueman L, Clay MG (1984) Histochemical identification of side chain substituted O-acylated sialic acids: the PAT-KOH-Bh-PAS and the PAPT-KOH-Bh-PAS procedures. Histochem J 16:623–639

42. Reid PE, Owen DA, Dunn WL, Ramey CW, Lazosky DA, Clay MG (1985) Chemical and histochemical studies of normal and diseased human gastrointestinal tract. III. Changes in the histochemical and chemical properties of the epithelial glycoproteins in the mucosa close to colonic tumours. Histochem J 17:171–181

43. Hanski C, Bornhoeft G, Topf N, Hermann U, Stein H, Riecken EO (1990) Detection of a mucin marker for the adenoma-carcinoma sequence in human colonic mucosa by monoclonal antibody AM-3. J Clin Pathol 43:379–384

44. Pilbrow SJ, Hertzog PJ, Linnane AW (1992) The adenoma-carcinoma sequence in the colorectum—early appearance of a hierarchy of small intestinal mucin antigen (SIMA) epitopes and correlation with malignant potential. Br J Cancer 66:748–757

45. Richman PI, Bodmer WF (1987) Monoclonal antibodies to human colorectal epithelium: markers for differentiation and tumour characterization. Int J Cancer 39:317–328

46. Hughes NR, Walls RS, Newland RC, Payne JE (1986) Gland to gland heterogeneity in histologically normal mucosa of colon cancer patients demonstrated by monoclonal antibodies to tissue-specific antigens. Cancer Res 46:5993–5999

47. Hughes NR, Walls RS, Newland RC, Payne JE (1986) Antigen expression in normal and neoplastic colonic mucosa: three tissue-specific antigens using monoclonal antibodies to isolated colonic glands. Cancer Res 46:2164–2171

48. Milton JD, Eccleston D, Parker N, Raouf A, Cubbin C, Hoffman J, Hart CA, Rhodes JM (1993) Distribution of O-acetylated sialomucin in the normal and diseased gastrointestinal tract shown by a new monoclonal antibody. J Clin Pathol 46:323–329

49. Jass JR, Allison LM, Edgar S (1994) Monoclonal antibody TKH2 to the cancer-associated epitope sialosyl Tn shows cross-reactivity with variants of

144   J.R. Jass

normal colorectal goblet cell mucin. Pathology 26:418–422

50. Cooper HS, Malecha MJ, Bass C, Fagel PL, Steplewski Z (1991) Expression of blood group antigens H-2, Le^y, and sialylated-Le^a in human colorectal carcinoma: an immunohistochemical study using double-labeling techniques. Am J Pathol 138:103

51. Jass JR, Allison LJ, Stewart SM, Lane MR (1994) *Dolichos biflorus* agglutinin binding in hereditary bowel cancer. Pathology 26:110–114

52. Yuan M, Itzkowitz SH, Palekar A, Shamsuddin AM, Phelps PC, Trump BF, Kim YS (1985) Distribution of blood group antigens A, B, H, Lewis^a, and Lewis^b in human normal, fetal, and malignant colonic tissue. Cancer Res 45:4499–4511

53. Sugihara K, Jass JR (1986) Colorectal goblet cell sialomucin heterogeneity: its relation to malignant disease. J Clin Pathol 39:1088–1095

54. Campbell F, Appleton MAC, Fuller CE, Williams GT, Williams ED (1993) Racial variation in O-acetylation of human colonic mucosa. J Pathol 174:169–174

55. Fuller CE, Davies RP, Willams GT, Williams ED (1990) Crypt restricted heterogeneity of goblet cell mucus glycoprotein in histologically normal human colonic mucosa: a potential marker of somatic mutation. Br J Cancer 61:382–384

56. Yonezawa S, Tachikawa T, Shin S, Sato E (1992) Sialosyl-Tn antigen: its distribution in normal human tissues and expression in adenocarcinomas. Am J Clin Pathol 98:167–174

57. Cooper HS, Marshall C, Ruggerio F, Steplewski Z (1987) Hyperplastic polyps of the colon and rectum: an immunohistochemical study with monoclonal antibodies against blood groups antigens (sialosyl-Le^a, Le^b, Le^x, Le^y, A, B, H). Lab Invest 57:421–428

58. Young GP, MaCrae FA, Gibson PR, Alexeyeff M, Whitehead RH (1992) Alimentary tract and pancreas: brush border hydrolases in normal and neoplastic colonic epithelium. J Gastroenterol Hepatol 7:347–354

59. Zweibaum A, Hauri H-P, Sterchi E, Chantret I, Haffen K, Bamat J, Sordat B (1984) Immunohistological evidence, obtained with monoclonal antibodies, of small intestinal brush border hydrolases in human colon cancers and foetal colons. Int J Cancer 34:591–598

60. Wiltz O, O'Hara CJ, Steele GDJ, Mercurio AM (1991) Expression of enzymatically active sucrase-isomaltase is a ubiquitous property of colon adenocarcinomas. Gastroenterology 100:1266–1278

61. Real FX, Xu M, Rosa Vila M, De Bolos C (1992) Intestinal brush-border associated enzymes: coordinated expression in colorectal cancer. Int J Cancer 51:173–181

62. Agawa S, Jass JR (1990) Sialic acid histochemistry and the adenoma-carcinoma sequence in colorectum. J Clin Pathol 43:528–532

63. Sata T, Roth J, Zuber C, Stamm B, Heitz PU (1991) Expression of α2,6-linked sialic acid residues in neoplastic but not in normal human colonic mucose: a lectin-gold cytochemical study with *Sambucus nigra* and *Maackia amurensis* lectins. Am J Pathol 139:1435–1448

64. Sakiyama T, Yamashita K, Ihida K, Nishimata H, Arima T, Murata F (1995) *Trichosanthes japonica* agglutinin I staining of human colonic carcinoma: a comparative study using monoclonal antibody against sialosyl-Tn antigen. Acta Histochem Cytochem 28:155–162

65. Cordon-Cardo C, Lloyd KO, Sakamoto J, McGroarty ME, Old LJ, Melamed MR (1986) Immunohistologic expression of blood-group antigens in normal human gastrointestinal tract and colonic carcinoma. Int J Cancer 37:667–676

66. Sakamoto J, Furukawa K, Cordon-Cordo C, Ying BWT, Rettig WJ, Oettgen HF, Old LJ, Lloyd KO (1986) Expression of Lewis^a, Lewis^b, x, and y blood group antigens in human colonic tumors and normal tissue and in human tumor-derived cell lines. Cancer Res 46:1553–1560

67. Schoentag R, Primus FJ, Kuhns W (1987) ABH and Lewis blood group expression in colorectal carcinoma. Cancer Res 47:1695–1700

68. Hindsgaul O, Norberg T, Le Pendu J, Lemieux RU (1982) Synthesis of type 2 human blood-group antigenic determinants: the H, X, and Y haptens and variations of the H type 2 determinant as probes for the combining site of the lectin 1 of *Ulex europaeus*. Carbohydr Res 109:109–142

69. Nakayama J, Ota M, Honda T, Katsuyama T (1987) Histochemical demonstration of sugar residues by lectin and immunocytochemical techniques for blood group antigens in human colon. Histochem J 19:454–464

70. Lee Y-S (1988) Lectin expression in neoplastic and non-neoplastic lesions of the rectum. Pathology 20:157–165

71. Calderó J, Campo E, Ascaso C, Ramos J, Panadés MJ, René JM (1989) Regional distribution of glycoconjugates in normal, transitional and neoplastic human colonic mucosa: a histochemical study using lectins. Virchows Arch [A] 415:347–356

72. Watanabe M, Ohtani H, Tanaka M, Ikehara H (1992) Appearance of *Ulex europaeus* agglutinin-1 and *Griffonia simplicifolia* agglutinin-1 binding sites on cancer cells in sigmo-rectal polyps. Acta Pathol Jpn 42:800–806

73. Jass JR, Allison LJ, Stewart SM (1993) *Ulex europaeus* agglutinin-1 binding in hereditary bowel cancer. Pathology 25:114–119

74. Kellokumpu I, Karhi K, Andersson LC (1986) Lectin-binding sites in normal, hyperplastic, adenomatous and carcinomatous human colorectal mucosa. Acta Pathol Microbiol Immunol Scand [A] 94:271–280

75. Campo E, Condom E, Palacin A, Quesada E, Cardesa A (1988) Lectin binding patterns in normal and neoplastic colonic mucosa: a study of *Dolichos biflorus* agglutinin, peanut agglutinin, and wheat germ agglutinin. Dis Colon Rectum 31:892–899

76. Schachter H, McQuire EY, Roseman S (1971) Sialic acids. XIII. A uridine diphosphate D-galactose: mucin galactosyl-transferase from porcine submaxillary gland. J Biol Chem 246:5312–5328

77. Kurosaka A, Nakayima H, Fuwakoshi I, Matsuyama M, Nagayo T, Yamashiwa I (1983) Structures of major oligosaccharides from a human rectal adenocarcinoma glycoprotein. J Biol Chem 285:11594–11598

78. Filipe MI (1979) Mucins in the human gastrointestinal epithelium: a review. Invest Cell Pathol 2:195–216

79. Pilbrow SJ, Hertzog PJ, Pinczower GD, Linnane AW (1992) Expression of a novel family of epitopes on small intestinal mucins in colorectal cancers, adjacent and remote mucosa. Tumor Biol 13:251–267

80. Lorenzsonn V, Trier JS (1968) The fine structure of human rectal mucosa: the epithelial lining of the base of the crypt. Gastroenterology 55:88–100

81. Kaye GI, Fenoglio CM, Pascal LRR, Lane N (1973) Comparative electron microscopic features of normal, hyperplastic and adenomatous human colonic epithelium. Gastroenterology 64:926–945

82. Chang WWL, Leblond CP (1971) Renewal of the epithelium in the descending colon of the mouse. I. Presence of three cell populations: vacuolated-columnar, mucous and argentaffin. Am J Anat 131:73–100

83. Brown A, Ellis IO, Embleton MJ, Baldwin RW, Turner DR, Hardcastle JD (1984) Immunohistochemical localization of Y hapten and the structurally related H type-2 blood-group antigen on large-bowel tumours and normal adult tissues. Int J Cancer 33:727–736

84. Itzkowitz SH, Yuan M, Fukushi Y, Pakelar A, Phelps PC, Shamsuddin AM, Trump BF, Hakomori S, Kim YS (1986) Lewis^x- and sialylated Lewis^x-related antigen expression in human malignant and nonmalignant colonic tissues. Cancer Res 46:2627–2632

85. Yuan M, Itzkowitz SH, Ferrell LD, Fukushi Y, Palekar A, Hakomori S, Kim YS (1987) Expression of Lewis^x and sialylated Lewis^x antigens in human colorectal polyps. J Natl Cancer Inst 78:479–488

86. Jass JR, England J, Miller K (1986) Value of mucin histochemistry in follow up surveillance of patients with long standing ulcerative colitis. J Clin Pathol 39:393–398

87. Veh RW, Meessen D, Kuntz D, May B (1982) Colonic carcinogenesis. In: Malt RA, Williamson RCN (eds). MTP, Lancaster, UK, pp 355–365

88. Eide TJ, Nielsen K, Solberg S (1987) Dysplasia in colorectal adenomas related to the presence of O-acetylated sialic mucin and to morphometric measurements. APMIS 95:365–369

89. Jass JR, Filipe MI, Abbas E, Falcon CA, Wilson Y, Lovell D (1984) A morphologic and histochemical study of metaplastic polyps of the colorectum. Cancer 53:510–515

90. Hutchins JT, Reading CL, Giavazzi R, Hoaglund J, Jessup JM (1988) Distribution of mono-, di-, and tri-O-acetylated sialic acids in normal and neoplastic colon. Cancer Res 48:483–489

91. Itzkowitz SH, Yuan M, Ferrell LD, Palekar A, Kim YS (1986) Cancer-associated alterations of blood group antigen expression in human colorectal polyps. Cancer Res 46:5976–5984

92. Kim YS, Yuan M, Itzkowitz SH, Sun Q, Kaizu T, Palekar A, Trump BF, Hakomori S (1986) Expression of Le^y and extended Le^y blood group-related antigens in human malignant, premalignant, and nonmalignant colonic tissues. Cancer Res 46:5985–5992

93. Itzkowitz SH, Bloom EJ, Lau T-S, Kim YS (1992) Mucin associated Tn and sialosyl-Tn antigen expression in colorectal polyps. Gut 33:518–523

94. Jass JR, Faludy J (1985) Immunohistochemical demonstration of IgA and secretory component in relation to epithelial cell differentiation in normal colorectal mucosa and metaplastic polyp: a semiquantitative study. Histochem J 17:373–380

95. Jeevaratnam P, Cottier DS, Browett PJ, Van de Water NS, Pokos V, Jass JR (1996) Familial giant hyperplastic polyposis predisposing to colorectal cancer: a new hereditary bowel cancer syndrome. Pathology 179:20–25

96. Burmer GC, Rabinovitch PS, Haggitt RC, Crispin DA, Brentnall TA, Kolli VR, Stevens AC, Rubin CE (1993) Neoplastic progression in ulcerative colitis: histology, DNA content and loss of a *p53* allele. Gastroenterology 103:1602–1610

97. Isaacson P, Attwood PRA (1979) Failure to demonstrate specificity of the morphological and histochemical changes in mucosa adjacent to colonic carcinoma (transitional mucosa). J Clin Pathol 32:214–218

146   J.R. Jass

98. Williams GT (1985) Transitional mucosa of the large intestine. Histopathology 9:1237–1243

99. Pilbrow SJ, Hertzog PJ, Linnane AW (1993) Differentiation-associated changes in mucin glycoprotein antigenicity in mucosa adjacent to rare gastrointestinal tract tumours of non-mucosal origin. J Pathol 169:259–267

100. Itzkowitz SH, Marshall A, Kornbluth A, Harpaz N, McHugh JBD, Ahnen D, Sachar DB (1995) Sialosyl-Tn antigen: initial report of a new marker of malignant progression in long-standing ulcerative colitis. Gastroenterology 109:490–497

101. Nakamori S, Ota DM, Cleary KR, Shirotani K, Irimura T (1994) MUC1 mucin expression as a marker of progression and metastasis of human colorectal carcinoma. Gastroenterology 106:353–361

102. Hanski C (1995) Is mucinous carcinoma of the colorectum a distinct genetic entity? Br J Cancer 72:1350–1356

103. Schwartz B, Bresalier RS, Kim YS (1992) The role of mucin in colon-cancer metastasis. Int J Cancer 52:60–65

104. Hoff SD, Irimura T, Matsushita Y, Ota DM, Cleary KR, Hakomori S (1990) Metastatic potential of colon carcinoma. Arch Surg 125:206–209

105. Kawakami H, Ito M, Miura Y, Hirano H (1992) Lectin-histochemical studies on the process of liver metastasis of mouse colon carcinoma (colon 26) cells. Acta Histochem Cytochem 25:577–582

Critical Determinants of Human Colon Cancer Metastasis

Isaiah J. Fidler

Summary. By the time of diagnosis, human colorectal carcinomas are heterogeneous and contain a large number of subpopulations of cells with diverse biological properties that include invasion and metastasis. The tumor cell heterogeneity is directed by both genetic and epigenetic events and may also be modulated by cell-to-cell interactions and tissue microenvironments. To produce metastasis, tumor cells must complete a series of sequential, interrelated, selective steps that include growth, vascularization, invasion into host stroma and entrance into the circulation, survival in the circulation and adhesion to capillary endothelial cells, extravasation into the organ parenchyma, response to local growth factors, proliferation, and induction of vascularization. All of these sequential steps must be completed by tumor cells if a metastasis is to develop. Although some of the steps in this process contain stochastic elements, metastasis as a whole favors the survival and growth of a few subpopulations of tumor cells that preexist within the heterogeneous parent neoplasm. Metastases can have a clonal origin, and different metastases can originate from the proliferation of single cells. Because each of the discrete steps in the pathogenesis of a metastasis is regulated by one or several independent genes, the identification of cells with metastatic potential in heterogeneous primary human tumors requires multiparametric–multivariate analysis of gene expression. The pathogenesis of metastasis depends on multiple favorable interactions of metastatic cells with host homeostatic mechanisms. Interruption of one or more of these interactions can lead to the inhibition or eradication of cancer metastasis. For many years, all of our efforts to treat cancer have concentrated on the inhibition or destruction of tumor cells. The recent advancements in our understanding of the biologic basis of cancer metastasis recommend that metastases could be eradicated by both treatment of the tumor cells and modulation of the host environment.

The major cause of death from colonic or rectal carcinoma is metastases that are resistant to conventional therapy [1]. For this reason, once colon cancer is diagnosed, the urgent question is whether the cancer is localized or has already spread to the regional lymph nodes and distant organs. The major obstacle to treatment of metastasis is the biologic heterogeneity of neoplasms. By the time of diagnosis, a malignant tumor contains multiple cell populations with various properties, such as growth rate, karyotype, cell surface properties, antigenicity, immunogenicity, marker enzymes, sensitivity to various cytokines and cytotoxic drugs, and the ability to invade and produce metastasis [1–6]. A second obstacle to therapy is the finding that different organ environments can modify a metastatic tumor cell's response to therapy [7, 8]. Understanding the mechanisms responsible for the development of biologic heterogeneity in primary cancers and metastases and the process by which tumor cells invade local tissues and spread to distant organs is a primary goal of cancer research. A better understanding of these processes should allow the design of more effective therapy for colon cancer and improvements in the way oncologists deal with disseminated cancer. In this chapter, I review recent data on the biology of human colon cancer metastasis and the host factors that influence this process.

Pathogenesis of a Metastasis

The process of cancer metastasis consists of a series of sequential steps, each of which can be rate-limiting [1]. After the initial transforming event, whether unicellular or multicellular, the growth of

Department of Cell Biology, The University of Texas M. D. Anderson Cancer Center, 1515 Holcombe Boulevard, Houston, TX 77030, U.S.A

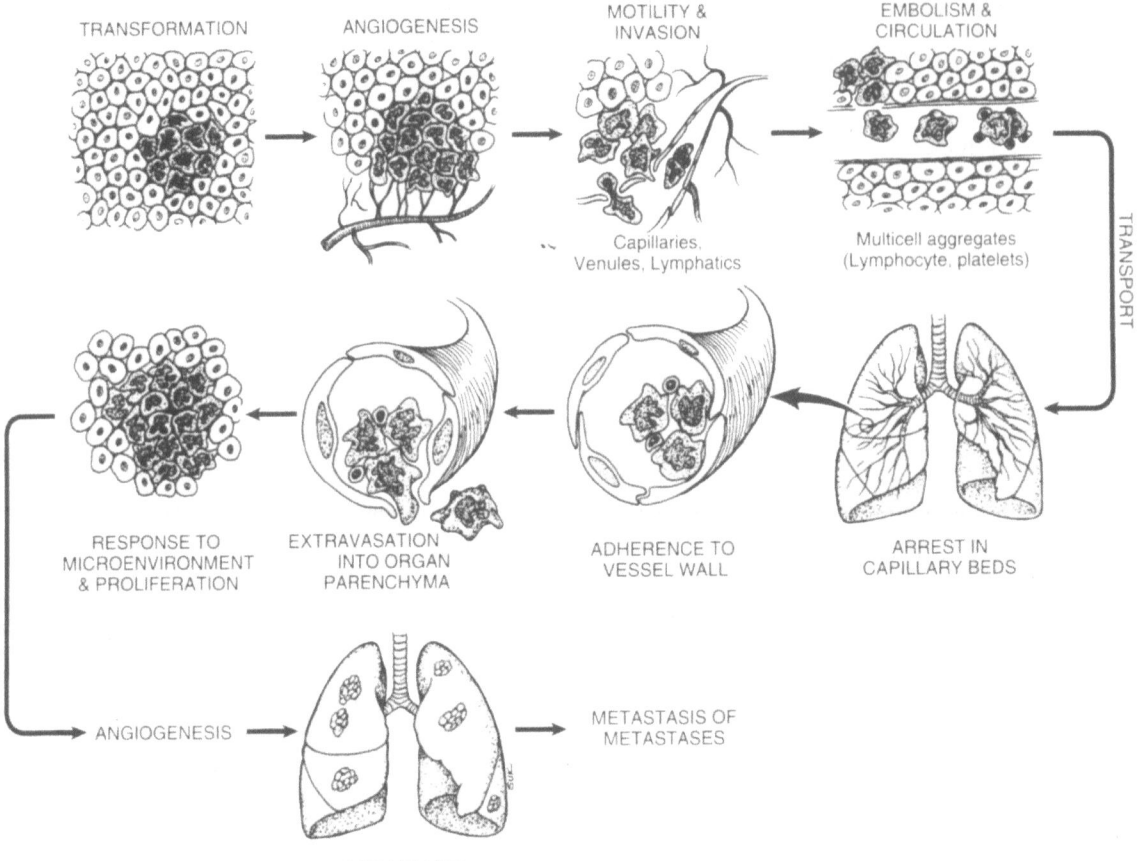

Fig. 1. Pathogenesis of cancer metastasis. To produce metastasis, tumor cells must detach from the primary tumor, invade the stroma to enter the circulation, survive in the circulation to arrest in the capillary bed, adhere to subendothelial basement membrane, extravasate into the organ parenchyma, respond to paracrine growth factors, proliferate and induce angiogenesis, and evade host defenses. To produce a metastasis, tumor cells must complete every step in the process. If they fail to complete one step, the cells are eliminated. The outcome of these multiple sequential, selective, and interdependent steps depends on the interaction of tumor cells with homeostatic factors

neoplastic cells must be progressive. Extensive vascularization must occur if a tumor mass is to exceed 2 mm in diameter [9]. Local invasion of the host stroma by some tumor cells, the next step, could occur by several mechanisms that are not mutually exclusive [10]. For example, thin-walled venules, like lymphatic channels, offer little resistance to penetration by tumor cells and provide the most common pathways for tumor cell entry into the circulation. Although clinical observations have suggested that carcinomas frequently metastasize and grow via the lymphatic system and that malignant tumors of mesenchymal origin (e.g., melanoma) more often spread by the hematogenous route, the presence of numerous venolymphatic anastomoses invalidates this belief [11]. Detachment and embolization of small tumor cell aggregates occur next, and tumor cells that survive the circulation must arrest in the capillary beds of organs. Extravasation is the next step, probably occuring by the same mechanisms that influence initial invasion; and proliferation within the organ parenchyma completes the metastatic process. To produce detectable lesions, the metastases must develop a vascular network, evade the host immune system, and respond to organ-specific factors that influence their growth [7]. Once they do so, the cells can invade host stroma, penetrate blood vessels, and enter the circulation to produce secondary metastases, the so-called metastasis of metastases [2, 3, 12] (Fig. 1).

Growth at Primary Site and Angiogenesis

The growth and survival of cells depend on an adequate supply of oxygen, growth factors, and the removal of toxic molecules. Oxygen can diffuse radially from capillaries for only 150 to 200 μm. When distances exceed this limit, cell death follows [13]. Thus the expansion of tumor masses beyond 2 mm in diameter depends on the development of an adequate blood supply (i.e., angiogenesis) [14].

The induction of angiogenesis is mediated by multiple molecules that are released by both tumor cells and host cells. Among these molecules are members of the fibroblast growth factor family, vascular endothelial cell growth factor (VEGF) also called vascular permeability factor (VPF), interleukin-8, angiogenin, angiotropin, epidermal growth factor, fibrin, platelet-derived endothelial cell growth factor, transforming growth factors alpha (TGF-α) and beta (TGF-β), and tumor necrosis factor-alpha (TNF-α) [13–18]. Angiogenesis consists of sequential steps: Endothelial cells must proliferate, migrate, and penetrate host stroma and the extracellular matrix (ECM). To yield a capillary, the endothelial cells must also undergo morphogenesis. The vasculature of many solid tumors is not identical to that in normal tissues, with differences in cellular composition, permeability, vessel stability, and regulation of growth [19]. The extent of angiogenesis is determined by the balance between factors that stimulate and those that inhibit new blood vessel growth. In many normal tissues the inhibitory influence predominates [9]. In contrast, many neoplastic cells switch from an angiogenesis-inhibiting to an angiogenesis-stimulating phenotype, which coincides with the loss of the wild-type allele of the p53 tumor suppressor gene and is the result of reduced production of antiangiogenic factor TSP-1 [20].

In rodent and human colonic epithelial cells, transformation by activated *ras* oncogenes has been shown to up-regulate the activity of the angiogenic molecule VEGF [21]. Because the human VEGF/VPF promoter contains four potential AP1 sites that are key components of the *ras* sig-

nal pathway, mutant *ras* genes may up-regulate angiogenic activity via direct transcriptional control of VEGF/VPF. Hence the transformation by a dominant oncogene can contribute to tumorigenicity by up-regulation of growth factor or receptor activity and up-regulation of angiogensis [20, 21].

Benign neoplasms are sparsely vascularized and tend to grow slowly, whereas malignant neoplasms are highly vascular and fast-growing [1]. The increase in vasculature also increases the probability that tumor cells will enter the circulation and produce metastasis [22–24]. Many [25–29] but not all [30, 31] studies have concluded that increased microvessel density in the areas of most intense neovascularization is a significant and independent prognostic indicator for early-stage breast cancer. Studies with other neoplasms, such as prostate cancer [32, 33], melanoma [34], ovarian carcinoma [35], gastric carcinoma [36], and colon carcinoma [37], also support the conclusion that the angiogenesis index is a useful prognostic factor.

Tumor Cell Invasion

After initial growth in the mucosa, colon carcinomas grow mainly in the transverse axis leading to circumferential tumors [38–40]. A tumor that traverses the muscularis mucosa and infiltrates the submucosa is termed invasive. As the tumor penetrates the gut wall, it can invade neighboring structures; adjacent organ involvement occurs in 10% of patients [39–41]. An additional pattern of local spread is perineural invasion, or spread along the perineural spaces that may reach as far as 10 cm from the primary tumor [42].

At least three nonmutually excluding mechanisms can be involved in tumor cell invasion of tissues. First, mechanical pressure produced by rapidly proliferating neoplasms may force cords of tumor cells along tissue planes of least resistance [43–45].

Second, increased cell motility can contribute to tumor cell invasion. Most tumor cells possess the necessary cytoplasmic machinery for active locomotion [46–48], and increased tumor cell motility is preceded by a loss of cell-to-cell cohesive forces. In epithelial cells the loss of cell-to-cell contact is associated with down-regulation of the expression of E-cadherin, a cell surface glycoprotein involved in calcium-dependent homotypic cell-to-cell adhesion [49, 50]. E-cadherin is located at the epithelial junction complex and is responsible for the organization, maintenance, and morphogenesis of epithelial tissue [50, 51]. Reduced levels of E-cadherin are associated with a decrease in cellular and tissue differentiation and the increased grade of various epithelial neoplasms [50–56]. Many differentiated carcinomas express high levels of E-cadherin mRNA, as do adjacent normal epithelial cells, whereas poorly differentiated carcinomas do not [55, 56]. Mutations in the E-cadherin gene [57] and abnormalities of α-catenin, which is an E-cadherin-associated protein, have been associated with the transition of cells from the noninvasive to the invasive phenotype [58, 59]; and the transfection of E-cadherin-encoding cDNA into invasive cancer cells has been shown to inhibit their motility and invasiveness [60, 61]. The motility of tumor cells is associated with the alteration of cytoskeletal elements and the response to the cytokine automotility factor [62–66], scatter factor [67, 68], thromboplastin [69], extracellular matrix [70], and monocyte-derived monokines [71].

Third, invasive tumor cells secrete enzymes capable of degrading basement membranes, which constitute a barrier between epithelial cells and the stroma. Epithelial cells and stromal cells produce a complex mixture of laminin, collagens, proteoglycans, and other molecules; this mixture contains ligands for adhesion receptors and is permeable to molecules but not to cells [72–78]. Colon cancer cells also produce and secrete basement membrane components such as laminin [79]. Well-differentiated human colon carcinomas produce a large amount of laminin, whereas poorly differentiated colon carcinomas produce discontinuous basement membranes that are low in laminin [80]. A decrease in laminin content has also been demonstrated in basement membranes of dysplastic adenomatous polyps, but discontinuity of basement membranes was noted only in colon carcinomas [79–82]. Proteoglycans, including chondroitin sulfate, heparan sulfate, hyaluronate, and heparin, comprise another major constituent of the ECM, whose major function may be a reservoir for growth factors [83] that can be released in an active form by degradation of the ECM [84].

To invade the basement membrane, a tumor cell must first attach to ECM components by a receptor–ligand interaction. One group of such cell surface receptors are the integrins. Some members of the integrin family specifically bind cells to laminin, collagen, or fibronectin [85, 86]. Many integrins that bind to components of the extracellular matrix are expressed on the surface of human colon carcinoma cells [86–88]. Tumor progression has been associated with a gradual decrease of integrin expression, suggesting that the loss of integrins may facilitate detachment from a primary neoplasm [87].

Another group of proteins that bind to ECM components are the lectins. Normal intestinal epithelial cells contain two highly conserved galactins of 31.0 and 14.5 kDa [89, 90]. The expression of the 31-kDa lectin is increased in carcinomas, absent in adenomas, and weak in normal epithelium. Its intramural content is significantly associated with carcinoembryonic antigen (CEA) [91]. CD44, a receptor responsible for lymphocyte homing [92, 93], binds to ECM components and to CEA [93, 94]. It is expressed as a 90-kDa protein in lymphocytes and as a 150- to 180-kDa protein in epithelial cells [94]. The production of CD44 gene transcript is markedly increased in human colon cancer cells as compared with normal adjacent mucosa [95]. CD44 may regulate migration through the ECM, and an abnormal pattern of activity of the CD44 gene has been reported in metastatic human colon carcinomas [96].

Subsequent to binding, tumor cells can degrade connective tissue ECM and basement membrane components [97]. Metastatic tumor cells produce various proteases and glucosidases capable of degrading extracellular matrix components. The production of enzymes such as type IV collagenase (gelatinase, matrix metalloproteinase) and heparinase in metastatic tumor cells correlates with the invasive capacity of human colon cancer cells. Type IV collagenolytic metalloproteinases with apparent molecular masses of 98, 92, 80, 68, and 64 kDa have been detected in highly metastatic cells. Poorly metastatic cells, on the other hand, appear to secrete low amounts of only the 92-kDa metalloproteinase [98].

Under experimental conditions collagenase activity can be stimulated by purified mucin products that are associated with poor prognosis [99]. Human colon cancer cells also secrete a plasminogen activator, urokinase, which activates the serine protease plasmin from plasminogen. Plasmin induces basement membrane (laminin) degradation and invasion. It further degrades the basement membrane by activation of collagenase type

IV, which in turn depletes the membrane of both laminin and collagen type IV [100]. Furthermore, plasmin acts as a chemoattractant for tumor cells [101].

Metastasis by Direct Extension

Intraluminal spread occurs by the release of viable cells from the mucosal surface of the primary tumor and their distal implantation, usually at the site of a denuded surface, such as a fistula, ulcer, or hemorrhoid. Serosal cell shedding accounts for intraperitoneal seeding and carcinomatosis seen even in the absence of lymphatic or hematogeneous spread. Other forms of implantation are related to surgical manipulations. The incidence of suture line recurrence is about 10%. About half of these recurrences are believed to be the result of cell shedding or inadequate excision during surgery [102]. Tumors can also develop in an abdominal scar [103] or at the mucocutaneous margin of a colostomy [104].

Lymphatic Metastasis

Early clinical observations suggested that carcinomas frequently spread and grow in the lymphatic system, whereas metastatic tumors of mesenchymal origin spread by means of the bloodstream [105–107]. This division is arbitrary because the two routes are interlinked. Cancer cells may invade the lymphatics directly or may gain access to them via blood vessels. Tumor cells can readily pass from blood to lymphatic channels and back again, indicating that venolymphatic communications via the interstitial spaces of lymph nodes and other tissues exist [108–110]. Rather than depending on the tissue of origin, the pattern of lymph node involvement (growth of tumor cells within a lymph node) depends on the site of the primary tumor and its lymphatic drainage [111–113]. Microscopic examinations of serial sections of blocks of tissues between a primary tumor and the regional lymph node draining the site demonstrated that lodging of tumor cell emboli in lymph vessels is responsible for lymphatic metastasis [113]. Tumor emboli may be trapped in the first lymph node encountered on their route; alternatively, they may traverse lymph nodes or even bypass them to form distant nodal metastases (the "skip"

metastasis) [113]. That lymphatic metastases may grow in distant rather than proximal lymph nodes even when the regional lymph nodes are not grossly involved had been recognized by Paget as early as 1889 [114] but was ignored when surgical approaches to cancer were considered.

Whether regional lymph nodes can retain tumor cells and serve as a temporary barrier for cell dissemination has been a controversial issue. This question has significant clinical implications regarding the extent of surgical resection and lymph node dissection required for colon cancer treatment. Answering this question experimentally is not simple because in experimental models normal lymph nodes are usually subjected to a sudden challenge with a large number of tumor cells, a situation that may not be analogous to small numbers of cancer cells that reach the lymph nodes continuously [115].

Hematogenous Metastasis

The most common site of hematogenous metastasis for colon carcinoma is the liver, followed by the lung. In 40% of autopsies the liver has been the only site involved. Involvement of other sites in the absence of metastases in the liver or lung is rare [116]. During hematogenous metastasis, metastatic cells must survive transport in the circulation, adhere to small blood vessels or capillaries, and invade the vessel wall to enter the parenchyma. Therefore the presence of tumor cells in the circulation does not constitute a metastasis because most circulating cells die rapidly [116–119]. Using radiolabeled mouse B16 melanoma cells, we found that by 24 hours after entry into the circulation fewer than 1% of the cells were still viable and fewer than 0.1% of these tumor cells eventually produced metastases [118]. Therefore the greater the number of cells released by a primary tumor, the greater is the probability that some cells survive to form metastases, as most cells are obviously destroyed in the bloodstream. The development of necrosis and hemorrhage in large tumors facilitates tumor cell entry into the circulation [117]. The rapid death of most circulating tumor cells is probably due to simple mechanical factors, such as blood turbulence or host defense mechanisms, including immune cells and nonimmune cells (e.g. endothelial cells) or production of nitric oxide [118, 119]. Tumor cell survival can be increased if tumor cells aggregate with each other [120, 121] or with host cells such as platelets [122] or lymphocytes [123]. Once metastatic cells reach the microcirculation, they interact with cells of the vascular endothelium. These interactions include nonspecific mechanical lodgement of tumor cell emboli and formation of adhesions to the endothelial cells. These properties of tumor cells, in part, determine their organ distribution [124, 125].

Tumor Cell Arrest, Adhesion, and Extravasation into the Organ Parenchyma

Tumor emboli must attach firmly (as contrasted with passive lodgement) to the internal layer of the intima of a vessel; and after attachment the successful tumor cells must penetrate the vessel wall to reach and grow in extravascular tissues [126–128]. The rapid turnover and shedding of endothelial cells from the capillary wall is a normal and continuous physiologic event. Thus the wear and tear of endothelium may lead to temporary gaps that expose the basement membrane. Tumor cells can attach firmly to a vessel wall if the endothelium is damaged or contains gaps [128, 129]. Because tumor cells can interact with platelets during transport in the circulation [121], any damage to endothelium may lead to adherence of platelets, which is enhanced by early deposition of fibrinogen on the endothelial cell surface [130, 131]. The initial arrest there of a tumor–platelet–lymphocyte clump could be the crucial first step in lodgement and could occur via the adherence of platelets associated with tumor cells to platelets adhering to the damaged endothelium [129–131]. The formation of fibrin clots at sites of tumor cell arrest in the microcirculation can damage blood vessels [132]. The increased coagulability often observed in the blood of patients with cancer may be related to the high levels of thromboplastin found in certain tumors, the production of high levels of procoagulant-A activity [133], or the presence of phosphatidylserine in the outer leaflet of tumor cell membranes [134].

Other factors, such as mechanical trapping of large tumor cell aggregates in small-diameter vessels, must also be considered. If the resulting emboli are large, a larger proportion of implanted cells survive to produce metastases [23, 119]. Tumor cells with high metastatic potential tend to aggregate with each other (homotypic clumps) or with lymphocytes and platelets (heterotypic clumps) [135]. Clumps of tumor cells can be arrested in the vasculature simply by a wedging process [128]. Tumor cell attachment in the microvasculature can also be enhanced by localized trauma. Tissue damaged physically, chemically, or even by reduced oxygen tension provides a better site for attachment [136].

The adhesion of tumor cells to the vascular endothelium is regulated by mechanisms similar to those used by leukocytes. The initial attachment of leukocytes to vascular endothelial cells is regulated by the selectin family of adhesion molecules, which consists of three closely related cell surface molecules [137]. E-selectin, which is expressed by endothelial cells, mediates the initial attachment of lymphocytes (and tumor cells) by interaction with specific carbohydrate ligands that contain sialylated fucosylated lactosamines [138]. The expression of mucin-type carbohydrates on the surface of human colon carcinoma has been correlated with their metastatic potential [139], perhaps through differential interaction with E-selectins expressed on specific endothelial cells [130, 140]. The development of firm adhesion requires the interaction of other adhesion molecules, another selective process during metastasis. Several classes of cell-to-cell adhesion molecules regulate this adhesion, including the hyaluronate receptor CD44 and its splice variants [141–144], the integrins $\alpha 5\beta 1$, $\alpha 6\beta 1$, and $\alpha 6\beta 4$ [145–147], and the galactoside-binding galectin-3 [148]. The arrest of tumor cells in capillary beds leads to the retraction of endothelial cells [149] and exposure of tumor cells to the ECM. The adhesion of metastatic cells to components of the ECM (e.g., fibronectin, laminin, and thrombospondin) facilitates metastasis to specific tissues [150, 151], and peptides containing sequences of these components of the ECM can reduce formation of hematogenous metastases [138, 151].

After they arrest or adhere, tumor cells may traverse the vessel wall to reach extravascular tissues. Tumor cells can grow and destroy the surrounding vessel, invade by penetrating the endothelial basement membrane, or follow migrating white blood cells [106]. Malignant cells frequently penetrate thin-walled capillaries but rarely invade arteries or arteriole walls, which are rich in elastin fibers [106, 107]. The extravasation of malignant cells at particular secondary sites also involves their responses to tissue or organ factors. Tumor cells can recognize tissue-specific motility factors that direct their movement and invasion [152].

Growth

The final step in metastasis is tumor cell proliferation at secondary sites. During the interaction of metastatic cells with host tissues, signals from autocrine, paracrine, or endocrine pathways influence tumor cell proliferation, with growth dependent on the net balance of positive and negative signals [1]. The presence of stimulatory or inhibitory growth factors in a tissue can correlate with site-specific metastasis [153]. To date, only a few organ-derived growth factors have been isolated and purified to homogeneity. A potent growth-stimulatory factor was isolated from lung-conditioned medium [154]; and stromal cells in the bone have been shown to produce a factor that stimulates the growth of human prostatic carcinoma cells [155]. Conversely, a number of tissue-specific inhibitors have been isolated and purified, including TGF-β [156], mammastatin [157], and amphiregulin [158].

Different concentrations of hormones in individual organs, differentially expressed local factors, or paracrine growth factors may influence the growth of malignant cells at particular sites [153, 159]. Specific peptide growth factors are concentrated in different tissues. For example, insulin-like growth factor-I (IGF-I) is synthesized in most mammalian tissue with the highest concentration in the liver [160]. IGF-1 stimulates cell growth by controlling cell cycle progression through G_1 [161]. The growth of carcinoma cells metastatic to the liver is stimulated by hepatocyte-derived IGF-I, correlating with IGF-I receptor density on the cells [162]. Another example is TGF-β. Many transformed cells produce increased levels of TGF-β and become refractory to its growth-inhibitory effects [163]. Clonal stimulation ·or inhibition of human colon and renal carcinoma cells by TGF-$β_1$ has been reported in correlation with differential expression of its receptors [164].

Autocrine or paracrine host growth factors that control organ repair and regeneration may also affect the proliferation of malignant tumor cells. We have completed transplantation experiments on human colon cancers and human renal cell carcinomas in nude mice subjected to hepatectomy, nephrectomy, or abdominal surgery (used as a trauma control) [1, 165]. After partial hepatectomy the liver undergoes rapid cell division. This process of liver regeneration involves quantitative changes in hepatocyte gene expression. TGF-α has been shown to be one regulator of liver regeneration [166–168] and proliferation of normal colonic epithelial cells [169, 170]. TGF-α exerts its effect through interaction with the epidermal growth factor receptor (EGF-R), a plasma membrane glycoprotein that contains within its cytoplasmic domain a tyrosine-specific protein tyrosine kinase (PTK) activity. The binding of TGF-α to the EGF-R stimulates a series of rapid responses, including phosphorylation of tyrosine residues within the EGF-R itself and within many other cellular proteins, hydrolysis of phosphatidyl inositol, release of Ca^{2+} from intracellular stores, elevation of cytoplasmic pH, and morphologic changes [171]. After 10 to 12h in the continuous presence of EGF or TGF-α, cells are committed to synthesize DNA and to divide [171, 172]. Human colon cancer cells implanted subcutaneously demonstrated accelerated growth in partially hepatectomized mice but not in nephrectomized mice. Human renal cell carcinoma cells established as micrometastases in the lungs of nude mice underwent significant growth acceleration subsequent to unilateral nephrectomy but not hepatectomy [1, 165]. Similar data have been reported for rat colon carcinoma cells injected intraportally. The incidence and size of liver metastases were significantly increased in hepatectomized rats compared to that in sham-operated controls [173]. These results indicate that metastatic cells can respond to physiologic signals produced when homeostasis is disturbed, and that tumor cells that originate from or have an affinity for growth in a particular organ can also respond to these physiologic signals.

One possible mechanism to explain the accelerated growth of human colon cancer in hepatectomized mice is the production of organ-specific growth factors. Liver regeneration that follows major hepatectomy involves quantitative changes in hepatocyte gene expression [174]. TGF-α mRNA has been shown to increase approximately twofold in rat hepatocytes during the first 8 to 24 h after partial hepatectomy, coinciding with an increase in EGF-R mRNA and down-regulation of these receptor proteins, as well as a loss of EGF-R protein kinase activity [167, 175]. These results suggest that TGF-α is a physiologic regulator of liver regeneration by means of an autocrine mechanism [167]. Moreover, TGF-α production by hepatocytes might also have a paracrine role, stimulating proliferation of adjacent nonparenchymal cells or tumor cells [176].

Hepatocyte growth factor (HGF), another liver mitogen, is synthesized and secreted by nonparenchymal liver cells (endothelial and Kupffer cells). Subsequent to liver damage, a rapid increase is observed in HGF mRNA in Kupffer cells [177], paralleling the down-regulation of its receptor, the *c-met* proto-oncogene, in hepatocytes. Similar to EGF-R, the receptor for HGF (*c-met*) belongs to the tyrosine kinase family of receptors [178]. HGF is a potent mitogen for hepatocytes, melanocytes, and prostate cells; and it enhances the invasive capacity of carcinomas [179]. Levels of TGF-β mRNAs increase in normal nonparenchymal liver cells coincidentally with hepatocyte DNA replication and mitosis; and TGF-β inhibits EGF-stimulated DNA synthesis, implying that it may be a component of a paracrine regulatory loop controlling hepatocyte replication at the late stages of liver regeneration [180]. Therefore when the liver is damaged, growth factors are likely to be released and stimulate the proliferation of receptive malignant tumor cells (i.e., cells that possess the appropriate receptors).

The EGF-Rs are present on many normal and tumor cells [171, 172]. Increased levels or amplification of EGF-R have been found in many human tumors and cell lines, including breast cancer [181], gliomas [182], lung cancer [183], bladder cancer [184], epidermoid carcinoma [185], and colon carcinoma [186]. These results suggest a physiologic significance of inappropriate expression of the EGF-R tyrosine kinase in abnormal cell growth control. We assessed the genes encoding for growth factor receptors of low- and high-metastatic human colon cancer variants [187, 188]. Analyses of human colon cancer cells from nonselected surgical specimens that differed in malignant potential showed no amplification or rearrangements in the genes encoding EGF-R. In contrast, highly metastatic human colon cancer

variants (Dukes' stage D or variant cells selected in nude mice from a Dukes' stage B2 tumor) expressed significantly increased EGF-R mRNA transcripts when compared with low-metastatic human colon cancer cell types [188]. The in vitro growth stimulation of cells with high- or low-metastatic potential to TGF-α demonstrated the functional significance of increased EGF-R numbers on specific cell types.

The EGF-Rs expressed on metastatic human colon cancer (HCC) cells were functional based on in vitro growth stimulation assays using picogram concentrations of TGF-α and specific as shown by neutralization with anti-EGF-R or anti-TGF-α antibodies. Moreover, EGF-R-associated PTK activity paralleled the observed EGF-R levels. Immunohistochemical analysis of the low metastatic parental HCC cells demonstrated heterogeneity in the EGF-R-specific staining pattern, with fewer than 10% of the cells in the population staining intensely for EGF-R, whereas the in vivo selected highly metastatic cells exhibited uniform, intense staining. Western blotting confirmed the presence of higher EGF-R protein levels in the metastatic cell lines than in the low-metastatic cell line. Finally, isolation of the top and bottom 5% of EGF-R-expressing cells by fluorescence-activated cell sorting confirmed the association between levels of EGF-R on human colon cancer cells and the production of liver metastases [188].

The analyses described show a direct correlation between EGF-R on variant cell lines isolated from HCC and the ability to produce liver metastases in nude mice. These findings are likely to be more generalized because in our analysis of formalin-fixed paraffin-embedded colon carcinoma surgical specimens for EGF-R-transcripts using a rapid calorimetric in situ mRNA hybridization (ISH) technique [189] we found that cell-surface hybridization with EGF-R-antisense hyperbiotinylated oligonucleotide probes in primary and metastatic colon carcinoma specimens directly correlated with immunohistochemistry and northern blot analyses.

Related to but distinct from the EGF-R is the *c-met* proto-oncogene, whose encoded protein is the receptor for HGF [190]. In human tissues the highest levels of *c-met* mRNA expression are found in the liver, kidney, stomach, and thyroid. Studies with anti-*c-met* antibodies have revealed that receptor protein levels are high in hepatocytes and in gastric and intestinal epithelium (including colon and rectum), indicating a role for

HGF and *c-met* in the growth and turnover of epithelial tissues [190]. Preliminary studies from our laboratory indicate high levels of *c-met* expression in colon cancer cell lines that have been adapted to grow in culture from Dukes' stage B2 or D or from liver metastases. Analyses of mRNA isolated directly from human colon cancer specimens and normal colon mucosa also suggest increased *c-met* transcripts in the tumor tissues [187].

To produce clinically detectable lesions, the metastases must develop a vascular network and evade the host immune system. Tumor cells can also invade host stroma, penetrate blood vessels, and enter the circulation to produce secondary metastases, the "metastasis of metastases" [191–193].

Biologic Heterogeneity of Neoplasms

Most tumor cells in a primary neoplasm fail to complete one or more steps in the metastatic process, explaining why only a few cells in a primary tumor can give rise to a metastasis. These data raised the question of whether the development of metastases represents the chance survival and growth of a few neoplastic cells or the selective growth of unique subpopulations of malignant cells endowed with special properties [1, 4]. Most data now show that neoplasms are biologically heterogeneous, and that the process of metastasis is highly selective. Cells obtained from individual tumors have been shown to differ with respect to many properties, including morphology, growth rates, karyotypes, metabolic characteristics, antigenic or immunogenic potential, production of extracellular matrix proteins, cell surface receptors, adhesion molecules, hormone receptors, drug and radiation sensitivities, invasiveness, and the ability to metastasize [1].

Many human neoplasms, including colon carcinoma, have a clonal origin [194, 195]; nevertheless, by the time of diagnosis the neoplasms have become heterogeneous and consist of multiple subpopulations of cells with different metastatic potential [1]. Data from our laboratory and many others clearly demonstrate that the process of metastasis is selective and favors the survival of unique metastatic cells that preexist within the parental neoplasm [196, 197].

The first experimental proof for the preexistence of metastatic cells in heterogeneous neoplasms was provided in 1977 by Fidler and Kripke in their work with murine melanoma [196]. Using a modification of the fluctuation assay [198], they showed that different tumor cell clones, each derived from an individual cell isolated from the parent tumor, varied dramatically in their ability to produce lung tumor nodules following intravenous inoculation. Control subcloning procedures demonstrated that the observed diversity was not a consequence of the cloning procedure [196]. The finding that preexisting tumor cell subpopulations exhibit heterogeneous metastatic potential has since been confirmed in numerous laboratories using a wide range of experimental animal tumors of different histories and histologic origins [for review, ref. 1]. In addition, studies using nude mice as models for metastasis of human neoplasms have shown that many human tumor lines and freshly isolated tumors, such as melanoma, breast carcinoma, prostate carcinoma, colon carcinoma, and renal carcinoma, are biologically heterogeneous and contain subpopulations of cells with widely differing metastatic properties [199–204].

Models for Human Colon Cancer Metastases

Appropriate animal models are necessary for advancing our understanding of the biology of colon cancer metastasis. We have developed a model of regional lymph node metastases by injecting colon cancer cells into the apical lymphoid follicle of the cecum in mice [115]. Dye distribution studies have shown rapid distribution of the injected material in the lymphatic channels, and the procedure has yielded a high incidence of mesenteric lymphatic metastases [115].

To develop a reproducible model of hepatic metastasis, we implanted tumor cells into the spleens of nude mice [205]. Splenic injections are easier to perform than portal or mesenteric vein injections; access to the portal bloodstream is gained from the spleen, and tumor cells can then reach the liver to proliferate into experimental liver metastases [206]. Merely implanting tumor cells in the spleen did not guarantee liver metastasis. Metastatic human renal cell carcinoma, for example, injected into the spleen produces only spleen tumors, but these cells produce extensive lung metastases when they are injected into the kidney [203]. Also, orthotopic implantation of

HCC cells in nude mice produces liver metastases, depending on the nature of the tumor cells [204]. In our study we were able to distinguish between HCC cells with low or high malignant potentials. Specifically, intrasplenically injected cells isolated from liver metastases in colon cancer patients produced rapidly growing liver lesions and the mice became moribund within 30 days, whereas cells from Dukes' stage B2 primary tumors produced only a few visible tumor foci by 90 days [202].

We also carried out a series of orthotopic implantation experiments to select and isolate cells with increased liver-metastasizing potential from heterogeneous primary human colon cancers. Cells derived from a surgical specimen of a primary human colon cancer, classified as Dukes' stage B2, were immediately established in culture or were injected directly into the subcutis, spleen (for liver metastasis), or cecal wall of nude mice. Progressively growing tumors were excised, enzymatically dissociated, and then established in culture. Subsequent implantation into the cecal wall or spleen of nude mice produced only a few hepatic metastases. Human colon cancer cells from these rare liver metastases were recovered, expanded in culture, and then injected into the spleens of nude mice, thus allowing further cycles of selection. With each successive in vivo selection cycle, the metastatic ability of the isolated-propagated cells increased. After four cycles of selection, we obtained cell lines with high liver-colonizing efficiency in nude mice [202].

As stated above, human colon carcinomas are heterogeneous for a variety of biologic properties that include invasion and metastasis. The presence of a small subpopulation of cells with a highly metastatic phenotype has important clinical implications for diagnosis and therapy of cancer. For this reason, it is important to develop animal models for the selection and isolation of metastatic variants from human colon cancers and for testing the metastatic potential of these cells. We have implanted cells from more than 100 surgical specimens of human colon and rectal carcinomas into various organs of nude mice. Regardless of their malignant potential in the patient, the human colon cancers did not metastasize unless they were implanted orthotopically: Only when they were injected into the cecum or spleen of nude mice did they yield hepatic metastases. These metastsaes were populated by highly metastatic cells [207]. Collectively, the results demonstrate that the orthotopic implantation of human colon cancer is mandatory for studying the biology of human colon cancer.

Homeostatic Mechanisms and Metastasis: "Seed and Soil" Hypothesis

The search for mechanisms that regulate the pattern of metastasis is not new. In 1889 Stephen Paget asked, "What is it that decides what organs shall suffer in a case of diseminated cancer" [114]? Paget's study was motivated by the discrepancy between consideration of blood flow and the frequency of metastases in various organs. He examined the autopsy records of hundreds of women who died of breast cancer and many other patients with different neoplasms. He noted the high frequency of breast cancer metastasis to the ovaries and the different incidence of skeletal metastases produced by different primary tumors. These findings were not compatible with the dogma that metastatic spread was due to "a matter of chance" or that tissues "played a passive role" in the process. To the contrary, Paget concluded that metastases were produced only when certain favored tumor cells (the "seed") had a special affinity for the growth milieu provided by specific tissues or organs (the "soil"). In other words, formation of metastasis required interaction of the right cells with the compatible organ environment [114].

In 1928 Ewing challenged Paget's seed and soil theory and suggested that metastatic dissemination occurs by purely mechanical factors that are a result of the anatomic structure of the vascular system [208]. These explanations are not mutually exclusive because common *regional* organ colonization or lymphatic drainage to regional lymph nodes could indeed be due to anatomic considerations, but *distant* organ metastases occur independent of blood flow [2].

A current definition of the seed and soil hypothesis includes two principles. First, the process of metastasis is selective for cells that succeed in producing angiogenesis, motility, invasion, embolization, survival in the circulation, arrest in a distant capillary bed, and extravasation into and multiplication within the organ parenchyma. Although some of the steps in this process contain stochastic elements [209], as a whole the process of metastasis favors the survival and growth of a few subpopulations of cells that preexist within the parent neoplasm [196, 197]. Second, the outcome of metastasis depends on multiple interactions of metastatic cells with host homeostatic factors [7].

Clinical observations of cancer patients and studies with experimental tumor systems have concluded that tumors metastasize to specific organs independently of the number of tumor cells that reach an organ. Tumor cells can reach the microvasculature of many organs, but growth in the organ parenchyma occurs only in some [118]. Experimental data supporting the seed and soil hypothesis of Paget were derived from studies comparing the metastatic potential of human tumor cells implanted in orthotopic or ectopic sites in nude mice [203, 204]. This may well be due in part to differences in responses to organ-specific growth factors [153, 210]. Depending on the physical location of cells within growing tumors and metastases, tumor cells are exposed to different miceoenvironments created by gradients of pH, oxygen, nutrients, and cell waste products that develop within tumors [211].

The introduction of peritoneovenous shunts for palliation of malignant ascites provided an opportunity to study some of the factors affecting metastatic spread in humans. Tarin and colleagues described the outcome in patients with malignant ascites draining into the venous circulation, with the resulting entry of viable tumor cells into the jugular veins [212]. Good palliation with minimal complications was reported for 29 patients with different neoplasms. The autopsy findings in 15 patients substantiated the clinical observations that the shunts do not significantly increase the risk of metastasis. In fact, despite continuous entry of millions of tumor cells into the circulation, metastases in the lung (the first capillary bed encountered) were rare [212]. These results provide compelling verification of the venerable seed and soil hypothesis.

Regulation of Angiogenesis by the Microenvironment

Our laboratory demonstrated that the organ microenvironment can directly contribute to the induction and maintenance of the angiogenic factors bFGF [213, 214] and interleukin-8 (IL-8) [215]. The production of these angiogenic factors by tumor cells or host cells or the release of ang-

iogenic molecules from the ECM induces the growth of endothelial cells and formation of blood vessels. For example, in renal cell carcinoma patients the expression of basic fibroblast growth factor (bFGF) inversely correlates with survival [216], as do elevated levels of bFGF in the serum and urine of patients [217]. Studies from our laboratory have concluded that bFGF expression (at the mRNA and protein levels) is influenced by the organ microenvironment. Human renal cancer cells implanted into different organs of nude mice had different metastatic potentials: Those implanted in the kidney produced a high incidence of lung metastasis, whereas those implanted subcutaneously were not metastatic [213]. Histopathologic examination of the tissues revealed that the tumors growing in the subcutis of nude mice had few blood vessels, whereas the tumors in the kidney had many [213]. The subcutaneous (or intramuscular) tumors had a lower level of mRNA transcripts for bFGF than did continuously cultured cells, whereas tumors in the kidney of nude mice had 10- to 20-fold the levels of bFGF mRNA and protein level.

Interleukin-8 induces proliferation, migration, and invasion of endothelial cells and hence neovascularization [218]. Several organ-derived cytokines (produced by inflammatory cells) can up-regulated expression of IL-8 in normal and tumorigenic cells, indicating that specific organ microenvironments can influence the expression of IL-8 in melanoma cells [219]. Constitutive expression of IL-8 directly correlates with the metastatic potential of human melanoma cells [215]. IL-8 expression was up-regulated in co-culture of melanoma cells with keratinocytes (skin), whereas it was inhibited in cells co-cultured with hepatocytes (liver). Similar results were obtained with conditioned media from keratinocyte and hepatocyte cultures. These data suggest that organ-derived factors (e.g., IL-1 and TGF-β) can modulate the expression of IL-8 in human melanoma cells [219].

Several factors that down-regulate or inhibit angiogenesis have already been incorporated into clinical trials, the most widely studied being interferon-alpha (IFN-α). Chronic daily administration of low-dose IFN-α has been shown to induce regression of fatal hemangiomas in infants [220] and highly vascular Kaposi's sarcoma [221]. We tested the ability of IFN-α to down-regulate bFGF mRNA expression and protein production in human carcinoma cell lines [214]. We found that IFN-α or IFN-β down-regulated the steady-state mRNA expression and protein production of bFGF in human rencal cancer cells by mechanisms independent of antiproliferation. The inhibition of bFGF mRNA and protein production required long-term exposure (>4 days) of cells to IFNs. Moreover, once IFN was withdrawn, cells resumed production of bFGF [214]. These observations were consistent with the clinical experience that IFN-α must be given for many months to bring about involution of hemangiomas [220]. Because IFN-β is not found in all tissues and is produced only by differentiated cells, the data suggest that modulation of the organ environment can lead to alterations in angiogensis.

Regulation of the Invasive Phenotype of Metastatic Colon Carcinoma Cells by the Microenvironment

The metastatic capacity of human colon cancer cells growing in orthotopic tissues of nude mice directly correlates with the level of collagenase type IV activity [73, 74, 222, 223]. Histologic examination of human colon carcinomas growing in the subcutis, wall of the colon, or kidney of nude mice revealed a thick pseudocapsule around the subcutaneous tumors but not the cecal or kidney tumors [201, 202, 224]. These differences suggested that the organ environment could influence the ability of metastatic cells to invade host stroma and hence produce metastasis. We found a strong correlation between the type IV collagenase activity of HCC cells and production of liver metastases [224]. We also found significant differences in the levels of secreted type IV collagenases between human colon carcinomas growing subcutaneously or in the cecum of nude mice. In the medium conditioned by human colon cancers growing subcutaneously, we detected only a latent form of the 92-kDa type IV collagenase. In contrast, both latent and active forms of the 92-kDa type IV collagenase were found in culture medium conditioned by human colon cancers growing in the cecum. Moreover, human colon cancers growing in the cecum secreted more than twice as much enzyme as the subcutaneous tumors [224, 225].

The invasive ability of HCC cells was directly influenced by organ-specific fibroblasts. Primary cultures of nude mouse fibroblasts, lung, and colon were established. Invasive and metastatic HCC cells were cultured alone or with the fibroblasts. The cancer cells grew on monolayers of all three fibroblast cultures but did not invade through skin fibroblasts [226]. Cancer cells growing on plastic and on colon or lung fibroblasts produced significant levels of latent and active forms of type IV collagenase, whereas colon cancer cells co-cultivated with nude mouse skin fibroblasts did not. Fibroblasts from the skin produce IFN-β, whereas those from the kidney or colon do not. The incubation of HCC cells [226] and human renal cancer cells [227] with IFN-β significantly reduced the expression and activity of collagenase type IV MMP-2 and MMP-9 independent of antiproliferative activity. Improvement in the use of IFNs for treatment of colon cancer is dependent on a better understanding of the mechanisms by which IFNs regulate different functions of tumor cells, perhaps through the invasive and angiogenic phenotypes.

Microenvironmental Regulation of Colon Cancer Cell Response to Chemotherapy

Clinical observations have suggested that the organ environment can influence the response of tumors to chemotherapy. For example, in women with breast cancer, lymph node and skin metastases respond better than lung or bone metastases [228]. Experimental systems suggested a basis for this observation [229–232]. Studies from our laboratory have shown that a mouse fibrosarcoma growing subcutaneously in syngeneic mice was sensitive to systemic administration of doxorubicin (DOX), whereas lung metastases were not [232]. We obtained similar results with the CT-26 murine colon cancer: Subcutaneous tumors were sensitive to DOX, whereas metastases growing in the liver or lung were not [233].

Several intrinsic properties of tumor cells can render them resistant to chemotherapeutic drugs, including increased expression of the *mdr* genes [234–236], leading to overproduction of the transmembrane transport protein P-gp [235–237]. Increased levels of P-gp can be induced by selecting tumor cells for resistance to natural product amphiphilic anticancer drugs [233–237]. Elevated expression of P-gp accompanied by development of the multidrug resistance (MDR) phenotype has also been found in many solid tumors of the colon, kidney, and liver that had not been exposed to chemotherapy [238, 239]. Because the development of MDR in tumor cells is a major obstacle to the therapy of cancer, understanding the mechanisms that control this process has been the goal of many researchers. Most of the present knowledge of drug resistance in tumor cells is derived from examining tumor cells growing in culture, but the relevance of these findings to in vivo growing tumors has been uncertain.

We investigated whether different organ environments influenced the response of tumor cells to chemotherapy and if this response was regulated by the expression level of P-gp in the tumor cells. In this study, murine CT-26 colon cancer cells growing in the lung of syngeneic mice were refractory to systemic administration of DOX, whereas the same cells growing subcutaneously were sensitive to the drug. CT-26 cells harvested from lung metastases exhibited increased resistance to DOX compared with cells harvested from subcutaneous tumors or parental cells maintained in culture. The resistance to DOX was reversed by the addition of verapamil. All the CT-26 cells, however, demonstrated similar sensitivity to 5-fluorowracil (5-FU). We found a direct correlation between the increased resistance to DOX (in vivo and in vitro) of CT-26 cells and expression levels of mdr-1 mRNA transcripts and P-gp. The drug resistance and accompanying elevated expression of mdr-1 found for cells growing in the lung were dependent on interaction with the specific organ environment. Once removed from the lung, the cells reverted to a sensitive phenotype similar to that of the parental cells [240].

The increased resistance to DOX in the CT-26 cells in lung metastases was not due to selection of resistant subpopulations. We based this conclusion on the results of the crossover experiment. Once implanted into the subcutis of syngeneic mice, CT-26 cells from lung metastases produced tumors that were sensitive to DOX. In parallel studies, DOX-sensitive CT-26 cells from subcutaneous tumors became resistant to the drug when they were inoculated intravenously and grew in the lung parenchyma as metastases. P-gp levels directly correlated with the drug resistance phenotype in these experiments. Moreover, the increased resistance to DOX and elevated levels of

mdr-1 mRNA and P-gp were all transient in CT-26 cells growing in the lung. Subsequent to growth in culture for more than 7 days, mdr-1 mRNA and P-gp reverted to the baseline levels of CT-26 parental cells [240].

The finding of an organ-specific response to DOX is not restricted to CT-26 cells. Previous reports from our laboratory with UV-2237 fibrosarcoma cells [232] and human KM12 colon carcinoma cells [241] also showed significant differences in resistance to DOX (but not 5-FU) between subcutaneous tumors (sensitive) and lung or liver metastases (resistant). Similarly, in patients with colon carcinoma, high level P-gp expression is found on the invasive edge of the primary tumor (growing in the colon) in lymph node, lung, and liver metastases [239, 242]. Whether this finding is due to selection or adaptation is still unclear.

In any event, we have shown that the in vivo sensitivity of colon carcinoma cells to DOX depends on the organ environment. The organ environment can induce the P-gp-associated MDR phenotype in tumor cells. The expression of P-gp is transient: Once removed from the environment (lung), the cells' resistance reverts to that of the sensitive parent cells. This environmental regulation of the MDR phenotype may explain, in part, the polarized expression of mdr-1 in colon carcinomas [243] and the discrepancy between in vitro and in vivo expression levels of the MDR phenotype [236, 237, 244, 245]. In any event, the model described here can be used to investigate molecular mechanisms that regulate the in vivo expression of the mdr-1 gene.

Predicting the Malignant Potential of Human Carcinomas

To produce a clinically relevant metastasis, metastatic cells must complete all the steps outlined in Fig. 1. The failure of most tumor cells to produce a metastasis is due to different single or multiple deficiencies, such as the inability to invade host stroma, inability to arrest in the capillary bed, and failure to grow in a distant organ's parenchyma. Searching for a uniform factor that prevents tumor cells from producing metastasis is therefore unproductive. Each discrete step of metastasis (e.g., invasion or extravasation) can be regulated by transient or permanent changes at the DNA or RNA level in different genes or by the activation or deactivation of many specific genes [246–248]. The identification of tumor cells capable of producing metastasis therefore requires a multiparametric analysis.

We developed a rapid technique for detecting the activity of genes involved in the formation of metastasis: vascularization, invasion, adhesion, and proliferation. This technique, colorimetric in situ hybridization (ISH), can detect specific mRNA transcripts in cultured cells, frozen tissues, and formalin-fixed, paraffin-embedded specimens [189, 249]. The expression level of several genes that regulate different steps of the metastatic process correlated with the metastatic potential of human colon carcinoma cells. The mRNA expression level for EGF-R (growth), bFGF and IL-8 (angiogenesis), type IV collagenase (invasion), E-cadherin (cohesion), CEA (adhesion), and multidrug resistance (mdr)-1 (drug resistance) in the human colon carcinoma cell lines and clones with different metastatic potential was measured by northern blot analysis and ISH. Highly metastatic cells growing in culture uniformly expressed high levels of EGFR, bFGF, and CEA mRNA, whereas cultures of low metastatic cells displayed heterogeneous patterns [250].

We next examined the expression of metastasis-related genes in surgical specimens of human colon carcinomas. Dukes' stages C and D tumors exhibited a higher level of expression for EGF-R, bFGF, type IV collagenase, and mdr-1 mRNA than Dukes' stage B tumors. The expression level of E-cadherin did not correlate with the stage of disease. The ISH technique revealed intertumoral heterogeneity for expression of several genes among Dukes' stage B neoplasms. Moreover, we found intratumoral heterogeneous staining for bFGF and type IV collagenase in some Dukes' stage B tumors, with the highest expression level at their invasive edge. In Dukes' stages C and D tumors, the expression of these genes was more uniform [250].

In the final set of experiments, we examined the expression level of EGF-R, bFGF, type IV collagenase, E-cadherin, and mdr-1 in formalin-fixed, paraffin-embedded archival specimens of primary human colon carcinomas from patients with at least 5 years of follow-up. The ISH technique revealed inter- and intratumoral heterogeneity for expression of the metastasis-related genes. The expression of bFGF, collagenase type IV, EGF-R, and mdr-1 mRNA was higher in Dukes' stage D than in Dukes' stage B tumors.

Among the 22 Dukes' stage B neoplasms, five specimens exhibited a high expression level of EGF-R, bFGF, and collagenase type IV. Clinical outcome data (5-year follow-up) revealed that all five patients with Dukes' stage B tumors developed distant metastasis (recurrent disease), whereas the other 17 patients with Dukes' stage B tumors expressing low levels of the metastasis-related genes were disease-free. Multivariate analysis identified high levels of expression of collagenase type IV and low levels of expression of E-cadherin as independent factors significantly associated with metastasis or recurrent disease. More specifically, metastatic or recurrent disease was associated with a high ratio of expression of collagenase type IV to E-cadherin. Collectively, these data show that multiparametric ISH analysis for metastasis-related genes may predict the metastatic potential, and hence the clinical outcome, of individual lymph node-negative human colon cancers.

We also found an inverse correlation between expression of collagenase type IV and E-cadherin in formalin-fixed, paraffin-embedded specimens of human gastric carcinoma by an in situ mRNA hybridization (ISH) technique. The ISH technique revealed intertumoral heterogeneity for expression of E-cadherin and collagenase among 12 cases of early gastric cancer and 13 cases of advanced gastric cancer. In most of the tumors, we found an inverse relation between the reactivities of E-cadherin and collagenase type IV. Specifically, E-cadherin was expressed at higher levels in the center of the neoplasms than in their periphery, whereas collagenase type IV was expressed at a higher level on the periphery (invasive edge) than in the center. Advanced gastric cancers with high levels of expression for collagenase type IV on the periphery had a higher incidence of distant lymph node metastasis than those with low expression. The data show an inverse relation between E-cadherin (involved in cell-to-cell adhesion) and collagenase type IV (involved in invasion) in different zones of human gastric carcinoma and suggest that the relative expression of these independent genes may be involved in local invasion and metastasis [251].

Acknowledgments. Supported in part by Cancer Center Support Core grant CA 16672 and grant R35 CA42107 from the National Cancer Institute, National Institutes of Health.

References

1. Fidler IJ (1990) Critical factors in the biology of human cancer metastasis: twenty-eighth GHA Clowes memorial award lecture. Cancer Res 50: 6130–6138

2. Sugarbaker EV (1979) Cancer metastasis: a product of tumor–host interactions. Curr Probl Cancer 3:1–59

3. Weiss L (1985) Principles of metastasis. Academic, San Diego

4. Fidler IJ, Hart IR (1982) Biological diversity in metastatic neoplasms: origins and implications. Science 217:998–1003

5. Heppner G (1984) Tumor heterogeneity. Cancer Res 44:2259–2265

6. Radinsky R, Aukerman SL, Fidler IJ (in press) The heterogeneous nature of metastatic neoplasms: relevance to biotherapy. In: Oldham RK (ed) Principles of cancer biotherapy, 3rd edn. Marcel Dekker, New York

7. Fidler IJ (1995) Modulation of the organ microenvironment for the treatment of cancer metastasis. J Natl Cancer Inst 84:1588–1592 (editorial)

8. Jain RK (1994) Barriers to drug delivery in solid tumors. Sci Am 271:58–65

9. Folkman J (1995) Angiogenesis in cancer, vascular, rheumatoid and other disease. Nature Med 1:27–31

10. Liotta LA, Stetler-Stevenson WG (1991) Tumor invasion and metastasis: an imbalance of positive and negative regulation. Cancer Res (suppl) 51: 5054s–5059s

11. Fisher B, Fisher ER (1966) The interrelationship of hematogenous and lymphatic tumor cell dissemination. Surg Gynecol Obstet 122:791–797

12. Poste G, Fidler IJ (1988) The pathogenesis of cancer metastasis. Nature 283:139–146

13. Gimbrone M, Cotran R, Folkman J (1974) Tumor growth and neovasculatrization: an experimental model using rabbit cornea. J Natl Cancer Inst 52:413–427

14. Folkman J (1986) How is blood vessel growth regulated in normal and neoplastic tissue? GHA Clowes memorial award lecture. Cancer Res 46: 467–473

15. Auerbach W, Auerbach R (1994) Angiogenesis inhibition: a review. Pharmacol Ther 63:265–311

16. Fidler IJ, Ellis LM (1994) The implications of angiogenesis for the biology and therapy of cancer metastasis. Cell 79:185–188

17. Folkman J, Klagsbrun M (1987) Angiogenic factors. Science 235:444–447

18. Nagy JA, Brown LF, Senger DR, Lanir N, Van de Water L, Dvorak AM, Dvorak HF (1989) Pathogenesis of tumor stroma generation: a critical role for leaky blood vessels and fibrin deposition. Biochim Biophys Acta 948:305–326

19. Folkman J, Cotran R (1976) Relation of vascular proliferation to tumor growth. Int Rev Exp Pathol 16:207–248

20. Dameron KM, Volpert OV, Tainsky MA, Bouk N (1994) Control of angiogenesis in fibroblasts by p53 regulation of thrombospondin-1. Science 265: 1502–1504

21. Rak J, Mitsuhashi Y, Bayko L, Filmus J, Shirawawa S, Sasazuki T, Kerbel RS (1995) Mutant *ras* oncogenes upregulate VEGF/VPF expression: implications for induction and inhibition of tumor angiogenesis. Cancer Res 55:4575–4580

22. Liotta LA, Kleinerman J, Saidel GM (1974) Quantitative relationships of intravascular tumor cells, tumor vessels, and pulmonary metastases following tumor implantation. Cancer Res 34:997–1004

23. Liotta LA, Kleinerman J, Saidel GM (1976) The significance of hematogenous tumor cell clumps in the metastatic process. Cancer Res 36:889–893

24. Liotta LA, Steeg PS, Stetler-Stevenson WG (1991) Cancer metastasis and angiogenesis: an imbalance of positive and negative regulation. Cell 64:327–336

25. Weidner N, Semple JP, Welch JR, Folkman J (1991) Tumor angiogenesis and metastasis—correlation in invasive breast cancer. N Engl J Med 324:1–8

26. Weidner N, Folkman J, Pozza F, Bevilacqua P, Allred E, Mili S, Gasparini G (1992) Tumor angiogenesis: a new significant and independent prognostic indicator in early stage breast carcinoma. J Natl Cancer Inst 84:1875–1887

27. Gasparini G, Harris AL (1995) Clinical importance of the determination of tumor angiogenesis in breast carcinoma: much more than a new prognostic tool. J Clin Oncol 13:765–782

28. Obermair A, Czerwenka K, Kurz C, Laider A, Sevelda P (1994) Tumoral microvessel density in breast cancer and its influence on recurrence-free survival. Chirurgie 65:611–615

29. Toi M, Kashitani J, Tominaga T (1993) Tumor angiogenesis is an independent prognostic indicator in primary breast carcinoma. Int J Cancer 55:371–374

30. Hall N, Fish D, Hunt N, Goldin R, Guillou P, Monson J (1992) Is the relationship between angiogenesis and metastasis in breast cancer real? Surg Oncol 1:223–229

31. Van Hoef ME, Knox WF, Dhesi SS, Howell A, Schor AM (1993) Assessment of tumour vascularity as a prognostic factor in lymph node negative invasive breast cancer. Eur J Cancer 29A: 1141–1145

32. Weidner N, Carroll PR, Flax J, Flumenfeld W, Folkman J (1993) Tumor angiogenesis correlates

with metastasis in invasive prostate carcinoma. Am J Pathol 143:401–409

33. Fregene TA, Khanuja PS, Noto AC, Gehani SK, Van Egmont EM, Luz DA, Pienta FJ (1993) Tumor-associated angiogenesis in prostate cancer. Anticancer Res 13:2377–2382

34. Graham CH, Rivers J, Kerbel RS, Stankiewicz KS, White WL (1994) Extent of vascularization as a prognostic indicator in thin (<0.76 mm) malignant melanomas. Am J Pathol 145:510–514

35. Hollingsworth HC, Kohn EC, Steinberg SM, Rothenberg ML, Meriono MJ (1995) Tumor angiogenesis in advanced stage ovarian carcinoma. Am J Pathol 147:33–41

36. Maeda K, Chung Y-S, Takatsuka S, Ogawa Y, Onoda N, Sawada T, Kato Y, Nitta A, Arimoto Y, Kondo Y (1995) Tumour angiogenesis and tumour cell proliferation as prognostic indicators in gastric carcinoma. Br J Cancer 72:319–323

37. Takahashi Y, Kitadai Y, Bucana CD, Cleary K, Ellis LM (1995) Expression of vascular endothelial growth factor and its receptor, KDR, correlates with vascularity, metastasis, and proliferation of human colon cancer. Cancer Res 55:3964–3968

38. Black WS, Waugh JM (1948) The intramural extension of carcinoma of the descending colon, sigmoid, and rectosigmoid: a pathologic study. Surg Gynecol Obstet 87:457–464

39. Spratt JS Jr, Spjut HJ (1967) Prevalence and prognosis of individual clinical and pathologic variables associated with colorectal carcinoma. Cancer 20:1976–1983

40. Willett CG, Tepper JE, Cohen AM, Orlow E, Welch CE (1984) Failure patterns following curative resection of colonic carcinoma. Ann Surg 200:685–693

41. Curley SA, Carlson GW, Shumate CR, Winshow KT, Ames FC (1992) Extended resection for locally advanced colorectal carcinoma. Am J Surg 163:553–562

42. Seefeld PH, Bargen JA (1943) The spread of carcinoma of the rectum: invasion of lymphatics, veins, and nerves. Ann Surg 18:76–84

43. Gabbert H (1985) Mechanisms of tumor invasion: evidence from in vivo observations. Cancer Metast Rev 4:283–310

44. Mareel MM, Van Roy FM, Bracke ME (1993) How and when do tumor cells metastasize? Crit Rev Oncogene 4:559–594

45. Portella G, Liddell J, Crombie R, Haddow S, Clarke M, Stoler AB, Balmain A (1994–1995) Molecular mechanisms of invasion and metastasis during mouse skin tumour progression. Invasion Metast 14:7–16

46. Strauli P, Haemmerli O (1984) The role of cancer cell motility in invasion. Cancer Metast Rev 3:127–156

47. Volk T, Geiger B, Raz A (1984) Motility and adhesive properties of high and low-metastatic murine neoplastic cells. Cancer Res 44:811–817

48. Doyle GM, Sharief Y, Mohler JL (1992) Prediction of metastatic potential by cancer cell motility in the Dunning R-3327 prostatic adenocarcinoma in vivo model. J Urol 147:514–520

49. Takeichi M (1990) Cadherin cell adhesion receptors as a morphogenetic regulator. Science 251:1451–1455

50. Shimoyama Y, Hirohashi S, Hirano S, Noguchi M, Shimasato Y, Takeichi M, Abe O (1989) Cadherin cell adhesion molecules in human epithelial tissues and carcinomas. Cancer Res 49:2128–2133

51. Dorudi S, Sheffield JP, Poulsom R, Northover JMA, Hart IR (1993) E-cadherin expression in colorectal cancer: an immunocytochemical and in situ hybridization study. Am J Pathol 142:981–986

52. Umbas R, Schalken JA, Alders TW, Cater BS, Karthas HFM, Schaafsma HE, Debruyne FMJ, Issaca WB (1992) Expression of the cellular adhesion molecule E-cadherin is reduced or absent in high-grade prostate cancer. Cancer Res 52:510–5109

53. Mayer B, Johnson JP, Leitl F, Jauch KW, Heiss MM, Schildberg FW, Birchmeier W, Funke I (1993) E-cadherin expression in primary and metastatic gastric cancer: downregulation correlates with cellular dedifferentiation and glandular disintegration. Cancer Res 53:1690–1695

54. Oka H, Shiozaki H, Kobayashi H, Inoue M, Tahara H, Kobayashi T, Takatsuka Y, Matsuyoshi N, Hirano S, Tekeichi M, Mori T (1993) Expression of E-cadherin cell adhesion molecule in human breast cancer tissues and its relationship to metastasis. Cancer Res 53:1696–1701

55. Kadowaki T, Shiozaki H, Inoue M, Tamura S, Oka H, Doki Y, Iihara K, Matsui S, Iwazawa T, Nagafuchi A, Tsukita S, Mori T (1994) E-cadherin and α-catenin expression in human esophageal cancer. Cancer Res 54:291–296

56. Schipper JH, Frixen UH, Behrens J, Unger A, Jahnke K, Birchmeier W (1991) E-cadherin expression in squamous carcinomas of the head and neck: inverse correlation with tumor differentiation and lymph node metastasis. Cancer Res 51:6328–6337

57. Oda T, Kanai Y, Oyama T, Yoshiura K, Shimoyama Y, Birchmeier W, Sugimura T, Hirohashi S (1994) E-cadherin gene mutations in human gastric carcinoma cell lines. Proc Natl Acad Sci USA 91:1858–1862

58. Shiozaki H, Iihara K, Oka H, Kadowaki T, Matsui S, Gofuku J, Inoue M, Nagafuchi A, Tsukita S, Mori T (1994) Immunohistochemical detection of α-catenin expression in human cancers. Am J Pathol 144:667–674

59. Vermeulen SJ, Bruyneel EA, Bracke ME, De Bruyne GK, Vennekens KM, Vleminckx KL, Berx GJ, van Roy FM, Mareel MM (1995) Transition from the noninvasive to the invasive phenotype and loss of α-catenin in human colon cancer cells. Cancer Res 55:4722–4728

60. Frixen UH, Behrens J, Sachs M, Eberle G, Voss B, Warda A, Löchner D, Birchmeier W (1991) E-cadherin-mediated cell–cell adhesion prevents invasiveness of human carcinoma cells. J Cell Biol 113:173–185

61. Vleminckx K, Vakaet L Jr, Mareel M, Fiers W, Van Roy F (1991) Genetic manipulation of E-cadherin expression by epithelial tumor cells reveals an invasion suppressor role. Cell 66:107–119

62. Liotta LA, Stracke ML, Aznavoorian SA, Beckner ME, Schiffman E (1991) Tumor cell motility. Semin Cancer Biol 2:111–114

63. Silletti S, Paku S, Raz A (1996) Tumor autocrine motility factor responses are mediated through cell contact and focal adhesion rearrangement in the absence of new tyrosine phosphorylation in metastatic cells. Am J Pathol 148:1649–1660

64. Lotan R, Amos B, Watanabe H, Raz A (1992) Suppression of motility factor receptor expression by retinoic acid. Cancer Res 52:4878–4886

65. Watanabe H, Shinozaki T, Raz A, Chigira M (1993) Expression of autocrine motility factor receptor in serum- and protein-independent fibrosarcoma cells: implications for autonomy in tumor-cell motility and metastasis. Int J Cancer 53:689–697

66. Silletti S, Yao JP, Pienta KJ, Raz A (1995) Loss of cell-contact regulation and altered responses to autocrine motility factor correlate with increased malignancy in prostate cancer cells. Int J Cancer 63:100–105

67. Kenworthy P, Dowrick P, Baillie-Johnson H, McCann B, Tsubouche H, Arakatz N, Daikuhara Y, Warn RM (1992) The presence of scatter factor in patients with metastatic spread to the pleura. Br J Cancer 66:243–247

68. Giordano S, Zhen Z, Medico E, Gaudino G, Galimi F, Comoglio PM (1993) Transfer of mitogenic and invasive response to scatter factor/hepatocyte growth factor by transfection of human *MET* protooncogene. Proc Natl Acad Sci USA 90:649–653

69. Yabkowitz R, Mansfield PJ, Dixit VM, Suchard SJ (1993) Motility of human carcinoma cells in response to thrombospondin: relationship to metastatic potential and thrombospondin structural domains. Cancer Res 53:378–384

70. Ruoslahti E (1992) Control of cell motility and tumour invasion by extracellular matrix interactions—the Walter Herbert lecture. Br J Cancer 66:239–247

71. Jiang WG, Puntis MCA, Hallett MB (1993) Monocyte-conditioned media possess a novel factor which increases motility of cancer cells. Int J Cancer 53:426–432

72. Behrens J (1994–1995) Cell contacts, differentiation, and invasiveness of epithelial cells. Invasion Metast 14:61–70

73. Liotta LA (1986) Tumor invasion and metastasis—role of the extracellular matrix: Rhoads memorial award lecture. Cancer Res 46:1–7

74. Nakajima M, Chop AM (1991) Tumor invasion and extracellular matrix degradative enzymes: regulation of activity by organ factors. Semin Cancer Biol 2:115–235

75. Crawford HC, Matrisian LM (1994–1995) Tumor and stromal expression of matrix metalloproteinases and their role in tumor progression. Invasion Metast 14:234–245

76. Moscatelli D, Rifkin DB (1988) Membrane and matrix localization of proteinases: a common theme in tumor cell invasion and angiogenesis. Biochim Biophys Acta 948:67–85

77. Nicolson GL (1989) Metastatic tumor cell interactions with endothelium, basement membrane, and tissue. Curr Opin Cell Biol 1:1009–1019

78. Sloane BF (1990) Cathepsin B and cystatins: evidence for a role in cancer progression. Semin Cancer Biol 1:137–152

79. Forster SI, Talbot IC, Critchley DR (1984) Laminin and fibronectin in rectal adenocarcinoma: relationship to tumor grade, stage, and metastasis. Br J Cancer 50:51–58

80. Daneker GW Jr, Mercurio AM, Guerra L, Wolf B, Salem RR, Bagli DJ, Steele GD Jr (1987) Laminin expression in colorectal carcinomas varying in degree of differentiation. Arch Surg 122:1470–1476

81. Remy L, Lissitsky JC, Daemi N, Jacquier MF, Bailly M, Martin PM, Bignon C, Dore JF (1992) Laminin expression by two clones isolated from the colon carcinoma cell line LoVo that differs in metastatic potential and basement membrane organization. Int J Cancer 51:204–211

82. Mafune K, Ravikumar TS (1992) Anti-sense RNA of 32-kDa laminin-binding protein inhibits attachment and invasion of a human colon carcinoma cell line. J Surg Res 52:340–347

83. Andres JL, Ronnstrand L, Cheifetz J, Massague J (1991) Purification of the transforming growth factor-beta (TGF-β) binding proteoglycan betaglycan. J Biol Chem 266:23282–23289

84. Chakrabarty S, Fan D, Varani J (1990) Modulation of differentiation and proliferation in human colon carcinoma cells by transforming growth factor beta 1 and beta 2. Int J Cancer 46:493–501

85. Ruoslahti E (1991) Integrins. J Clin Invest 87:1–16

86. Koretz K, Schlag P, Boumsell L, Moller P (1991) Expression of VLA-alpha 2, VLA-alpha 6, and

VLA-beta 1 chains in normal mucosa and adenomas of the colon, and in colon carcinomas and their liver metastases. Am J Pathol 138:741–749

87. Pignatelli M, Smith MEF, Bodmer WF (1990) Low expression of collagen receptors in moderate and poorly differentiated colorectal adenocarcinomas. Br J Cancer 61:636–642

88. Hemler ME, Crouse C, Sonnenberg A (1989) Association of the VLA alpha 6 subunit with a novel protein: a possible alternative to the common VLA beta 1 subunit on certain cell lines. J Biol Chem 264:6529–6536

89. Leffler H, Masiarz FR, Barondes SH (1989) Soluble lactose-binding vertebrate lectins: a growing family. Biochemistry 28:9222–9229

90. Gabius HJ, Engelhardt R, Hellmann T (1987) Characterization of membrane lectins in human colon carcinoma cells by flow cytofluorometry, drug targeting and affinity chromatography. Anticancer Res 2:109–116

91. Byrn R, Medrek P, Thomas P (1985) Effect of heterogeneity of CEA on liver cell membrane binding and its kinetics of removal from circulation. Cancer Res 45:3137–3143

92. Culty M, Miyake K, Kincade PW, Sikorski E, Butcher EC, Underhill E, Silorski E (1990) The hyaluronate receptor is a member of the CD44 (H0CAM) family of cell surface glycoproteins. J Cell Biol 111:2765–2773

93. Jalkanen S, Jalkanen M (1992) Lymphocyte CD44 binds the COOH-terminal heparin-binding domain of fibronectin. J Cell Biol 116:817–825

94. Faassen AE, Schrager JA, Klein DJ, Oemega TR, Couchman JR, McCarthy JB (1992) A cell surface chondroitin sulfate proteoglycan, immunologically related to CD44, is involved in type I collagen-mediated melanoma cell motility and invasion. J Cell Biol 116:521–430

95. Stamenkovic I, Aruffo A, Amiot M, Seed B (1991) The hematopoietic and epithelial forms of DC44 are distinct polypeptides with different adhesion potentials for hyaluronate bearing cells. EMBO J 10:343–349

96. Matsumura Y, Tarin D (1992) Significance of CD44 gene products for cancer diagnosis and disease evaluation. Lancet 340:1053–1056

97. Nakajima M, Irimura T, Nicolson GL (1988) Heparanases and tumor metastasis. J Cell Biochem 36:157–167

98. Morikawa K, Walker SM, Nakajima M, Pathak S, Jessup JM, Fidler IJ (1988) Influence of organ environment on the growth, selection, and metastasis of human colon carcinoma cells in nude mice. Cancer Res 48:6863–6871

99. Schwartz B, Bresalier RS, Kim YS (1992) The role of mucin in colon-cancer metastasis. Int J Cancer 52:60–65

100. Boyd D, Ziober B, Chakrabarty S, Brattain MG (1989) Examination of urokinase protein/transcript levels and their relationship with laminin degradation in cultured colon carcinoma. Cancer Res 49:816–821

101. Terranova P, Maslow D, Markus G (1989) Directed migration of murine and human tumor cells to collagenase and other proteases. Cancer Res 49:4835–4841

102. Umpleby HC, Williamson RCN (1987) Anastomotic recurrence in large bowel cancer. Br J Surg 74:873–878

103. Pomeranz AA, Garlock JH (1955) Postoperative recurrence of cancer of colon due to desquamated malignant cells. JAMA 158:1434–1438

104. Mayo WJ (1913) Grafting and traumatic dissemination of carcinoma in the course of operations for malignant disease. JAMA 60:512–517

105. Coman DR (1953) Mechanisms responsible for the origin and distribution of blood-borne tumor metastasis: a review. Cancer Res 13:397–404

106. Zeidman I (1957) Metastasis: a review of recent advances. Cancer Res 17:157–164

107. Fisher ER, Fisher B (1967) Recent observations on concepts of metastasis. Arch Pathol 83:321–329

108. Fisher B, Fisher ER (1966) The interrelationship of hematogenous and lymphatic tumor cell dissemination. Surg Gynecol Obstet 122:791–797

109. Zeidman I (1961) The fate of circulating tumor cells. I. Passage of cells through capillaries. Cancer Res 21:38–43

110. Zeidman I, Buss JM (1952) Transpulmonary passage of tumor cell emboli. Cancer Res 12:731–737

111. Del Regato JA (1977) Pathways of metastatic spread of malignant tumors. Semin Oncol 4:33–49

112. Fisher B, Fisher ER (1967) The organ distribution of disseminated ^{51}Cr-labeled tumor cells. Cancer Res 27:412–418

113. Carr I (1983) Lymphatic metastasis. Cancer Metast Rev 22:307–338

114. Paget S (1889) The distribution of secondary growths in cancer of the breast. Lancet 1:571–573

115. Schackert H, Fidler IJ (1989) Development of an animal model to study the biology of recurrent colorectal cancer originating from mesenteric lymph system metastasis. Int J Cancer 44:177–181

116. Weiss L, Grundmann E, Torhorst J, Hartveit F, Eder M, Fenoglio-Preiser CM, Napier J, Horne CHW, Lopez MJ, Shaw-Dunn RI, Sugar J, Davies JO, Day DW, Hallows JP (1986) Hematogenous metastatic patterns in colonic carcinoma: an analysis of 1541 necropsies. J Pathol 150:195–203

117. Weiss L (1986) Metastatic inefficiency: causes and consequences. Cancer Rev 3:1–24

118. Fidler IJ (1970) Metastasis: quantitative analysis of distribution and fate of tumor emboli labeled with ^{125}I-5-iodo-2'-deoxyuridine. J Natl Cancer Inst 45:773–782

119. Fidler IJ (1973) The relationship of embolic homogeneity, number, size, and viability to the incidence of experimental metastasis. Eur J Cancer 9:223–227

120. Fidler IJ (1973) Selection of successive tumor lines for metastasis. Nature 242:148–149

121. Updyke TV, Nicolson GL (1986) Malignant melanoma lines selective in vitro for increased homotypic adhesion properties have increased experimental metastatic potential. Clin Exp Metast 4:231–237

122. Gasic GJ (1984) Role of plasma, platelets and endothelial cells in tumor metastasis. Cancer Metast Rev 3:99–127

123. Fidler IJ, Bucana CD (1977) Mechanism of tumor cell resistance to lysis by lymphocytes. Cancer Res 37:3945–3956

124. Naito S, Giavazzi R, Fidler IJ (1987) Correlation between the in vitro interaction of tumor cells with an organ environment and metastatic behavior in vivo. Invasion Metast 7:16–29

125. Nicolson GL, Dulski KM (1986) Organ specificity of metastatic tumor colonization is related to organ-selective growth properties of malignant cells. Int J Cancer 38:289–294

126. Weiss L, Orr FW, Honn KV (1988) Interactions of cancer cells with the microvasculature during metastasis. FASEB J 2:12–17

127. Nicolson GL (1988) Cancer metastasis: tumor cell and host organ properties important in metastasis to specific secondary sites. Biochim Biophys Acta 948:175–224

128. Weiss L (1994–1995) Cell adhesion molecules: a critical examination of their role in metastasis. Invasion Metast 14:192–197

129. El-Sabban ME, Pauli BU (1994–1995) Adhesion-mediated gap junctional communication between lung-metastatic cancer cells and endothelium. Invasion Metast 14:164–176

130. Karpatkin S, Pearlstein E, Ambrogio C, Coller BS (1988) Role of adhesive proteins in platelet tumor interaction in vitro and metastasis formation in vivo. J Clin Invest 81:1012–1018

131. Karpatkin S, Pearlstein E (1981) Role of platelets in tumor cell metastasis. Ann Intern Med 95:636–643

132. Dvorak HF, Seneger DR, Dvorak AM (1983) Fibrin as a component of the tumor stroma: origins and biological significance. Cancer Metast Rev 2:41–63

133. Cliffton EE, Grossi CE (1974) The rationale of anticoagulants in the treatment of cancer J Med 5:107–113

134. Fidler IJ (1985) Macrophages and metastasis—a biological approach to cancer therapy: presidential address. Cancer Res 45:4714–4726

135. Fidler IJ, Bucana C (1977) Mechanism of tumor cell resistance to lysis by syngeneic lymphocytes. Cancer Res 37:3945–3956

136. Nicolson GL (1982) Metastatic tumor cell attachment and invasion assay utilizing vascular endothelial cell monolayer. J Histochem Cytochem 30:214–221

137. Hofmann M, Rudy W, Zoller M, Tolg C, Ponta H, Jerrlich P, Gunthert U (1992) CD44 splice variants confer metastatic behavior in rats: homologous sequences are expressed in human tumor cell lines. Cancer Res 51:5292–5297

138. McCarthy JB, Skubitz APN, Lidy J, Mooradian DL, Wilke DS, Furcht LJ (1991) Tumor cell adhesive mechanisms and their relationship to metastasis. Semin Cancer Biol 2:155–167

139. Mareel M, Vleminckx K, Vermeulen S, Gao Y, Vakaet L Jr, Bracke M, Van Roy R (1992) Homotypic cell-cell adhesion molecules and tumor invasion. Prog Histochem Cytochem 26:95–106

140. Yamamura K, Kibbey MC, Kleinman HK (1993) Melanoma cells selected for adhesion to laminin peptides have different malignant properties. Cancer Res 53:423–429

141. Birch M, Mitchell S, Hart IR (1991) Isolation and characterization of human melanoma cell variants expressing high and low levels of CD44. Cancer Res 51:6660–6665

142. Matsumura Y, Tarin D (1992) Significance of CD44 gene products for cancer diagnosis and disease evaluation. Lancet 340:1053–1056

143. Friedrichs K, Franke F, Lisboa B-W (1995) CD44 isoforms correlate with cellular differentiation but not with prognosis in human breast cancer. Cancer Res 55:5424–5433

144. Ponta H, Sleeman J, Dall P, Moll J, Sherman L, Herrlich P (1994–1995) CD44 isoforms in metastatic cancer. Invasion Metast 14:82–86

145. Nesbit M, Herlyn M (1994–1995) Adhesion receptors in human melanoma progression. Invasion Metast 14:131–146

146. Ruiz P, Dunon D, Sonnenberg A, Imhof BA (1993) Suppression of mouse melanoma metastasis by EA-1, a monoclonal antibody specific for $\alpha6$ integrins. Cell Adhes Commun 1:67–81

147. Ruoslahti E (1994–1995) Fibronectin and its $\alpha_5\beta_1$ integrin receptor in malignancy. Invasion Metast 14:87–97

148. Xu X-C, El-Naggar AK, Lotan R (1995) Differential expression of galectin-1 and galectin-3 in thyroid tumors. Am J Pathol 147:815–822

149. Nicolson GL, Dulski K, Basson C, Welch DR (1985) Preferential organ attachment and invasion in vitro by B16 melanoma cells selected for differ-

ing metastatic colonization and invasive properties. Invasion Metast 5:144–152

150. Kim WH, Jun SH, Kibbey MC, Thompson EQ, Kleinman HK (1994–1995) Expression of β1 integrin in laminin-adhesion-selected human colon cancer cell lines of varying tumorigenicity. Invasion Metast 14:147–155

151. Terranova VP, Williams JE, Liotta LA, Martin GR (1984) Modulation of the metastatic activity of melanoma cells by laminin and fibronectin. Science 226:982–985

152. Hujanen ES, Terranova VP (1985) Migration of tumor cells to organ-derived chemoattractants. Cancer Res 45:3517–3522

153. Radinsky R (1993) Paracrine growth regulation of human colon carcinoma organ-specific metastases. Cancer Metast Rev 12:345–361

154. Cavanaugh PG, Nicolson GL (1989) Purification and some properties of a lung-derived growth factor that differentially stimulates the growth of tumor cells metastatic to the lung. Cancer Res 49:3928–3933

155. Chung LWK (1991) Fibroblasts are critical determinants in prostatic cancer growth and dissemination. Cancer Metast Rev 10:263–275

156. Roberts AB, Thompson NL, Heine U, Flanders C, Sporn MB (1988) Transforming growth factor β: possible roles in carcinogenesis. Br J Cancer 57:594–600

157. Ervin PR, Kaminski MS, Cody RL, Wicha MS (1989) Production of mammastatin, a tissue-specific growth inhibitor, by normal human mammary cells. Science 244:1585–1587

158. Plowman GD, Green JM, McDonald VL, Neubauer MG, Disteche CM, Todaro GJ, Shoyab M (1981) The amphiregulin gene encodes a novel epidermal growth factor-related protein with tumor-inhibitory activity. Mol Cell Biol 10:1969–1981

159. Radinsky R (1991) Growth factors and their receptors in metastasis. Semin Cancer Biol 2:169–177

160. Zarrilli R, Bruni CB, Riccio A (1994) Multiple levels of control of insulin-like growth factor gene expression. Mol Cell Endocrinol 101:R1–R14

161. Stiles CD, Capone GT, Scher CD, Antoniades HN, Van Wyk JJ, Pledger WJ (1979) Dual control of cell growth by somatomedins and platelet-derived growth factor. Proc Natl Acad Sci USA 76:1279–1283

162. Long L, Nip J, Brodt P (1994) Paracrine growth stimulation by hepatocyte-derived insulin-like growth factor-1: a regulatory mechanism for carcinoma cells metastatic to the liver. Cancer Res 54:3732–3737

163. Roberts AB, Sporn MB, Assoian RK, Smith JM, Roche NS, Wakefield LM, Heine VI, Liotta LA,

Falanga V, Kehr LJM (1986) Transforming growth factor type B: rapid induction of fibrosis and angiogenesis in vivo and stimulation of collagen formation in vitro. Proc Natl Acad Sci USA 83:4167–4171

164. Fan D, Chakrabarty S, Seid C, Bell CW, Schackert H, Morikawa K, Fidler IJ (1989) Clonal stimulation or inhibition of human colon carcinomas and human renal carcinoma mediated by transforming growth factor-β1. Cancer Commun 1:117–125

165. Gutman M, Singh RK, Price JE, Fan D, Fidler IJ (1995) Accelerated growth of human colon cancer cells in nude mice undergoing liver regeneration. Invasion Metast 14:362–371

166. Grupposo PA, Mead JE, Fausto N (1990) Transforming growth factor receptors in liver regeneration following partial hepatectomy in the rat. Cancer Res 50:1464–1469

167. Mead JE, Fausto N (1989) Transforming growth factor α may be a physiological regulator of liver regeneration by means of an autocrine mechanism. Proc Natl Acad Sci USA 86:1558–1562

168. Noji S, Tashiro K, Koyama E, Nohno T, Ohyama K, Taniguchi S, Nakamura T (1990) Expression of hepatocyte growth factor gene in endothelial and Kupffer cells of damaged rat livers, as revealed by in situ hybridization. Biochem Biophys Res Commun 173:42–47

169. Malden L, Novak U, Burgess A (1989) Expression of transforming growth factor alpha messenger RNA in normal and neoplastic gastrointestinal tract. Int J Cancer 43:380–384

170. Markowitz SD, Molkentin K, Gerbic C, Jackson J, Stellato T, Willson JKV (1990) Growth stimulation by coexpression of transforming growth factor-α and epidermal growth factor receptor in normal and adenomatous human colon epithelium. J Clin Invest 86:356–362

171. Van der Geer P, Hunter T, Lindberg RA (1994) Receptor protein-tyrosine kinases and their signal transducation pathways. Annu Rev Cell Biol 10:251–337

172. Schlesinger J (1986) Allosteric regulation of the epidermal growth factor receptor kinase. J Cell Biol 103:2067–2072

173. Van Dale P, Galand P (1988) Effect of partial hepatectomy on experimental liver invasion by intraportally injected colon carcinoma cells in rats. Invasion Metast 8:217–227

174. Michalopoulos GK (1990) Liver regeneration: molecular mechanisms of growth control. FASEB J 4:176–187

175. Rubin RA, O'Keefe EJ, Harp HS (1982) Alteration of epidermal growth factor-dependent phosphorylation during rat liver regeneration. Proc Natl Acad Sci USA 79:776–780

176. Derynck R (1992) The physiology of transforming growth factor-α. Adv Cancer Res 58:27–56

177. Gherardi E, Stoker M (1991) Hepatocyte growth factor-scatter factor: mitogen, motogen, and *met*. Cancer Cells 3:227–232

178. Ullrich A, Schlessinger J (1990) Signal transduction by receptors with tyrosine kinase activity. Cell 61:203–212

179. Furlong RA (1992) The biology of hepatocyte growth factor/scatter factor. Bioessays 14:613–620

180. Grupposo PA, Mead JE, Fausto N (1990) Transforming growth factor receptors in liver regeneration following partial hepatectomy in the rat. Cancer Res 50:1464–1469

181. Sainsbury JRC, Sherbert GV, Farndon JR, Harris AL (1986) Epidermal growth factor receptors and oestrogen receptors in human breast cancer. Lancet 1:364–366

182. Libermann TA, Nusbaum HR, Razon N, Kris R, Lax I, Soreq H, Whittle H, Waterfield MD, Ullrich A, Schlessinger J (1985) Amplification, enhanced expression and possible rearrangement of EGF receptor gene in primary brain tumours of glial origin. Nature 313:144–147

183. Harris AL, Neal DE (1987) Epidermal growth factor and its receptor in human cancer. In: Sluyser M (ed) Growth factors and oncogenes in breast cancer. Ellis Horwoo, Chichester, UK, pp 60–90

184. Berger MS, Greenfield C, Gullick WJ, Haley J, Downward J, Neal DE, Harris AL, Waterfield MD (1987) Evaluation of epidermal growth factor receptors in bladder tumours. Br J Cancer 56:533–537

185. Ullrich AL, Coussens L, Hayflick JS, Dull TJ, Gray A, Tam AW, Lee J, Yarden Y, Libermann TA, Schlessinger J, Downward J, Whittle ELV, Waterfield MD, Seeburg PH (1984) Human epidermal growth factor receptor cDNA sequence and aberrant expression of the amplified gene in A431 epidermoid carcinoma cells. Nature 309:418–425

186. Gross ME, Zorbas MA, Daniels YJ, Garcia R, Gallick GE, Olive M, Brattain MG, Boman BM, Yeoman LC (1991) Cellular growth response to epidermal growth factor in colon carcinoma cells with an amplified epidermal growth factor receptor derived from a familial adenomatous polyposis patient. Cancer Res 51:1452–1459

187. Radinsky R, Fidler IJ (1992) Regulation of tumor cell growth at organ-specific metastases. In Vivo 6:325–332

188. Radinsky R, Risin S, Fan D, Dong Z, Bielenberg D, Bucana CD, Fidler IJ (1995) Level and function of epidermal growth factor receptor predict the metastatic potential of human colon carcinoma cells. Clin Cancer Res 1:19–31

189. Radinsky R, Bucana CD, Ellis LE, Sanchez R, Cleary KR, Brigati DJ, Fidler IJ (1993) A rapid colorimetric in situ messenger RNA hybridization technique for analysis of epidermal growth factor receptor in paraffin-embedded surgical specimens of human colon carcinomas. Cancer Res 53:937–943

190. Bottaro DP, Rubin JS, Faletto DL, Chan AM, Kmiecik TE, Vande-Woude GF, Aaronson SA (1991) Identification of the hepatocyte growth factor receptor as the *c-met* proto-oncogene product. Science 215:802–805

191. Sugarbaker EV, Cohen AM, Ketcham AS (1971) Do metastases metastasize? Am Surg 174:161–170

192. Fidler IJ, Nicolson G (1976) Organ selectivity for implantation survival and growth of B16 melanoma variant tumor lines. J Natl Cancer Inst 57:1199–1202

193. Hoover HC, Ketcham AS (1975) Metastasis of metastases. Am J Surg 130:405–411

194. Fialkow PJ, Gartler SN, Yoshida A (1967) Clonal origin of myelocytic leukemia in man. Proc Natl Acad Sci USA 59:1468–1473

195. Vogelstein B, Fearon ER, Hamilton SR (1985) Use of restriction fragment length polymorphisms to determine the clonal origin of human tumors. Science 227:642–645

196. Fidler IJ, Kripke ML (1977) Metastasis results from preexisting variant cells within a malignant tumor. Science 197:893–895

197. Fidler IJ, Gruys E, Cifone MA, Barnes Z, Bucana CD (1981) Demonstration of multiple phenotype diversity in a murine melanoma of recent origin. J Natl Cancer Inst 67:947–856

198. Luria SE, Delbruck M (1943) Mutations of bacteria from virus sensitivity to virus resistance. Genetics 28:491–511

199. Fidler IJ (1986) Rationale and methods for the use of nude mice to study the biology and therapy of human cancer metastasis. Cancer Metast Rev 5:29–49

200. Giavazzi R, Campbell DE, Jessup JM, Cleary K, Fidler IJ (1986) Metastatic behavior of tumor cells isolated from primary and metastatic human colorectal carcinomas implanted into different sites of nude mice. Cancer Res 46:1928–1933

201. Naito S, von Eschenbach AC, Giavazzi R, Fidler IJ (1986) Growth and metastasis of tumor cells isolated from a human renal cell carcinoma implanted into different organs of nude mice. Cancer Res 46:4109–4115

202. Morikawa K, Walker SM, Jessup JM, Fidler IJ (1988) In vivo selection of highly metastatic cells from surgical specimens of different human colon carcinomas implanted into nude mice. Cancer Res 48:1943–1948

203. Fidler IJ, Naito S, Pathak S (1990) Orthotopic implantation is essential for the selection, growth and metastasis of human renal cell cancer in nude mice. Cancer Metast Rev 9:149–165

204. Fidler IJ (1991) Orthotopic implantation of human colon carcinomas into nude mice provides a valuable model for the biology and therapy of cancer metastasis. Cancer Metast Rev 10:229–243

205. Giavazzi R, Jessup JM, Campbell DE, Walker SM, Filder IJ (1986) Experimental nude mouse model in human colorectal cancer liver metastases. J Natl Cancer Inst 77:1303–1308

206. Leduce EH (1959) Metastasis of transplantable hepatomas from the spleen to the liver in mice. Cancer Res 19:1091–1095

207. Jessup JM, Giavazzi G, Campbell D, Cleary K, Morkawa K, Fidler IJ (1988) Growth potential of human colorectal carcinomas in nude mice: association with the preoperative serum concentration of carcinoembryonic antigen. Cancer Res 48:1689–1692

208. Ewing J (1928) Neoplastic disease, 6th edn. Saunders, Philadelphia

209. Price JE, Aukerman SL, Fidler IJ (1986) Evidence that the process of murine melanoma metastasis is sequential and selective and contains stochastic elements. Cancer Res 46:5172–5178

210. Holmgren L, O'Reilly MS, Folkman J (1995) Dormancy of micrometastases: balanced proliferation and apoptosis in the presence of angiogenesis suppression. Nature Med 1:149–153

211. Sutherland RM (1988) Cell and environment interactions in tumor microregions: the multicell spheroid model. Science 240:177–180

212. Tarin D, Price JE, Kettlewell MGW, Souter RG, Vass ACR, Crossley B (1984) Clinicopathological observations on metastasis in man studied in patients treated with peritoneovenous shunts. BMJ 288:749–751

213. Singh RK, Bucana CD, Gutman M, Fan D, Wilson MR, Fidler IJ (1994) Organ site-dependent expression of basic fibroblast growth factor in human renal cell carcinoma cells. Am J Pathol 145:365–374

214. Singh RK, Gutman M, Bucana CD, Sanchez R, Llansa N, Fidler IJ (1995) Interferons alpha and beta downregulate the expression of basic fibroblast growth factor in human carcinomas. Proc Natl Acad Sci USA 92:4562–4566

215. Singh RK, Gutman M, Radinsky R, Bucana CD, Fidler IJ (1994) Expression of interleukin 8 correlates with the metastatic potential of human melanoma cells in nude mice. Cancer Res 54:3242–3247

216. Nanus DM, Schmitz-Drager BJ, Motzer RJ, Lee AC, Vlamis V, Cordon-Cardo C, Albino AP, Reuter VE (1994) Expression of basic fibroblast growth factor in primary human renal tumors: correlation with poor survival. J Natl Cancer Inst 85:1597–1599

217. Nguyen M, Watanabe H, Budson AE, Richie JP, Hayes DF, Folkman J (1994) Elevated levels of an angiogenic peptide, basic fibroblast growth factor, in the urine of patients with a wide spectrum of cancers. J Natl Cancer Inst 86:356–361

218. Leek RD, Harris AL, Lewis CE (1994) Cytokine networks in solid human tumors: regulation of angiogenesis. J Leukocyte Biol 56:423–435

219. Gutman M, Singh RK, Xie K, Bucana CD, Fidler IJ (1995) Regulation of IL-8 expression in human melanoma cells by the organ environment. Cancer Res 55:2470–2475

220. Ezekowitz RAB, Mulliken JB, Folkman J (1992) Interferon alfa-2a therapy for life-threatening hemangiomas of infancy. N Engl J Med 326:1456–1463

221. Real FX, Oettgen HF, Krown SE (1986) Kaposi's sarcoma and the acquired immunodeficiency syndrome: treatment with high and low doses of recombinant leukocyte interferon. J Clin Oncol 4:544–551

222. Liotta LA, Stetler-Stevenson WG (1990) Metalloproteinases and cancer invasion. Semin Cancer Biol 1:107–116

223. Stetler-Stevenson WG (1990) Type IV collagenase in tumor invasion and metastases. Cancer Metast Rev 9:289–303

224. Morikawa K, Walker SM, Nakajima M, Pathak S, Jessup JM, Fidler IJ (1988) Influence of organ environment on the growth, selection, and metastasis of human colon carcinoma cells in nude mice. Cancer Res 48:6863–6871

225. Nakajima M, Morikawa K, Fabra A, Bucana CD, Fidler IJ (1990) Influence of organ environment on extracellular matrix degradative activity and metastasis of human colon carcinoma cells. J Natl Cancer Inst 82:1890–1898

226. Fabra A, Nakajima M, Bucana CD, Fidler IJ (1992) Modulation of the invasive phenotype of human colon carcinoma cells by fibroblasts from orthotopic or ectopic organs of nude mice. Differentiation 52:101–110

227. Gohji K, Fidler IJ, Tsan R, Radinsky R, von Eschenbach AC, Tsuruo T, Nakajima M (1994) Human recombinant interferons-beta and -gamma decrease gelatinase production and invasion by human KG-2 renal carcinoma cells. Int J Cancer 58:380–384

228. Slack NH, Bross JDJ (1975) The influence of the site of metastasis on tumor growth and response to chemotherapy. Br J Cancer 32:78–86

229. Pratesi G, Manzotti C, Tortoreto M, Audisio RA, Zunino F (1991) Differential efficacy of flavone acetic acid against liver versus lung metastases

in a human tumour xenograft. Br J Cancer 663:71–74

230. Smith KA, Begg AC, Denekamp J (1985) Differences in chemosensitivity between subcutaneous and pulmonary tumors. Eur J Cancer Clin Oncol 21:249–256

231. Donelli MG, Russo R, Garattini S (1975) Selective chemotherapy in relation to the site of tumor transplantation. Int J Cancer 32:78–86

232. Staroselsky A, Fan D, O'Brian CA, Bucana CD, Gupta KP, Fidler IJ (1990) Site-dependent differences in response of the UV-2237 murine fibrosarcoma to systemic therapy with adriamycin. Cancer Res 40:7775–7780

233. Wilmanns C, Fan D, O'Brian CA, Bucana CD, Fidler IJ (1992) Orthotopic and ectopic organ environments differentially influence the sensitivity of murine colon carcinoma cells to doxorubicin and 5-fluorouracil. Int J Cancer 52:98–104

234. Germann UA, Pastan I, Gottesman MM (1993) P-glycoproteins: mediators of multidrug resistance. Semin Cell Biol 4:63–78

235. Tsuruo T (1988) Mechanisms of multidrug resistance and implication for therapy. Gann 79:285–296

236. Bradley G, Juranka PE, Ling V (1988) Mechanism of multidrug resistance. Biochim Biophys Acta 948:87–128

237. Kartner N, Riordan JR, Ling V (1983) Cell surface P-glycoprotein associated with multidrug resistance in mammalian cell lines. Science 221:1285–1288

238. Chabner BA, Foji A (1989) Multidrug resistance: P-glycoprotein and its allies—the elusive foes. J Natl Cancer Inst 81:910–913

239. Weinstein RS, Kuszak IR, Kluskens LF, Cons JS (1990) P-glycoprotein in pathology: the multidrug resistance gene family in humans. Hum Pathol 21:34–48

240. Dong Z, Radinsky R, Fan D, Tsan R, Bucana CD, Wilmanns C, Fidler IJ (1994) Organ-specific modulation of steady-state *mdr* gene expression and drug resistance in murine colon cancer cells. J Natl Cancer Inst 86:913–920

241. Wilmanns C, Fan D, O'Brian CA, Radinsky R, Bucana CD, Tsan R, Fidler IJ (1993) Modulation of doxorubicin sensitivity and level of P-glycoprotein expression in human colon carcinoma cells by ectopic and orthotopic environments in nude mice. Int J Oncol 3:412–422

242. Kitadai Y, Ellis LM, Takahashi K, Bucana CD, Anzai H, Tahara T, Fidler IJ (1995) Multiparametric in situ mRNA hybridization analysis to detect metastasis-related genes in surgical specimens of human colon carcinoma. Clin Cancer Res 1:1095–1102

243. Mizoguchi T, Yamada K, Furukawa T, Hidaka T, Hisatsugu H, Shimazu T, Tsuruo T, Sumizawa T, Akiyama S (1990) Expression of the *mdr1* gene in human gastric and colorectal carcinomas. J Natl Cancer Inst 82:1679–1683

244. Morrow CS, Cowan KH (1988) Mechanisms and clinical significance of multidrug resistance. Oncology 2:55–63

245. Bradley G, Sharma R, Rajalakshmi S, Ling V (1992) P-glycoprotein expression during tumor progression in the rat liver. Cancer Res 52:5154–5161

246. Fidler IJ, Radinsky R (1990) Genetic control of cancer metastasis. J Natl Cancer Inst 82:166–168 (editorial)

247. Liotta LA (1988) Gene products which play a role in cancer invasion and metastasis. Breast Cancer Res Treat 11:113–124

248. Collard JG, Roos E, La Riviere G, Habets GGM (1988) Genetic analysis of invasion and metastasis. Cancer Surv 7:691–710

249. Bucana CD, Radinsky R, Dong Z, Sanchez R, Brigati DJ, Fidler IJ (1993) A rapid colorimetric in situ mRNA hybridization technique using hyperbiotinilated oligonucleotide probes for analysis of *mdr1* in mouse colon carcinoma cells. J Histochem Cytochem 41:499–506

250. Kitadai Y, Bucana CD, Ellis LM, Anzai H, Tahara E, Fidler IJ (1995) In situ mRNA hybridization technique for analysis of metastasis-related genes in human colon carcinoma cells. Am J Pathol 147:1238–1247

251. Anzai H, Kitadai Y, Bucana CD, Sanchez R, Omoto R, Fidler IJ (1996) Intratumoral heterogeneity and inverse correlation between expression of E-cadherin and collagenase type IV in human gastic carcinomas. Differentiation 60:119–127

Abnormal *CD44* Gene Expression in Neoplasia: Biological and Clinical Implications

David Tarin

Summary. The CD44 gene is one of the most interesting and promising new candidate markers for early cancer detection and for the analysis of genetic disturbances involved in neoplasia. It a large gene that under normal circumstances produces a variety of heavily glycosylated cell surface proteins by alternative splicing of its exons. Severe abnormalities have been observed in its patterns of expression in many types of common human tumors by both protein and RNA analyses. They are manifested by markedly increased levels of unusual CD44 transcripts and proteins in many tumors compared to corresponding normal tissues. Also, inappropriate expression patterns of the alternatively spliced exons have been linked to both tumor growth and metastatic potential. A unique manifestation of aberrant CD44 gene expression is the retention of introns in mature mRNA transcripts in the nucleus and cytoplasm of tumor cells but not in their normal counterparts. This phenomenon would naturally result in abnormal or truncated protein products. The clinical relevance of these observations is demonstrated by the frequent detection of all these abnormalities in fresh tissue samples from tumors of many organs and by their presence in preinvasive and high risk precancerous lesions. It has also been possible to achieve noninvasive detection of malignancy by identifying aberrant CD44 expression in exfoliated cells in body fluids and waste products. This chapter reviews the molecular mechanisms that result in such profound misregulation of the expression of this gene in neoplasia and the biological and clinical implications of these changes for tumors of the gastrointestinal tract.

Nuffield Department of Pathology and Bacteriology, Oxford University, John Radcliffe Hospital, Headington, Oxford OX3 9DU, UK

This chapter is an account of current ideas and information on one of the most interesting and mysterious components in the mammalian genetic repertoire. It is still known only by the code name *CD44*, indicating that its products and functions are largely unknown, although it has leapt to the forefront of attention and curiosity because its expression is so strikingly unusual in many common types of cancer, including those of the gastrointestinal tract and because it appears to be involved in a large variety of biological processes that are unrelated to each other.

The group of proteins encoded by this locus first attracted interest as a result of efforts by several research laboratories to identify and characterize cell surface molecules on white blood cells that might be important in cell-mediated immunity. These investigations included studies to isolate molecules involved in organizing the recirculatory traffic of lymphocytes as they patrol the organs of the body on surveillance missions [1]. The work resulted in the raising of a number of monoclonal antibodies (mAbs), which were eventually recognized to bind to different epitopes on a family of structurally related proteins assigned the designation CD (cluster of differentiation) 44 by the Human Leukocyte Workshop.

Subsequent studies [2, 3] with these antibodies rapidly made it clear that the CD44 family of proteins are not confined to the surfaces of white blood cells, and that some of them appear to be ubiquitously distributed on all cell types. It also emerged almost simultaneously that they are involved not just in immunological activities but in a surprising diversity of biological processes [4, 5], although their exact role in these processes remains unclear. Some of the functions in which they have been implicated include the following.

- Lymphocyte recirculation
- T lymphocyte activation
- Adhesion to other cells and to the intercellular matrix

- Embryonic development
- Hyaluronan metabolism
- Signal transduction across the cell membrane
- Growth factor secretion

Shortly afterward various parts of the gene were cloned and sequenced by several groups [6–11], and it became evident that by alternative splicing of its exons it can produce a large variety of protein isoforms. It appears to be one of the most alternatively spliced genes yet found.

The human *CD44* gene has now been mapped to the chromosomal locus 11p13 and confirmed to encode a family of large transmembrane glycoproteins. It is composed of a stretch of approximately 60 kb comprising at least 21 exons, 10 of which (exons 1–5 and 16–20) are constantly expressed on all cell types as the standard form (CD44s). The remaining 11 can be alternatively spliced with the constant ones (Fig. 1) to generate a number of variant protein isoforms (CD44v), which can be further modified by differential posttranslational glycosylation.

The complexity of the processes in which this gene is involved in cell and tissue function was further revealed when it became apparent that its expression is characteristically and severely changed in many common types of neoplasia, and that such dysfunction is involved in the acquisition of metastatic ability in some circumstances. The following account summarizes current knowledge of the unusual patterns of CD44 expression in cancer and considers their clinical and biological implications.

Abnormalities of CD44 Expression in Neoplasia

The deduction from early studies leading to the identification of CD44 that it is involved in cell attachment phenomena, such as the binding of circulating lymphocytes to vascular endothelium and of sedentary epithelial and stromal cells to each other or to the intercellular matrix, induced curiosity about the status of these cell surface molecules in tumors. The initial studies, using Northern blotting [6, 12], suggested that fresh tumor tissues contained additional unusual CD44 transcripts relative to corresponding normal ones. Separate work on tumor cell lines [13, 14] indicated that cells with elevated levels of CD44 proteins were more capable of producing metastases in animal experiments. However, such investigations were labor-intensive, and the prevalence and degree of anomalous expression of this gene in many common tumor types could not be fully appreciated until the technique of reverse transcription polymerase chain reaction (RT-PCR) became available. This method revealed that there is overproduction of a striking array of unusual CD44 mRNA species [15] in a wide variety of tumor tissues relative to their normal counterparts. In the meantime, independent investigations on metastatic and nonmetastatic clones derived from a rat pancreatic carcinoma cell line had led to isolation of a new variant CD44 protein, which was necessary for metastasis of this cell type [16]. These two new findings were followed

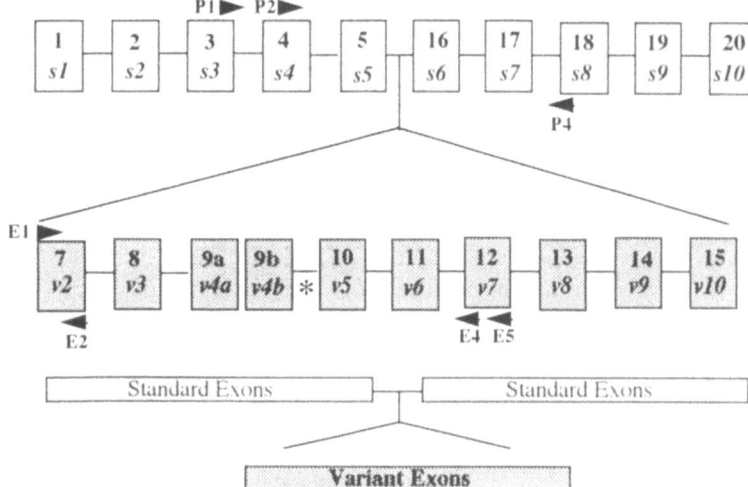

Fig. 1. Map of the human *CD44* gene. The nomenclature of exons, annealing positions of primers, and mode of splicing are shown. The *asterisk* marks the position of intron 9

by a large number of studies on CD44 gene expression in neoplasia that have established beyond reasonable doubt that misregulation of this gene and disorderly assembly of its products are hallmarks of this pathological process [17].

It remains unknown at present whether this disturbance is causally involved in cancer pathogenesis or is a consequence of this disease process. Although it is of considerable biological interest to resolve this uncertainty, it does not affect the promising implications of these findings for clinical cancer diagnosis, as is seen from the data presented below. Details of the changes observed in individual organ systems have been reviewed elsewhere [17], and the discussion that follows focuses on further developments and new considerations.

Abnormalities in Assembly of CD44 Transcripts

Although it has been reported by some groups that the level of expression of this gene can diminish in certain types of cancer, most publications [17] have described elevated CD44s and v transcription and translation in the most common types of cancers, including those of the stomach [18], colon [15], breast, bladder, and uterine cervix. RT-PCR consistently reveals an extensive array of amplicons of unusual sizes including many that are much larger than would be predicted from the known structure of the gene and the primers chosen for amplification (Fig. 2). Southern blot hybridization analysis with probes for several

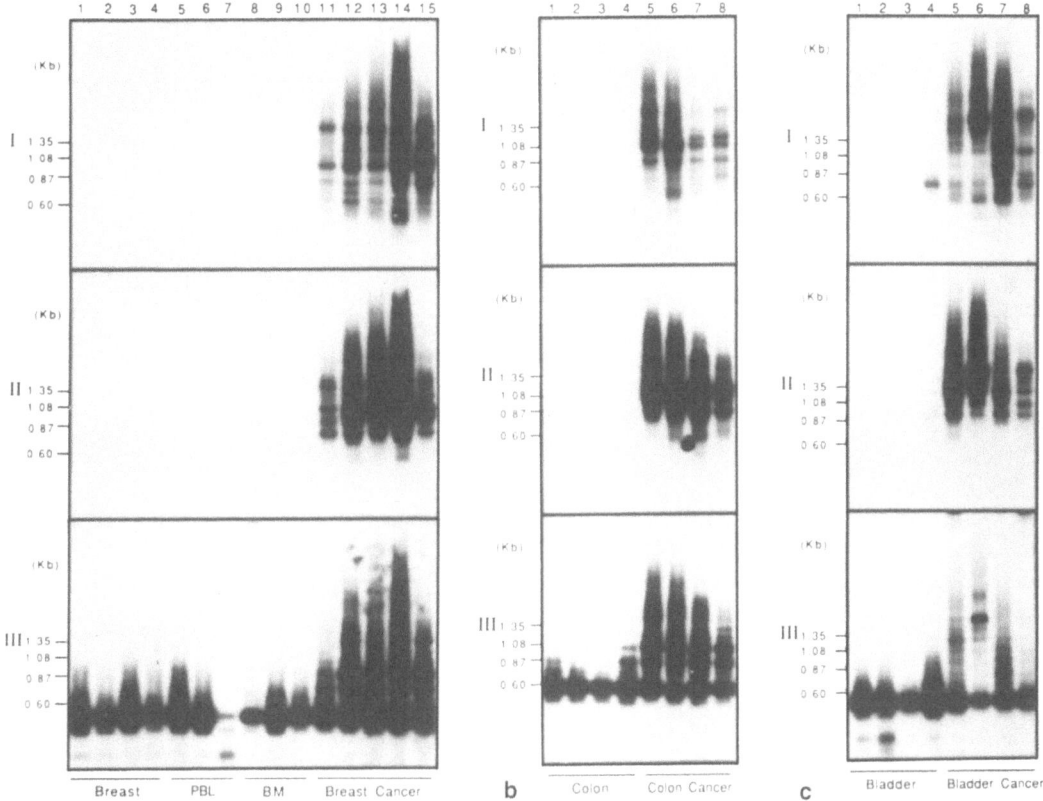

Fig. 2a–c. Autoradiograph of filters probed with oligonucleotide E2 (exposed for 1 day), E4 (exposed for 8 hours), and P2 (exposed for 2 hours) in rows I, II, and III, respectively, after amplification with primers P1 and P4. **a** Normal breast tissue (lanes 1–4), peripheral blood leukocytes from healthy volunteers (lanes 5–7), sternal bone marrow from patients with heart disease (lanes 8– 10), and breast cancer tissue (lanes 11–15). **b** Nonneoplastic colon tissue (lanes 1–4): normal tissue in lanes 1 and 3, inflamed colonic mucosa from Crohn's disease in lane 2, and ulcerative colitis in lane 4. Tissue from primary colonic cancer (lanes 5–8). **c** Normal bladder tissue (lanes 1–4) and primary bladder cancer tissue (lanes 5–8)

exons in the standard and variably expressed regions of the gene (Fig. 1) indicate that the abnormality is a global disorder affecting the expression of all exons studied, but it is clear that expression of the variant isoforms is particularly elevated. Detailed study of the results obtained from numerous tumors of several organs has led to the conclusion that there is no specific pattern of expression of any individual exon or of any detectable combination of exons that is characteristic of malignant neoplasia. Further analysis by PCR has revealed that the order of assembly of the exons in the transcript is also abnormal in tumors relative to comparable normal tissue, and that many variations can be seen in the same specimen (Goodison and Tarin, unpublished data). It is

therefore the overall irregular assembly of excessive amounts of large mRNA species in a given lesion that is itself the characteristic marker of malignancy.

The data available on early premalignant lesions, such as dysplastic areas in the bladder [10] and adenomas of the colon [19, 20], as well as on early-stage malignancies from carcinoma in situ to minimally invasive carcinomas indicate that the disorderly expression of this gene begins when the neoplasm is first forming and increases as the tumor becomes larger, invasive, and metastatic. However, observations on deeply invading late-stage tumors of the bladder [21] and of the colon (unpublished observations), where the tumor cells have reached the boundaries of the organ or have

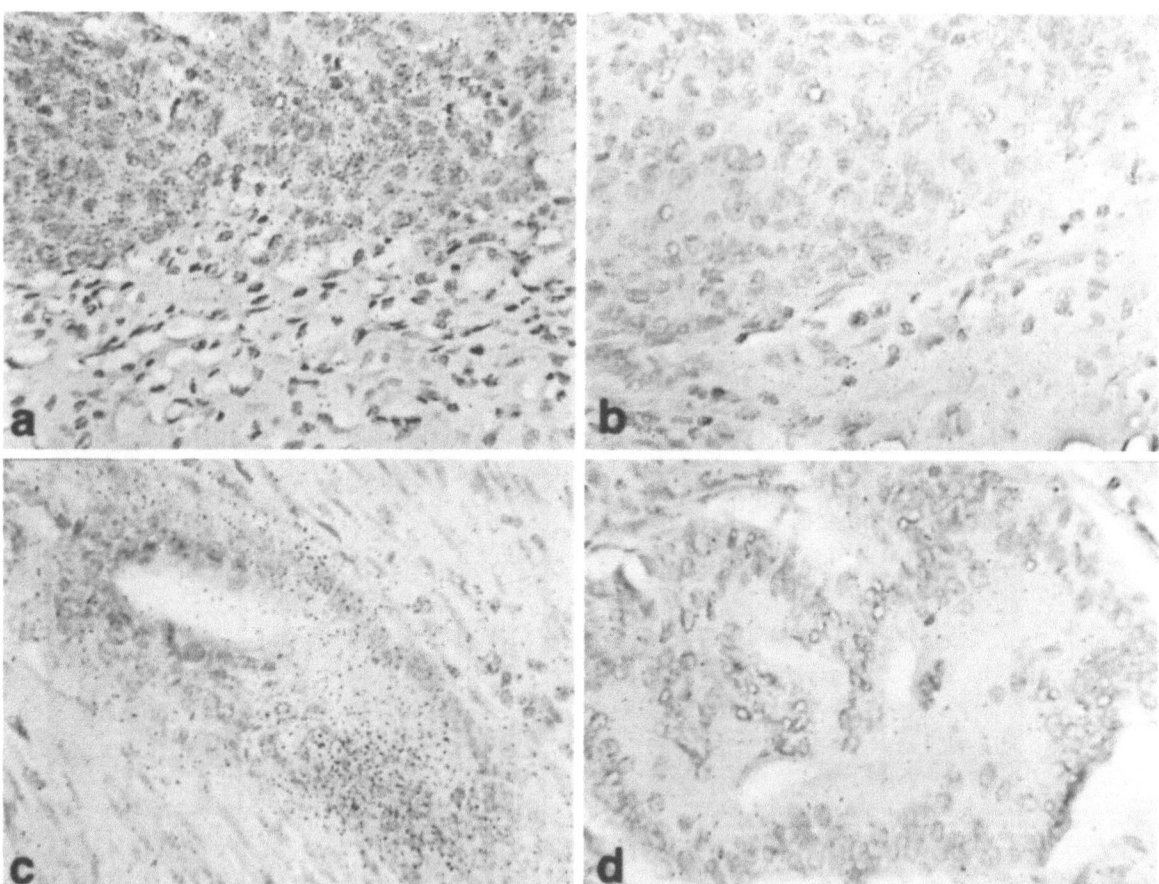

Fig. 3a–d. Paraffin wax sections of colonic carcinoma studied by in situ hybridization. **a** There is a detectable signal over carcinoma cells in a section hybridized with riboprobe complementary (anti-sense) to CD44s mRNA. **b** Section hybridized with sense riboprobe. **c** Detectable signal over carcinoma cells in a section hybridized with riboprobe complementary (antisense) to CD44v. **d** Section hybridized with sense riboprobe. Both sense hybridizations show only weak, nonspecific background grain density. (Original magnification ×400)

entered surrounding tissues, have shown that CD44 expression diminished to undetectable levels in the deepest areas of invasion.

In situ hybridization studies on histological sections of fresh frozen and formalin-fixed, paraffinembedded archival specimens of tumors and corresponding normal tissues [20–23] from the colon, breast, bladder, and cervix with anti-sense riboprobes that hybridize exclusively to CD44s or CD44v sequences have been performed. These studies confirmed that overexpression of this gene occurs only in the tumor cells, not in any reactive inflammatory cells that may be in the vicinity or in nonneoplastic resident cells of the supporting stroma (Fig. 3).

It is noteworthy that figures illustrating the results of Southern blot hybridization analysis of CD44 expression in tumors frequently show long, dense smears between the numerous individual bands that represent the predominant mRNA species in that specimen. These smears diminish if the autoradiograph is underexposed but do not disappear. Detailed analysis of this phenomenon in colon [24], stomach [25], bladder [11], and

breast cancers [26] has confirmed that these signals represent a smooth range of less prevalent alternatively spliced transcripts of intermediate sizes among which there are many incompletely spliced abnormal mRNA molecules containing introns. This interpretation has been proved by several converging lines of evidence including analysis with probes designed to hybridize to specific intron sequences (Fig. 4), amplifications with

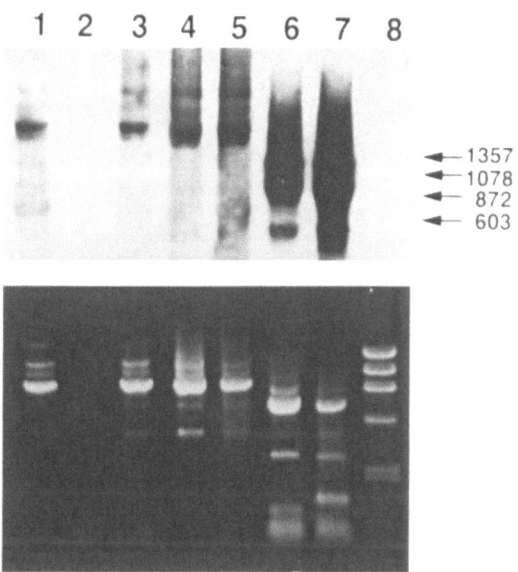

Fig. 5. Results of RNase and DNase digestion analysis of PCR products from HT29 human colon carcinoma cells are presented in lanes 1, 2, and 3. Lane 1: RT-PCR on untreated extracts; lane 2: RT-PCR following RNase digestion of extracts; lane 3: RT-PCR following DNase digestion of extracts. Poly(A)$^+$-selected RNA was digested with either RNase or DNase, followed by the RT-PCR reaction using primers P1 and P4. Southern blot analysis of the PCR products was performed using a probe for intron 9 for hybridization. Further analysis of the retention of intron 9 in mRNA transcripts in nuclear and cytoplasmic RNA fractions is presented in lanes 4–7. These experiments used 100 ng poly(A)$^+$-selected RNA from HT29 human colon carcinoma cells. Lanes 4 and 5: P1, P4 primer set was used for the RT-PCR reaction. Lanes 6 and 7: E1, E5 primer set was used for the RT-PCR reaction. Cytoplasmic RNA was used in lanes 4 and 6, and nuclear RNA was used in lanes 5 and 7, respectively. Ethidium bromide staining of the gel is presented below the Southern blot hybridization autoradiogram. The marker used was Phi × 174 HaeIII. The results show that the signal is abolished by RNase digestion of the extracts but not by DNase digestion, verifying that it is generated by amplification of mRNA transcripts containing the intron and that contamination with genomic DNA is excluded

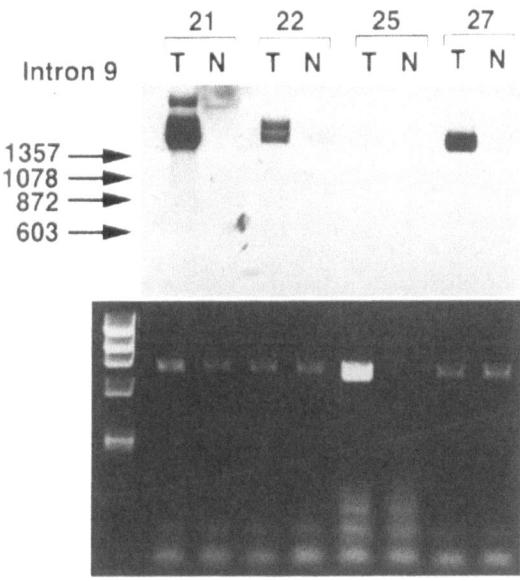

Fig. 4. Demonstration of abnormal retention of CD44 intron 9 in mRNA transcripts from human colon carcinoma tissues (*T*) and matched adjacent normal mucosa (*N*). Poly(a)$^+$ selected RNA (100 ng) was used for each RT-PCR reaction with E1, E5 primers. The estimated size of these amplicons containing both exon 9a and intron 9 is about 1.6 kb. Ethidium bromide staining of the gel is presented below the Southern blot hybridization autoradiogram. The marker used was Phi × 174 HaeIII

intron specific primers, DNAse digestion studies, and RNase digestion experiments (Fig. 5) [11, 24]. Similar studies conducted on normal tissues from the same organs rarely showed any signal with intron-specific probes, and when they were de-tected they were present in only trace amounts at the limit of detection.

Further experiments involving separation of nuclear and cytoplasmic components of HT 29 colon carcinoma cells and on RT112 bladder can-

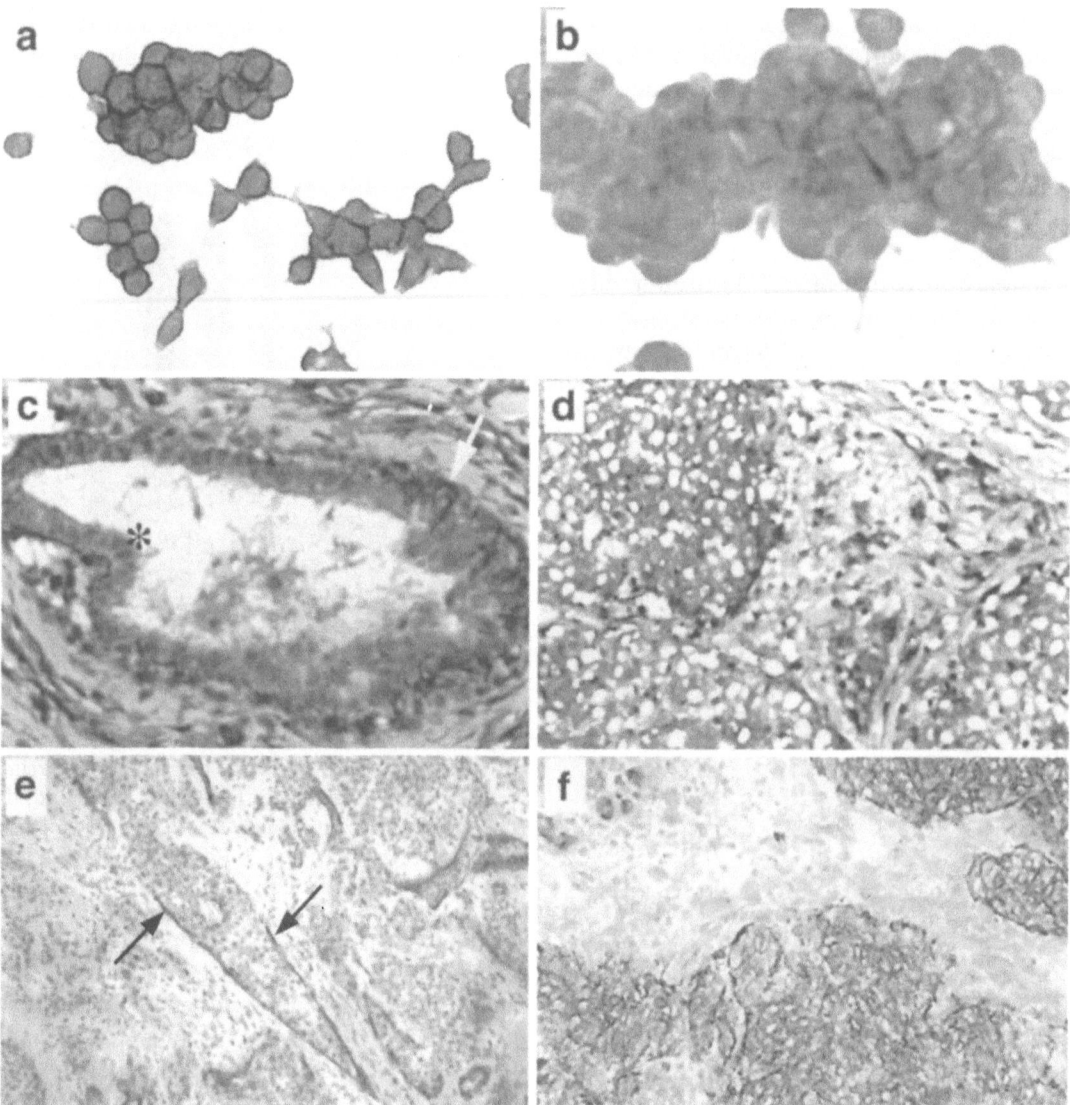

Fig. 6a–f. Immunocytochemical analysis of CD44 protein isoforms in ZR75-1 breast cancer cell line and in frozen sections of normal and malignant breast tissue. In ZR75-1 cells, strong membrane and cytoplasmic staining was observed with **a** MAb Hermes 3 (exon 5 epitope) which demonstrates all CD44 isoforms and **b** MAb 23.6.1 (exon 7 epitope) which reacts only with variant CD44 isoforms containing the peptide encoded by exon 7. **c–f** Representative immunohistochemical staining in normal and malignant tissues. **c** normal breast duct stained with Hermes-3 (exon 5 epitope); myoepithelial cells showing positive immunoreactivity are indicated by *arrows*, whereas negative ductal epithelial cells are marked with an *asterisk*. **d–f** Malignant breast tumors stained with Hermes-3, MAb 23.6.1 (exon 7 epitope) and MAb 2F10 (exon 11 epitope), respectively. The *arrow* in **e** shows residual positively stained myoepithelium and the *asterisks* mark the position of unstained tumor cells. The microscopical studies show that there is widespread gross over-expression of standard and variant CD44 proteins in the tumor cells and that there is regional heterogeneity of expression in different parts of the same tumor

cer cell line indicated that substantial quantities of the abnormal, intron-retaining transcripts enter the cytoplasm (Fig. 5), although such RNAs are virtually undetectable in nonneoplastic cells (e.g., urine cell sediments from patients with no evidence of neoplasia [11]). As with the previous hybridization studies using exon-specific probes, there does not appear to be any specific intron that is characteristically incorporated in cancer cells. The initial data on intron retention in CD44 transcripts in tumor cells were obtained using probes for intron 9, but subsequent work using probes for introns 14 and 18 on bladder and colorectal carcinomas, respectively (unpublished results), showed that these sequences, together or alone, are expressed in each specimen. These findings demonstrate that there are profound disturbances in assembly and processing of *CD44* gene transcripts in tumors that do not appear to affect transcription of at least some other alternatively spliced genes (Goodison and Tarin, unpublished data), but that none of these individual disorderly transcripts is diagnostic of cancer.

Abnormalities in Translation of CD44 Products

There have been several immunohistochemical investigations on *CD44* gene expression in a variety of cancers [20, 27–34] using monoclonal antibodies to epitopes encoded by several individual exons. These studies have confirmed that in many types of common cancers (with the apparent exception of squamous cell carcinomas of the head and neck and neuroblastomas) there is overexpression of CD44 protein isoforms in tumor tissues relative to nonneoplastic control tissues (Figs. 6–8). Such expression is not seen in every cancer cell but is limited to tumor cells and is heterogeneous throughout the tumor. An important exception has been observed in deeply invasive cells in late stage, advanced, aggressive cancers of the bladder [21] and colon (Yoshida and Tarin, unpublished data) that have reached the boundaries of the organ or penetrated surrounding tissues. These cells uniformly show little or no expression of any isoform.

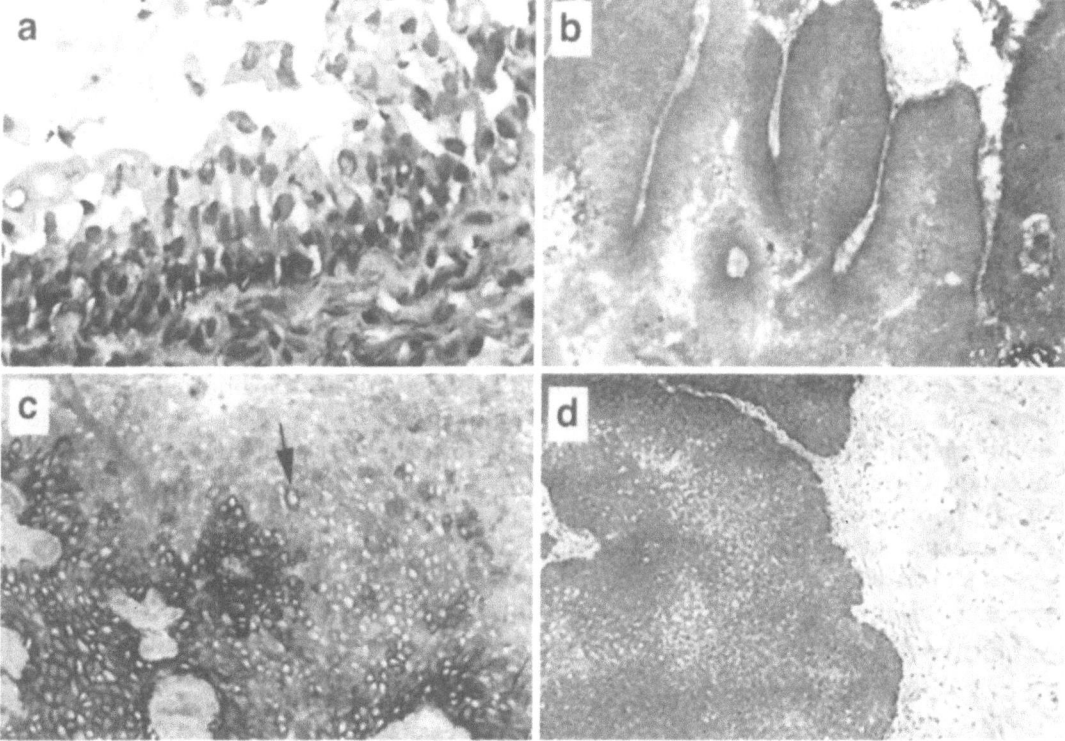

Fig. 7a–d. Immunohistochemical analysis of the distribution of CD44 protein isoforms in normal and neoplastic bladder. **a** Normal bladder stained with Hermes 3. **b–d** Malignant bladder tumor stained with Hermes 3, MAb 23.6.1, and MAb 2F10, respectively. The *arrow* in **c** identifies a cell showing strong immunoreactivity among others showing less, but still elevated, staining

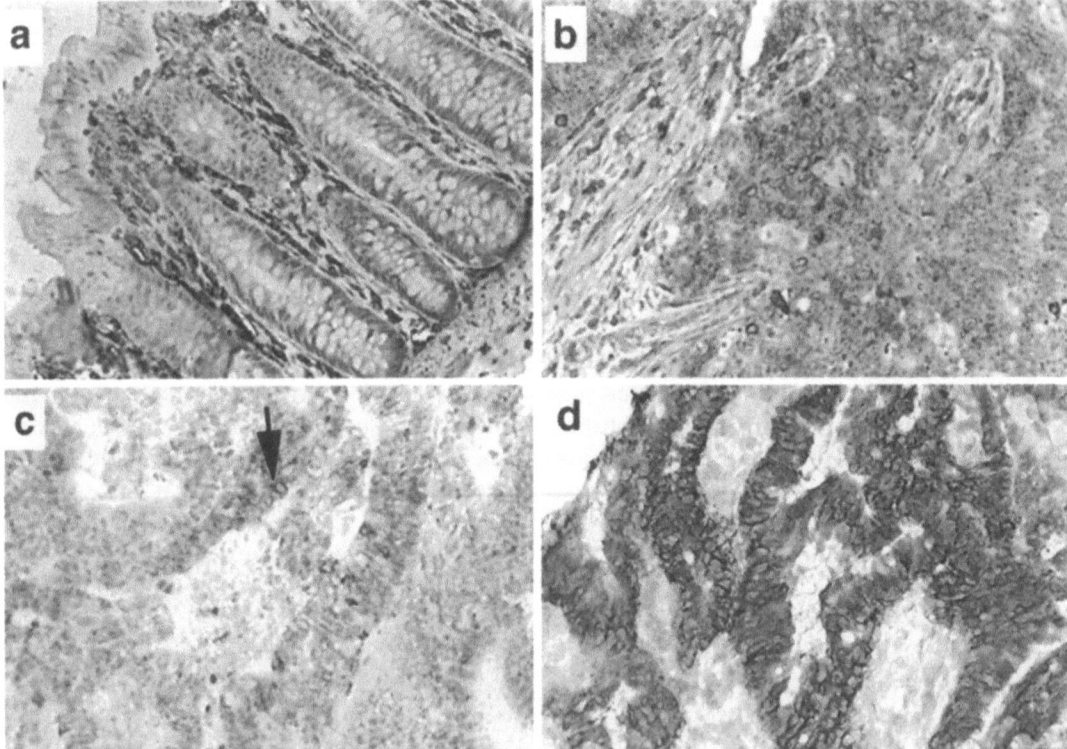

Fig. 8a–d. Distribution of CD44 protein isoforms in normal and neoplastic colonic mucosa. **a** Normal colon stained with Hermes 3. **b–d** Colon carcinoma stained with Hermes 3, MAb 23.6.1, and MAb 2F10, respec- tively. The *arrow* in **c** marks malignant cells exhibiting strong immunoreactivity with MAb 23.6.1. Widespread overexpression of all isoforms can be seen in many parts of the tumor

These immunohistochemical studies have re- vealed that there is not only an overall increase in the amount and diversity of CD44 protein produc- tion in tumors but also a marked alteration in the spatial location of these proteins within the indi- vidual cells involved and within the tissues in which the neoplasm is growing. Such changes are not seen in the cells of the nonmalignant stoma within the lesion. This finding implies that the abnormali- ties in the regulation of expression of this gene, which is known to have functions in cell adhesion and signal transduction, may contribute to the bi- zarre morphogenetic rearrangements of tissue components characteristic of malignant tumors.

Direct Comparison of CD44 Transcription and Translation in Tumor Cell Lines

Studies correlating CD44 mRNA and protein pro- files simultaneously in the same populations of tumor cells [34] have provided additional intrigu-

ing insights into the degree of misregulation of this gene in neoplasia. These investigations revealed that the production of transcripts and the transla- tion of these gene products appear to become un- coupled, resulting in the presence of many mRNA transcripts without corresponding proteins in the corresponding cells (Figs. 9, 10). In particular RT- PCR/Southern blot hybridization analysis with various probes showed that in each of the three cell lines studied (HT29 colon carcinoma and ZR- 75-1 and MDA435-4A4 breast cancer) many prominent bands did not have counterparts in the Western blots of cells harvested from the same dish analyzed with mAbs to epitopes encoded by the corresponding exons (Fig. 10). This discrep- ancy is unlikely to be the result of amplification of rare transcripts by PCR because some of the mRNA bands that were translated were no more prominent than those that were not. More prob- able is the interpretation that the retention of introns in some of the transcripts results in abro- gation or truncation of the translation process or in secretion and loss of products that may not have

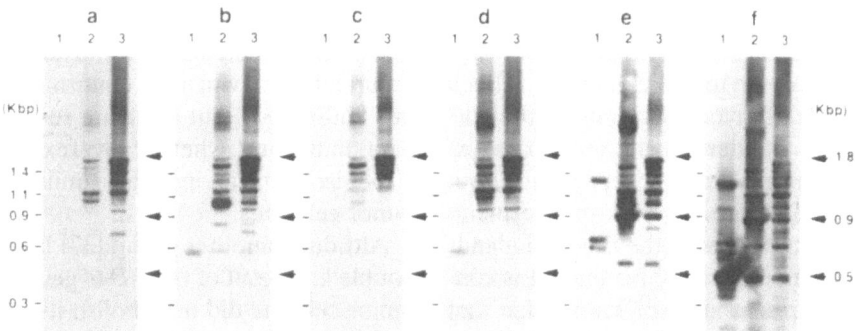

Fig. 9a–f. Autoradiographs of Southern hybridizations of RT-PCR products obtained from mRNA extracted from MDA-MB-435-4A4; (lane 1), HT29-1-2-H; (lane 2), and ZR75-1 (lane 3) cell lines. The blot was hybridized with probes specifically annealing to exon 7 (**a**), exon 8 (**b**), exon 10 (**c**), exon 11 (**d**), exon 15 (**e**) and standard exons (**f**) of the *CD44* gene. Between each hybridization, the filter was stripped to remove the previous probe

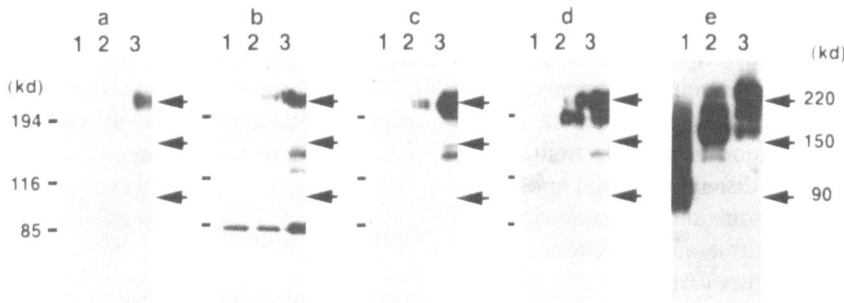

Fig. 10a–e. Western blot analysis of MDA-MB-435-4A4; (lane 1), HT29-1-2-H; (lane 2), and ZR75-1 (lane 3) cell lysates. The lysates (5 µg of protein per well) were probed with antibodies to epitopes encoded by CD44 exon 7 (23.6.1; **a**); exon 8 (3G5; **b**), exon 10 (VFF8; **c**), exon 11 (2F10; **d**), and Hermes-3 (**e**). Molecular weights are shown by the *arrows* depicting the positions of prestained protein markers

an anchoring trans-membrane domain. This viewpoint receives some support from the reports that soluble truncated forms of CD44 can be detected in culture media [34] and in elevated amounts in clinical samples of body fluids such as blood [35] and urine (Woodman and Tarin, unpublished data) from cancer patients.

Biological and Clinical Implications of Disturbances in CD44 Gene Expression

Biological Implications

Cell Differentiation, Turnover, and Tissue Organization

As mentioned above, an extensive body of work in many laboratories has implicated the CD44 family of proteins in a wide variety of cellular functions. Some of this research has demonstrated the prevalence of certain isoforms containing the products of exons 13–15 in many epithelia. From this and other work on the mechanisms of attachment of epithelial cell lines to hyaluran and other components of the intercellular matrix, it has been inferred that these CD44 isoforms are involved in the attachment of cells to each other and to the adjacent supporting connective tissue. Given the information from other unrelated studies that in certain circumstances CD44 proteins can also exercise signal transduction functions, the possibility emerges that this group of proteins may be active in epithelial mesenchymal interactions known to be essential for the establishment and maintenance of normal organotypic histological structure.

Histochemical analysis of the distribution of CD44 proteins in various tissues show that some isoforms are almost ubiquitous, whereas others are predominantly located in the basal layer or stem cell compartment of epithelia; still others are strictly localized to more superficial layers of a stratified epithelium or to individual special cell types elsewhere (e.g., myoepithelium). In the normal colon CD44 standard form protein is expressed on the stroma and the epithelium, but variant isoforms are detected only on the membranes of cells at the bases of the mucosal glands where cell replication occurs. This finding is consistent with the present state of knowledge that the gene has several functions, probably each executed at a different site by one of the several proteins it encodes. In carcinoma cell populations such orderly localization of expression is lost in favor of global haphazard overexpression associated with disorderly function of the tissue. Such immunohistochemical investigations also reveal that loss of the regular spatial patterns of CD44 expression is seen only in the tumor cells and not in the nonneoplastic cells of the supporting stroma. These changes in the patterns of activity of a multifunctional gene in a single tissue of an organ are expected to disrupt essential epithelial–mesenchymal interactions and thus contribute to the progressive structural and functional disorganization characteristic of cancer.

Tumor Metastasis

Metastasis is the defining and most intriguing characteristic of malignant tumors. It constitutes the major challenge to cancer biology and medicine. The initial indications that the products of the CD44 gene may have some involvement in metastasis came from studies on melanoma and lymphoma tumor cell lines inoculated into animals. Using a fluorescence activated cell sorter, Birch et al. [13] divided melanoma cells into populations that strongly expressed the 90 kDa form of the protein recognized by the Hermes 3 antibody and ones that did not. They found that the former were substantially more metastatic.

Almost simultaneously Sy et al. [14] described a moderate increase in metastatic capability of human lymphoma cells if they were transfected with the standard form of the gene but not if they were transfected with a construct coding for the epithelial variant. That same year Herrlich and colleagues [16] published a study identifying a new variant isoform of the CD44 gene that was expressed by a metastatic clone of a rat pancreatic carcinoma cell line but not by a nonmetastatic sister clone from the same parent cell line. The variant was cloned into an expression vector and

transfected into the nonmetastatic cell line, which then became metastatic. Further work by this group later convincingly confirmed and extended this finding [36], but there are so far no published data indicating whether overexpression of this CD44 isoform can induce a similar effect in other tumor cell lines.

Although another group [37] has reported that double knockout of the CD44 gene in a metastatic tumor cell line did not abolish its metastatic ability, the issue of whether expression of certain CD44 variant isoforms (containing exons 11, v6 and 12, v7) usually play an important role in natural tumor metastasis remains open. It remains formally possible that CD44v isoforms perform important functions during the process, but that these functions can be fulfilled by other related molecules in certain circumstances. It also cannot be excluded that inappropriate overexpression of CD44 might not induce metastasis because other important components with which it needs to interact to do so are absent.

Clinical Implications

Early Cancer Diagnosis

The profound misregulation of the expression of the CD44 gene in neoplasia identifies it as one of the most interesting and promising new candidate markers for early cancer detection. The clinical relevance of the observations described above is demonstrated by the frequent detection of all these abnormalities in fresh tissue samples from tumors of many organs and by their presence in preinvasive and high-risk precancerous lesions. With these techniques it has also been possible to achieve noninvasive detection of malignancy by identifying aberrant CD44 expression in exfoliated cells in body fluids and waste products.

For example, we [38] investigated whether colonic cancer cells that exfoliate into the lumen of the organ can be detected by identifying their abnormal CD44 gene products. Exfoliated cells were obtained by centrifugation of saline washouts of 27 surgically resected colon specimens obtained from 15 patients with carcinoma, 7 with ulcerative colitis, and 5 with Crohn's disease. After extracting cellular mRNA, amplification by the RT-PCR technique and analysis by Southern blot hybridization were performed to examine the levels and patterns of transcription of exons 11 (v6) and 12 (v7) and intron 9 of the CD44 gene.

We also examined the transcription of these CD44 components in snap-frozen solid tissue specimens from 11 of the above patients with colorectal carcinoma, 7 with ulcerative colitis, and 5 with Crohn's disease with RT-PCR. Abnormal expression of exons 11 (v6) and 12 (v7) was detected in exfoliated cells from 11 (73%) of 15 carcinoma cases but not in the cells from patients with inflammatory bowel disease (IBD). The retention of intron 9 in CD44 mRNA transcripts was detected in washings from 4 (27%) carcinoma cases but not in washings from nonmalignant specimens. It was confirmed that in solid tissue samples from the same carcinomas there was abnormal overexpression of numerous alternatively spliced CD44 species containing transcripts of exon 11 and 12 and retention of intron 9. Low-level expression of these exons was detected in tissue from inflammatory lesions from five of seven patients with ulcerative colitis and four of five with Crohn's disease, but the retention of an intron was not seen in normal mucosa or IBD tissue.

These findings suggest that abnormal expression of the variant exons and of intron 9 of the *CD44* gene in tumor cells that exfoliate into the colonic lumen may be helpful markers for early, noninvasive diagnosis of colorectal cancer. The clinical implication of this result is that modification of this technique to apply it to evacuated stool specimens could result in a noninvasive test for colorectal cancer. In preliminary experiments we have successfully detected abnormal CD44 expression, using RT-PCR on mRNA from exfoliated cells in stools from a small group of patients (6/11) with colorectal cancer but not in cells from normal subjects (Matsumura and Tarin, unpublished observations). For the sensitivity and specificity of this approach to be accurately evaluated, it is necessary to develop reliable techniques for retrieving viable exfoliated cells from evacuated stools. Clinical bowel preparation regimens that render the stools liquid and evacuate the lumen in preparation for surgery or radiological or endoscopic examination may be helpful for this purpose.

These results indicate that tests for this and other genetic abnormalities will probably soon revolutionize the diagnostic repertoire for early cancer detection in clinical gastroenterology. Traditional methods for noninvasive investigation or screening for bowel cancer are crude. Fecal occult blood (FOB) testing is unsatisfactory as a detection method for colorectal cancer. Most of the

carcinoma patients in the study had symptoms of anal bleeding or tested positive for FOB. Most of the IBD patients revealed the same symptoms, however, illustrating the difficulty of discriminating cancer patients from IBD patients. Cytology is a powerful, reliable method for identifying cancer cells, but it is labor-intensive, and expensive, and depends heavily on the quality of preservation of the cells in the sample. It has not been found useful for colorectal cancer diagnosis, but the data now accumulating indicate that molecular genetic analytical methods are poised to offer more specific and informative diagnostic alternatives.

As an aid to the evaluation of the clinical potential of using assays for abnormal *CD44* gene activity for early cancer diagnosis, all data published by this laboratory between 1992 and 1996 on this subject were compiled and statistically analyzed. The results are presented in Table 1 overleaf. This analysis clearly supports the interpretation that disorderly expression of the *CD44* gene is a characteristic feature of these common types of cancer and could therefore prove to be a useful diagnostic marker, but it is important to note that (1) the amalgamated figures have been obtained by pooling data from studies using different analytes and methods on samples of different types (e.g., solid tissues, exfoliated cells); and (2) the work has been done on a hospital-based population among whom the prevalence of disease is higher. Statistically, it is a fact that, as the prevalence of disease increases, the positive predictive value rises. Hence a test that is effective for diagnosis may be less valuable for screening and vice versa.

Prognostic Features

The science of evaluating the individual prognosis of patients with cancer is still in its infancy. Several studies have shown statistical associations between some of the clinical and molecular properties of tumors and the survival of the host, which in general correlates with the presence of metastases, but the ultimate goal of accurately evaluating the prognosis of individual patients so their treatment can be tailored accordingly is still out of reach.

Several groups have reported data indicating that overexpression of splice variants containing epitopes encoded by exon 11 (v6) of this gene assessed by immunohistochemistry correlates with a poor prognosis of patients with colorectal cancer [32], breast cancer [39], non-Hodgkin's lymphoma [40], and other neoplasms [17] as

Table 1. *CD44* gene expression in tumors of the bladder, breast, and colon; evaluation of CD44 as a diagnostic marker: 1992–1996

Part 1: Raw Data

Figures denote numbers of samples recorded as positive (numerator) over total number of samples studied (denominator). Criteria for positive results are given below. References to published work are given in brackets.

Bladder
   Solid tissues [15, 21]
      Cancer: 20[a]/25
      Controls: 0/8
      Technique: RT-PCR with probe for exon 12
   Urine: exfoliated cells [10, 11, 45]
      Cancer: 96[b]/121
      Controls: 8[c]/128
      Techniques: RT-PCR with probe for exon 12
               RT-PCR with probe for intron 9
               Western blotting with Hermes 3 antibody

Colon and rectum
   Solid tissues [10, 15, 24, 25]
      Cancer: 72/80
      Controls: 4[d]/47
      Techniques: RT-PCR with probe for exon 12
               RT-PCR with probe for intron 9
   Colon washings [38]
      Cancer: 11/15
      Controls: 0/12
      Technique: RT-PCR with probe for exon 12

Breast cancer
   Solid tissues [26, 46]
      Cancer: 42/42
      Controls: 3[e]/21
      Techniques: RT-PCR with probe for exon 12
               RT-PCR with probe for intron 9

Part 2: Statistical Analysis

Bladder
   Solid tissues
      Sensitivity = 20/25 = 80%
      Specificity = 8/8 = 100%
      Positive predictive value = 20/20 = 100%
   Urine
      Sensitivity = 96/121 = 79%
      Specificity = 120/128 = 94%
      Positive predictive value = 96/104 = 92%

Colon
   Solid tissues
      Sensitivity = 72/80 = 90%
      Specificity = 43/47 = 91%
      Positive predictive value = 72/76 = 95%
   Washings
      Sensitivity = 11/15 = 73%
      Specificity = 12/12 = 100%
      Positive predictive value = 11/11 = 100%

Breast
      Sensitivity = 42/42 = 100%
      Specificity = 18/21 = 86%
      Positive predictive value = 42/45 = 93%

RT-PCR, reverse transcription-polymerase chain reaction.

Note: This compilation does not include further unpublished data in our possession. Where more than one technique was used the figures represent amalgamated results from separate studies on separate specimens.

A positive result in RT-PCR studies using probes for exon 12 requires amplicons above 1 kb in size on autoradiographs. A positive result in RT-PCR studies using probes for intron 9 is recorded if any signal is seen on the autoradiograph of that sample. A positive result in Western blotting requires bands above 150 kDa reacting with Hermes 3 antibody.

We consider that a weak signal obtained from normal tissue in studies with an intron probe is easily recognized with the naked eye as different from the signal from a positive cancer sample. However, it is still a signal and we have recorded it as such. (The signal probably comes from pre-mRNA in the nucleus, which is in the process of being spliced.)

[a] The five cases that were negative were all deeply invasive advanced cancer. All early cancers and precancers were positive.

[b] Collated data from separate studies using different techniques as shown.

[c] All eight "false positives" resulted from weak signals in RT-PCR studies with exon 12. In the other studies the controls were all negative.

[d] All four "false positives" resulted from weak signals in RT-PCR studies with intron 9. In the other study all controls were negative.

[e] All three "false positives" resulted from very weak signals in RT-PCR studies with intron 9. In the other study all controls were negative.

judged by a more advanced tumor stage, the presence of metastases, or a shorter survival time. Results obtained by other groups using RT-PCR [15, 41, 42] and Northern blotting [43] supported these conclusions. On the other hand, a few contradictory reports describing either a lack of any such correlation in breast cancer [33] or downregulation of CD44 isoforms in pulmonary adenocarcinomas [44] have also been published. Collectively, most of the available evidence indicates that there are meaningful associations between abnormal expression of alternatively spliced CD44 isoforms, tumor metastasis, and reduced survival. However, the mode of evaluating histochemical staining results and Southern blot hybridizations is subjective and not quantitative. Therefore although the data show an overall general trend that the degree of CD44s and v misregulation correlates with the aggressiveness of the disease, it is presently not a sufficiently reliable indicator of the outcome of disease in an individual patient to use it when making treatment decisions. This situation might well change if an accurate, reliable method for measuring *CD44* gene overexpression becomes available.

References

1. Culty M, Miyake K, Kincade PW, Sikorski E, Butcher EC, Underhill C, Sikorski E (1990) The hyaluronate receptor is a member of the CD44 (H-CAM) family of cell surface glycoproteins. J Cell Biol 111:2765–2774
2. Picker LJ, Nakache M, Butcher EC (1989) Monoclonal antibodies to human lymphocyte homing receptors define a novel class of adhesion molecules on diverse cell types. J Cell Biol 109:927–937
3. Mackay CR, Terpe H-J, Stauder R, Marston WL, Stark H, Gunthert U (1994) Expression and modulation of CD44 variant isoforms in humans. J Cell Biol 124:71–82
4. Haynes BF, Telen MJ, Hale LP, Denning SM (1989) CD44—a molecule involved in leukocyte adherence and T-cell activation. Immunol Today 10:423–428
5. Lesley J, Hyman R, Kincade PW (1993) CD44 and its interaction with the extracellular matrix. Adv Immunol 54:271–335
6. Stamenkovic I, Amiot M, Pesando JM, Seed B (1989) A lymphocyte molecule implicated in lymph node homing is a member of the cartilage link protein family. Cell 56:1057–1062
7. Hofmann M, Rudy W, Zoller M, Tolg C, Ponta H, Herrlich P, Gunthert U (1991) CD44 splice variants confer metastatic behaviour in rats: homologous sequences are expressed in human tumour cell lines. Cancer Res 51:5292–5297
8. Screaton GR, Bell MV, Jackson DG, Cornelis FB, Gerth U, Bell JI (1992) Genomic structure of DNA encoding the lymphocyte homing receptor CD44 reveals at least 12 alternatively spliced exons. Proc Natl Acad Sci USA 89:12160–12164
9. Tolg C, Hofmann M, Herrlich P, Ponta H (1993) Splicing choice from ten variant exons establishes CD44 variability. Nucleic Acids Res 21:1225–1229
10. Matsumura Y, Hanbury D, Smith J, Tarin D (1994) Non-invasive detection of malignancy by identification of unusual CD44 gene activity in exfoliated cancer cells. BMJ 308:619–624
11. Matsumura Y, Sugiyama M, Matsumura S, Hayle AJ, Robinson P, Smith JC, Tarin D (1995) Unusual retention of introns in CD44 gene transcripts in bladder cancer provides new diagnostic and clinical oncological opportunities. J Pathol 177:11–20
12. Stamenkovic I, Aruffo A, Amiot M, Seed B (1991) The hematopoietic and epithelial forms of CD44 are distinct polypeptides with different adhesion potentials for hyaluronate-bearing cells. EMBO J 10:343–348
13. Birch M, Mitchell S, Hart IR (1991) Isolation and characterization of human melanoma cell variants expressing high and low levels of CD44. Cancer Res 51:6660–6667
14. Sy MS, Guo Y-J, Stamenkovic I (1991) Distinct effects of two CD44 isoforms on tumor growth in vivo. J Exp Med 174:859–866
15. Matsumura Y, Tarin D (1992) Significance of CD44 gene products for cancer diagnosis and disease evaluation. Lancet 340:1053–1058
16. Gunthert U, Hofmann M, Rudy W, Reber S, Zoller M, HauBmann I, Matzku S, Wenzel A, Ponta H, Herrlich P (1991) A new variant of glycoprotein CD44 confers metastatic potential to rat carcinoma cells. Cell 65:13–24
17. Tarin D, Bolodeoku J, Hatfill SJ, Sugino T, Woodman AC, Yoshida K (1995) The clinical significance of malfunction of the CD44 locus in malignancy. J Neurooncol 26:209–219
18. Yokozaki H, Ito R, Nakayama H, Kuniyasu H, Taniyama K, Tahara E (1994) Expression of CD44 abnormal transcripts in human gastric carcinomas. Cancer Lett 83:229–234
19. Imazeki F, Yokosuka O, Yamaguchi T, Ohto M, Isono K, Omata M (1996) Expression of variant CD44-messenger RNA in colorectal adenocarcinomas and adenomatous polyps in humans. Gastroenterology 110:362–368
20. Gorham H, Sugino T, Woodman AC, Tarin D (1996) Cellular distribution of CD44 gene tran-

scripts in colorectal carcinomas and in normal colonic mucosa. J Clin Pathol 49:482–488

21. Sugino T, Gorham H, Yoshida K, Bolodeoku J, Nargund V, Cranston D, Goodison S, Tarin D (1996) Progressive loss of CD44 gene expression in invasive bladder cancer. Am J Pathol 149:873–882

22. Orzechowski HD, Beckenbach C, Herbst H, Stolzel U, Riecken EO, Stallmach A (1995) Expression of CD44v6 is associated with cellular dysplasia in colorectal epithelial cells. Eur J Cancer 31A:2073–2079

23. Gorham H, Sugino T, Bolodeoku J, Yoshida K, Goodison S, Tarin D (1996) Distribution of CD44 messenger RNA in archival paraffin wax embedded tumours and normal tissues viewed by in situ hybridisation. J Clin Pathol Mol Pathol 49:M147–M150

24. Yoshida K, Bolodeoku J, Sugino T, Goodison S, Matsumura Y, Warren BF, Toge T, Tahara E, Tarin D (1995) Abnormal retention of intron 9 in CD44 gene transcripts in human gastrointestinal tumors. Cancer Res 55:4273–4277

25. Higashikawa K, Yokozaki H, Ue T, Taniyama K, Ishikawa T, Tarin D (1996) Evaluation of CD44 transcription variants in human digestive tract carcinomas and normal tissues. Int J Cancer 66:11–17

26. Bolodeoku J, Yoshida K, Sugino T, Goodison S, Tarin D (1996) Accumulation of immature intron-containing CD44 gene transcripts in breast cancer tissues. Mol Diag 1:175–181

27. Heider K-H, Hofmann M, Hors E, van den Berg F, Ponta H, Herrlich P, Pals ST (1993) A human homologue of the rat metastasis-associated variant of CD44 is expressed in colorectal carcinomas and adenomatous polyps. J Cell Biol 120:227–233

28. Wielenga VJM, Heider K-H, Offerhaus GJA, Adolf GR, van den Berg FM, Ponta H, Herrlich P, Pals ST (1993) Expression of CD44 variant proteins in human colorectal cancer is related to tumor progression. Cancer Res 53:4754–4756

29. Borgya A, Woodman A, Sugiyama M, Donie F, Kopetzki E, Matsumura Y, Tarin D (1995) Isolation and characterisation of antibodies which specifically recognise the peptide encoded by exon 7 (v2) of the human CD44 gene. J Clin Pathol Mol Pathol 48:M241–M250

30. Kawahara K, Yoshino T, Kawasaki N, Miyake K, Akagi T (1996) Abnormal expression of the human CD44 gene in early colorectal malignancy with special reference to variant exon 9 (9v). J Clin Pathol 49:478–481

31. Dall P, Heider K-H, Hekele A, von Minchwitz G, Kaufmann M, Ponta H, Herrlich P (1994) Surface protein expression and messenger RNA-splicing analysis of CD44 in uterine cervical cancer and normal cervical epithelium. Cancer Res 54:3337–3341

32. Mulder J-WR, Kruyt PM, Sewnath M, Oosting J, Seldenrijk CA, Weidema WF, Offerhaus GJA, Pals ST (1994) Colorectal cancer prognosis and expression of exon-v6-containing CD44 proteins. Lancet 344:1470–1472

33. Friedrichs K, Franke F, Lisboa B-W, Kugler G, Gille I, Terpe H-J, Holzel F, Maass H, Gunthert U (1995) CD44 isoforms correlate with cellular differentiation but not with prognosis in human breast cancer. Cancer Res 55:5424–5433

34. Woodman AC, Sugiyama M, Yoshida K, Sugino T, Borgya A, Goodison S, Matsumura Y, Tarin D (1996) Analysis of anomalous CD44 gene expression in human breast, bladder and colon cancer and correlation with observed mRNA and protein isoforms. Am J Pathol 149:1519–1530

35. Guo Y-J, Liu G, Wang X, Jin D, Wu M, Ma J, Sy M-S (1994) Potential use of soluble CD44 in serum as indicator of tumor burden and metastasis in patients with gastric or colon cancer. Cancer Res 54:422–426

36. Rudy W, Hofmann M, Schwartz-Albiez R, Zoller M, Heider K-H, Ponta H, Herrlich P (1993) The two major CD44 proteins expressed on a metastatic rat tumor cell line are derived from different splice variants: each one individually suffices to confer metastatic behavior. Cancer Res 53:1262–1268

37. Driessens MH, Stroeken PJ, Rodriguez-Erena NF, van-der-Valk MA, van Rijthoven EA, Roos E (1995) Targeted disruption of CD44 in MDAY-D2 lymphosarcoma cells has no effect on subcutaneous growth or metastatic capacity. J Cell Biol 131:1849–1855

38. Yoshida K, Sugino T, Bolodeoku J, Warren BF, Goodison S, Woodman A, Toge T, Tahara E, Tarin D (1996) Detection of exfoliated carcinoma cells in colonic luminal washings by identification of deranged patterns of expression of the CD44 gene. J Clin Pathol 49:300–305

39. Kaufmann M, Heider K-H, Sinn H-P, von Minckwitz G, Ponta H, Herrlich P (1995) CD44 variant exon epitopes in primary breast cancer and length of survival. Lancet 345:615–619

40. Koopman G, Heider K-H, Horst E, Adolf GR, van den Berg F, Ponta H, Herrlich P, Pals ST (1993) Activated human lymphocytes and aggressive non-Hodgkin's lymphomas express a homologue of the rat metastasis-associated variant of CD44. J Exp Med 177:897–904

41. Finn L, Dougherty G, Finley G, Meisler A, Becich M, Cooper DL (1994) Alternative splicing of CD44 pre-mRNA in human colorectal tumors. Biochem Biophys Res Commun 200:1015–1022

42. Lee J-H, Kang YS, Kim BG, Park SY, Lee KH, Park KB (1995) Expression of the CD44 adhesion molecule in primary and metastatic gynecologic malignancies and their cell lines. Int J Gynecol Cancer 5:193–199

43. Takeuchi K, Yamaguchi A, Urano T, Goi T, Nakagawara G, Shiku H (1995) Expression of CD44 variant exons 8–10 in colorectal cancer and its relationship to metastasis. Jpn J Cancer Res 86:292–297

44. Clarke MR, Landreneau RJ, Resnick NM, Crowley R, Dougherty GJ, Cooper DL, Yousem SA (1995) Prognostic significance of CD44 expression in adenocarcinoma of the lung. J Clin Pathol Mol Pathol 48:M200–M204

45. Sugiyama M, Woodman A, Sugino T, Crowley S, Ho K, Smith J, Matsumura Y, Tarin D (1995) Noninvasive detection of bladder cancer by identification of abnormal CD44 proteins in exfoliated cancer cells in urine. J Clin Pathol Mol Pathol 48:M142–M147

46. Tarin D, Matsumura Y (1993) Deranged activity of the CD44 gene and other loci as biomarkers for progression to metastatic malignancy. J Cell Biochem 17G:173–185

Molecular Diagnosis of Gastrointestinal Cancer

Wataru Yasui, Hiroshi Yokozaki, and Eiichi Tahara

Summary. Multiple genetic alterations of oncogenes, tumor-suppressor genes, and DNA repair genes are involved in the conversion of normal cells to clinical cancers. These genetic alterations can be applied in a multistep mechanism of development and progression of gastrointestinal cancers, although common and distinct genetic changes are observed in esophageal, gastric, and colorectal carcinomas. Inactivation of the *p53* gene, reactivation of telomerase, and anomalous CD44 expression are common events that serve as genetic markers for the differential diagnosis of cancer. Amplification of the cyclin D1 gene is preferentially found in esophageal cancer, whereas amplification of c-*met* is common in gastric cancer. The cyclin E gene amplification is frequently associated with both gastric and colorectal cancers. Deletion of the cyclin-dependent kinase inhibitor gene is often found in esophageal carcinoma cell lines. The scenario of multiple genetic alterations differs depending on the two histological types of gastric cancer, suggesting that they may have different genetic pathways. By applying these observations to routine clinical practice, we can facilitate and improve the differential diagnosis of cancer, obtain information of the grade of malignancy, foresee patient prognosis, identify patients at high risk for developing multiple cancers, and discover novel therapies for cancer. The molecular diagnosis of gastrointestinal cancers, which has been performed at Hiroshima City Medical Association Clinical Laboratory, may provide a new approach to cancer diagnosis for the twenty-first century. These advances raise a number of questions concerning the ethics of molecular diagnosis and treatment. The practical and ethical implications of identifying carriers of hereditary cancer should be considered in clinical and nonclinical contexts.

Introduction

It has become clear that the precise molecular mechanisms of the development and uncontrolled proliferation of gastrointestinal cancers involve abnormalities of oncogenes, tumor-suppressor genes, and growth factor/receptor systems [1–4]. The significance of cell cycle regulation, the genetic instability and DNA repair system, and human telomerase in the pathogenesis of cancers has been under discussion [5–11]. Among various genetic events, common and distinct genetic or epigenetic alterations are observed in gastrointestinal cancers [2–12]. The points at which genetic changes occur are different. The genetic instabilities and inactivation of tumor-suppressor genes mainly confer an early step of tumorigenesis, whereas gene amplification of growth factor receptor or cyclin is frequently associated with advanced cancers, indicating the causative role in cancer progression [2, 13–15].

New techniques in molecular biology and genetics enable us to detect specific alterations in cancer and precancerous tissues that have been obtained during surgery or from biopsies [16, 17]. We can analyze various genetic alterations, such as point mutations, loss of heterozygosity, genetic instabilities, gene amplification, and overexpression, even in formalin-fixed paraffin-embedded specimens obtained for the purpose of histopathological diagnosis. By transferring this knowledge and the techniques to practice, we can make powerful cancer diagnoses to differentiate cancers from benign lesions, foresee the grade of malignancy or the patient's prognosis, and identify individuals at high risk for developing cancer.

The purpose of this chapter is to describe the concepts and principles of molecular diagnosis and introduce the strategy and markers of diag-

First Department of Pathology, Hiroshima University School of Medicine, 1-2-3 Kasumi, Minami-ku, Hiroshima 734, Japan

nostic molecular pathology on gastrointestinal lesions that have been routinely implemented at the Hiroshima City Medical Association Clinical Laboratory since 1993. Cost–benefit and ethical concerns are also discussed.

Concept of Molecular Diagnosis of Cancer

Molecular diagnosis, also called DNA diagnosis or genetic diagnosis, entails analyzing genetic alterations that participate in the development and progression of cancer using clinical materials and introducing these results to clinical diagnosis and treatment. The role of molecular diagnosis of cancer is to predict susceptible individuals preclinically, determine if cancer is present, make a precise differential diagnosis, obtain information about the grade of malignancy, and so on (Table 1). By analyzing the gene abnormalities related to carcinogenesis, an objective differential diagnosis between the benign state and malignancy is possible. In the case of hematopoietic tumors, specific genetic changes or chromosomal aberrations suggest subtyping of the diseases [18]. Detection of genetic alterations related to proliferation, invasion, and metastasis can be utilized to obtain information about the biological behavior of the cancer. Chemosensitivity can be studied by analyzing multidrug-resistant gene status [19]. Identification of gene carriers in kindreds of familial or hereditary cancer prior to clinical manifestation can be done only by analyzing the status of the causative genes [20, 21]. In the case of molecular diagnosis of gastrointestinal lesions, the main purpose is to make a precise differential diagnosis

and to obtain information about the grade of malignancy because materials are usually taken from the suspicious lesions endoscopically. Genetic instabilities monitored by replication error is a good indicator for high susceptibility to multiple cancers [22].

Methods and Materials for Molecular Diagnosis

In general, the materials for molecular diagnosis are the same as for clinical examinations. For the purpose of determining the presence of the tumor, blood, urine, bile, and pancreatic juice are analyzed. For preclinical prediction of hereditary diseases, such as familial polyposis coli (FAP) and hereditary nonpolyposis colorectal cancer (HNPCC), lymphocytes or normal-looking mucosa are used because germline mutations of causative genes are sought. In the case of solid tumors, tissue samples obtained by surgery, endoscopic removal, or biopsy are used. Although the most suitable samples for genetic analyses are fresh or frozen, various genetic alterations can be analyzed on formalin-fixed paraffin-embedded tissues, as shown in Table 2 [23]. To obtain clear results, however, the period between removal and fixation should be minimized.

The DNA can be extracted from paraffin-embedded tissue prepared for routine histopathological examination [16]. Formylation of nucleic acids produces Schiff bases on free amino groups

Table 1. Clinical implications of molecular diagnosis of cancer

Clinical implication	Object
Diagnosis of existence of cancer	General cancer
Objective differential diagnosis	General cancer
Information on grade of malignancy	General cancer
Identification of gene carrier	Hereditary cancer
Subclassification of cancer	Hematopoietic cancer
Prediction of susceptibility to multiple cancer	Solid cancer
Sensitivity to chemotherapy	General cancer

Table 2. Application of molecular techniques to formalin-fixed paraffin-embedded material

Method	Application
Slot blot analysis	Gene amplification
PCR-SSCP method	Screening of gene mutation
PCR-sequencing method	Identification of gene mutation
PCR-RFLP method	Loss of heterozygosity
Microsatellite method	Replication error (genetic instability)
In situ hydridization	Localization of mRNA expression
Immunohistochemistry	Protein expression and accumulation

PCR, polymerase chain reaction; SSCP, single-strand conformation polymorphism analysis; RFLP, restriction fragment length polymorphism.

of nucleotides, and exposure of nucleoproteins to formaldehyde results in the formation of cross-links between proteins and DNA. These processes are reversible in aqueous solution, implying that DNA can be recovered from formalin-fixed tissues. Although DNA extracted in this way is not intact, it is double-stranded, is cleaved with restriction endonucleases, can be hybridized with labeled probes, and can be amplified using the polymerase chain reaction (PCR). The paraffin-embedded sections were deparaffinized by sequential incubation in xylene and ethanol as conventional deparaffinization for histological staining. After cutting out the portion of interest from the sections, it is digested with proteinase K and sodium dodecyl sulfate (SDS). DNA is extracted with phenol-chloroform-isoamyl alcohol. The most important cause of failure to recover nearly intact DNA is the use of inadequately fixed tissues.

Amplification of known genes is detected by Southern blot analysis or dot-blot analysis [16]. Although the latter can be applied to paraffin-embedded tissues, the specificity of hybridization should be carefully checked. Amplification is determined by comparing the signal intensity by densitometry of equal parallel samples hybridized with a single-copy gene such as β-actin and the gene of interest. Southern blot analysis in combination with adequate restriction enzymes and DNA probes (restriction fragment length polymorphism, or RFLP) can also detect loss of heterozygosity (LOH). The altered mobility of restriction fragments on the gel is detected with a labeled probe. Variable numbers of tandem repeats (VNTRs) are available as RFLP markers.

The PCR is a powerful technique for analyzing small amounts of DNA (e.g., that extracted from paraffin-embedded sections). PCR allows specific in vitro DNA amplification by synthetic oligonucleotide primers. The basic PCR cycle involves heat denaturation of DNA followed by primer annealing and then DNA synthesis, which can be achieved simply by altering the temperature of the reaction. After the sequences of interest are amplified and labeled by PCR, point mutations can be screened by single-strand conformation polymorphism (SSCP) analysis [16]. Most of the single-base changes in fragments of up to 200 bases can be detected as mobility shifts. Because this analysis cannot determine the precise position or the exact nature of the base changes, sequencing analysis of the shifted band is

recommended to identify the base substitutions. If information on the polymorphic site in genes of interest is available, target sequences amplified by PCR are digested with adequate restriction enzymes, and RFLP can be undertaken to detect LOH.

Genetic instability in the form of replication errors (RER) at microsatellite loci is monitored by microsatellite assay [9]. Microsatellite loci are composed of simple repeated sequences, such as (CA)n, (GA)n, and (A)n, scattered in the human genome and represent polymorphism. These nucleotide repeats may be inserted or deleted at a certain rate by the phenomenon of "slippage" during DNA replication. Alteration of the number of these repeats, called RER, reflect a genetically unstable status. DNA extracted even from paraffin-embedded sections is amplified by PCR with labeled primers of microsatellite loci, and the products are analyzed on polyacrylamide gel or an autosequencer. The autosequencer is useful, as it can analyze many samples (many loci) at a time for short periods. This method is also applied to detect LOH because microsatellite loci sometimes show polymorphism.

Immunohistochemistry can detect overexpression or abnormal accumulation of gene products on paraffin-embedded sections. This method can identify the site of the protein, and Western blot analysis can suggest the molecular abnormalities, which appear as altered migration on gels. A fresh or frozen sample is necessary for the latter. Fluorescence in situ hybridization (FISH) can determine the loss or gain of the genes of interest in paraffin-embedded sections.

Biomarkers for Molecular Diagnosis of Gastrointestinal Cancer

Esophageal Carcinoma

Esophageal squamous cell carcinoma has a poorer prognosis than that of gastric or colorectal carcinomas not only because the anatomical location of the tumor is difficult to approach by the surgeon but also because the esophageal tumor may show highly malignant behavior. The genetic abnormalities of tumor-suppressor genes or oncogenes implicated in the development and progression of esophageal cancer are summarized in Table 3. These abnormalities include the amplification and overexpression of the epidermal

Table 3. Genes altered in esophageal cancer

Gene and molecule	Abnormality	Incidence (%)
Tumor suppressor genes		
p53(17p13)	LOH, mutation	30–50
APC(5q21)	LOH	40–70
RB(13q14)	LOH	40–50
MTS1/CDK4/(9p21)	Loss, mutation	50
3p, 9q, 10p, 17q, 18q, 19q, 21q	LOH	>30
Oncogenes		
cyclin D1/hst-1/int-2(11q13)	Amplification	Primary: 40–50
		Metastasis: 100
erbB (EGF receptor)	Amplification	10
	Overexpression	50–80
Growth factors		
EGF	Overexpression	30
TGF-α	Overexpression	80

LOH, loss of heterozygosity; EGF, epidermal growth factor; TGF-α, transforming growth factor-α.

growth factor (EGF) receptor gene [24, 25], amplification of the cyclin D1 gene [26, 27], LOH at multiple chromosomal loci (e.g., 3p, 5q, 9p, 9q, 13q, 17p, 17q) [28, 29], mutation of the p53 gene [30], total deletion or mutation of the MTS1 gene [31], and overexpression of growth factors.

Among these alterations, LOH and mutation of the p53 gene at chromosome 17p13 occur at an early stage of esophageal carcinogenesis, such as dysplasia and carcinoma in situ [30]. About 40% of esophageal carcinomas show mutations of the p53 gene, most of which are missense mutations with amino acid changes. Considering the base substitution spectrum, G:C to T:A transversion is common in esophageal carcinomas, similar to that in carcinomas of the lung and liver [30, 32]. This situation is different from the observation that colorectal carcinomas frequently share transition of CpG to TpG. This evidence suggests that different environmental or intrinsic factors may affect the tumorigenesis between the esophageal carcinomas and colorectal carcinomas. Because a half-life of mutant p53 protein is much longer than that of the wild type, abnormal accumulation of p53 protein can be easily detected by immunohistochemistry. About 60% of esophageal carcinomas are immunohistochemically positive for p53.

Wild-type p53 functions as a transcription factor for several genes, such as p21$^{WAF1/CIP1}$, GADD45, and BAX [33–35]. The promoters of these genes have a p53 binding site, and the transcription is activated by wild-type p53 but not mutated p53.

p21$^{WAF1/CIP1}$ is a negative regulator of the cell cycle through inhibition of enzyme activity of various cyclins/cyclin-dependent kinase (CDK) complexes [36, 37]. GADD45 binds to proliferating cell nuclear antigen (PCNA), a normal component of CDK complexes, and is involved in DNA replication and repair [34]. BAX makes a heterodimer with BCL-2 protein and positively regulates with the induction of apoptosis [35]. Taken together with this evidence, p53 gene alterations may confer esophageal carcinogenesis through abnormalities in cell cycle progression, DNA repair, and cell survival. Although microsatellite instability is frequently observed in Barrett's-associated adenocarcinoma, it is rare in squamous cell carcinomas of the esophagus [38].

Abnormalities in cell cycle progression are important determinants in developing a variety of carcinomas [5, 6]. Cyclins and CDKs regulate cell cycle progression through key checkpoints in mammalian cells [6, 7]. The enzyme activity of several cyclin–CDK complexes is modulated by a group of cellular CDK inhibitors, such as p21$^{WAF1/CIP1}$, p16$^{INK4A/MTS1}$, p15$^{INK4B/MTS2}$, and p27^{KIP1} [36–44]. Because the loss of these inhibitors would lead to unbridled cell proliferation, they should be candidates for tumor-suppressor genes. The p15 and p16 genes, both located on chromosome 9p21, encode related proteins that primarily inhibit the activities of cyclin D/CDK4 and cyclin D/CDK6 [39–41]. The mutations and homozygous deletions of the p16 gene have been reported in cell lines from many tumor types, including the esophageal origin [39–41]. We have also confirmed that homozygous deletion of the *p16* gene is closely correlated with the increased expression of cyclin D1 and CDK4 in the esophageal carcinoma cell lines [45]. Although alterations of the *p16* gene are less common in primary tumors than in the cell lines, *p16* gene mutations are found in 50% of the primary esophageal carcinomas [31].

On the other hand, we have discovered the co-amplification of *hst*-1 and *int*-2 genes, both of which are located on chromosome 11q13, in approximately 50% of primary tumors and in 100% of metastases of esophageal squamous cell carcinomas [46]. Gene amplification, however, is not accompanied by overexpression of the two genes. Subsequently, cyclin D1 gene, an important target of *p15* and *p16*, has been located on the same chromosomal locus as *hst*-1 and *int*-2 genes [47]. The amplicon of this locus found in esophageal carcinomas has been demonstrated to include these three genes. We also confirmed frequent co-amplification of the cyclin D1, *hst*-1, and *int*-2 genes in esophageal carcinomas, accompanied by enhanced expression of cyclin D1 [27]. No amplification can be detected in dysplasia of the esophagus. The amplification of the cyclin D1 gene is closely correlated with tumor staging, depth of tumor invasion, and distant metastasis [27]. Cyclin D1 binds to RB protein and stimulates its phosphorylation [48]. Unregulated phosphorylation of RB in response to overexpressed cyclin D1 could lead to loss of growth control. LOH at the *RB* gene locus (13q14) frequently occurs in esophageal carcinomas [28, 29].

Overexpression of EGF, transforming growth factor-α (TGF-α), and EGF receptor is frequently associated with esophageal carcinoma. They are found in 30%, 80%, and 50%, respectively, of the primary tumors by Northern blot analysis [25]. Amplification of the EGF receptor gene (*erb*B) occurs in 10% of primary tumors [24]. Furthermore, the number of EGF receptors is about 10 times greater than that of the gastric carcinomas, and EGF receptor levels are correlated with metastatic potential and patient prognosis [49]. In in vitro examinations, EGF and TGF-α produced by tumor cells function as autocrine growth factors for esophageal carcinoma cells [50]. In addition, EGF and TGF-α stimulate the production of matrix metalloproteinases (MMPs) such as interstitial collagenase (MMP-1) and stromelysin (MMP-3), which promote tumor cell invasion [25].

These findings indicate that the detection of *p53* alterations can be used to differentiate between the benign state and malignancy. Amplification and overexpression of the cyclin D1 gene and inactivation of *p15* and *p16* genes, as well as overexpression of the EGF receptor system, are valuable biomarkers for a high-grade of malignancy of esophageal carcinomas.

Gastric Carcinoma

Gastric carcinoma displays multiple genetic alterations of oncogenes, tumor-suppressor genes, cell cycle regulators, and DNA repair genes and genetic instability. The scenarios of multiple gene changes found in gastric cancer differ depending on the histological type, suggesting that the two types (well-differentiated and poorly differentiated adenocarcinoma) may have different genetic pathways [2, 4, 12]. The molecular mechanism of the development and progression of gastric cancer is described in detail in the chapter by H. Yokozaki and E. Tahara in this volume. Genetic alterations in gastric cancer and the possibility of their being genetic markers for a molecular diagnosis are discussed briefly.

Genetic instability, chromosomal instability (telomere reduction), and immortality (reactivation of telomerase) may be involved in the first step of stomach carcinogenesis [13, 14, 51]. The amplification and aberrant expression of the c-*met* gene, inactivation of the *p53* gene, and anomalous expression of *CD44* are common events of both well differentiated and poorly differentiated gastric cancers [52–54]; cyclin E gene amplification is frequently observed regardless of histological type [55]. Decreased expression of p21$^{WAF1/CIP1}$ occurs mostly independent of the *p53* gene status [56, 57]. Reduced expression of p27^{KIP1} is associated with advanced stage and invasiveness [58]. On the other hand, K-*ras* mutations, c-*erb*B2 gene amplification, LOH and mutations of the *APC* gene, LOH of the *bcl*-2 gene, and LOH at the *DCC* locus are preferentially associated with the well-differentiated type [2]. Precancerous lesions, such as intestinal metaplasia and adenoma, share genetic changes found in well-differentiated cancers, which are similar to those of colorectal cancer [13]. Reduction or loss of cadherin and catenins, K-*sam* gene amplification, and c-*met* gene amplification are necessary for the development and progression of poorly differentiated or scirrhous-type carcinoma [2]. An interaction between cell-adhesion molecules in the c-*met*-expressing tumor cells and hepatocyte growth factor (HGF) from stromal cells is implicated in the morphogenesis of the two types of gastric cancer [59]. Multiple autocrine loops of growth factors/cytokines, such as EGF, TGF-α, and interleukin-1α (IL-1α) confer the progression of gastric cancer [60, 61]. Reduced expression of *nm23* may participate in the metastatic potential of gastric cancer cells [62].

Therefore inactivation of tumor-suppressor genes such as *p53* and *APC*, genetic instability, and telomerase activity could be useful markers for the early detection and differential diagnosis of gastric cancer. The gene amplification and overexpression of c-*met*, c-*erb*B2, K-*sam*, and cyclin E and the overexpression of multiple growth factors are indicators of high grade malignancy.

Colorectal Carcinoma

The accumulation of multiple genetic alterations in tumor-suppressor genes and oncogenes takes place during colorectal carcinogenesis [63]. LOH at chromosomes 5q, 17p, and 18q and K-*ras* mutation occur during the course of the malignant progression from normal mucosal cells through adenomas (adenoma–carcinoma sequence) [63]. Tumor-suppressor genes *APC*, *p53*, and *DCC* have been identified at 5q, 17p, and 18q, respectively [64–66]. DNA mismatch repair genes have been identified as responsible for genetic instability found in hereditary nonpolyposis colorectal cancer (HNPCC) [67]. The molecular mechanism for development and progression of colorectal cancer is illustrated in Fig. 1.

The *APC* gene, first isolated as a causative gene for familial adenomatous polyposis (FAP), encodes a large protein of 2843 amino acids, which forms a complex with α- and β-catenins and may mediate cell adhesion, cytoskeletal anchoring, and signal transduction [64, 68, 69]. The *APC* gene is abnormal in the germline of FAP patients [20]. In addition, LOH and mutations of the *APC* gene occur in 60% of sporadic colorectal adenomas and adenocarcinomas [70]. These tumors usually show loss of the *APC* gene in one allele and mutation of the gene in the remaining allele, supporting the two-hits theory of carcinogenesis proposed by Knudson [71]. The characteristic of the mutation is the base substitution to make a stop codon (nonsense mutation), which occurs in about 70% of FAP kindred [20]. The *APC* alterations are found even in small adenomas (<3 mm in diameter) with mild atypia [72]. Therefore *APC* gene mutation may play a major role in the early development of colorectal adenomas.

Mutation in K-*ras* oncogene is involved in the progression from small adenoma with mild atypia to large adenoma with severe atypia. About 40% to 50% of large adenomas with severe atypia and adenocarcinomas show K-*ras* point mutations at codon 12 or 13, whereas fewer than 10% of small adenomas with mild atypia do [63, 73–75]. On the other hand, the frequency of K-*ras* mutations is

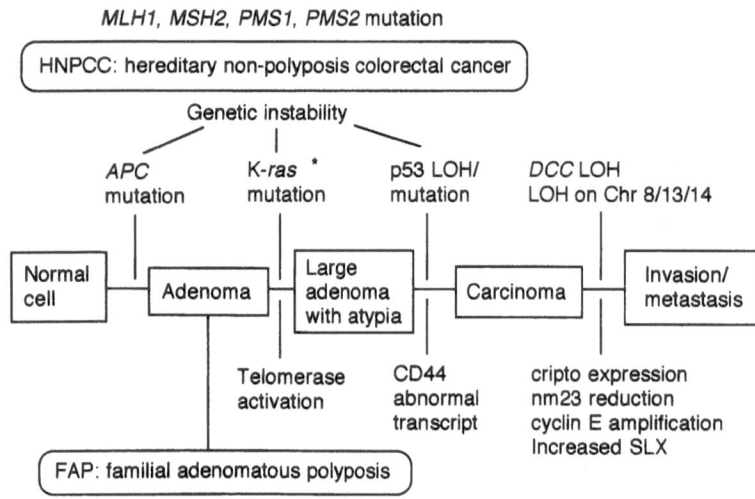

Fig. 1. Molecular mechanism of colorectal carcinogenesis. *K-*ras* mutation is infrequent in superficial-type (flat) adenomas

lower (<10%) in superficial-type or flat adenomas with considerable atypia than in polypoid adenomas [76, 77]. Jen et al. [78] have reported that K-*ras* mutations alone are common in small nondysplastic (hyperplastic) lesions that apparently have a limited potential to progress to larger tumors, whereas *APC* mutations alone are closely associated with adenomatous polyps. Therefore the nature and order of genetic changes have a specific impact on tumor morphology and the likelihood of tumor progression.

Loss of heterogeneity of the *p53* gene locus is found in about 80% of colorectal adenocarcinomas, and most of them show inactivation of the *p53* gene in both alleles (LOH and mutation of the remaining allele) [63, 79, 80]. Because only 5% to 20% of the adenomas have *p53* inactivation it must play a crucial role in the transition from adenoma to adenocarcinoma [63, 79, 80]. There are hot spots for point mutations in the highly conserved region of the gene, such as codon 175, 248, and 273, where G:C to A:T transition occurs [79]. Furthermore, the incidence of LOH of the *p53* gene among colorectal adenocarcinomas increases as the tumor stage progresses [81]. Abnormal accumulation of p53 protein detected by immunohistochemistry is frequently associated with deeply invasive carcinomas and carcinomas with metastatic lesions [82]. Colon cancer patients with a *p53* mutation have a poorer prognosis [83]. The *p53* abnormalities thus participate not only in the development of colorectal carcinomas but in the malignant behavior of the cancer cells. The expression of p21$^{WAFI/CIPI}$, a CDK inhibitor, is not necessarily correlated with *p53* gene status in colorectal carcinomas, suggesting the importance of p53-independent induction of p21.

The *DCC* (deleted in colorectal cancer) gene encodes protein that is highly homologous to a cell adhesion molecule, the neural cell adhesion molecule (N-CAM) [66, 84]. LOH of the *DCC* gene on chromosome 18q is rare in adenomas but frequent (about 70%) in adenocarcinomas of the colorectum [66, 84]. LOH of *DCC* increases as the tumor cells invaded deeply, and almost all the metastatic liver tumors show this LOH [85].

The colorectal carcinomas express multiple growth factors, such as EGF and TGF-α and their receptors, to make autocrine loops [86]. The *cripto* gene was originally identified in undifferentiated human embryonal carcinoma cells and encodes an 188-amino-acid protein containing a 37-amino-acid region that shares structural homology with other members of the EGF family, although the cripto protein cannot bind EGF receptor [87]. Expression of cripto is detected in 40% of tubular adenomas and 80% of adenocarcinomas [88]. The level of cripto is closely related to the tumor stage [89]. Amphiregulin (AR) is another member of the EGF family that utilizes EGF receptor as an acceptor [90]. About half of the colorectal carcinomas express AR [88]. It has been confirmed that cripto and AR act as autocrine growth stimulators for colorectal cancer cell lines [91]. The amplification of c-*erb*B2 gene, which is common in gastric well differentiated adenocarcinoma, is observed in 5% of colorectal carcinomas. The amplification of cyclin E gene, a positive regulator of the cell cycle progression, occurs in about 10% of colorectal carcinomas [92]. The incidence of overexpression of cyclin E is significantly higher in adenocarcinomas (20%) than in adenomas (5%) [82]. Among adenomas, a significant correlation is detected between cyclin E expression and the grade of atypia [82]. Overexpression of cyclin E is prominent in carcinomas invading the submucosa or deeper compared to those limited to the mucosal layer. These factors are thus candidates for molecular markers to predict high grade malignancy.

The *CD44* gene is expressed not only in lymphocytes but in a variety of epithelial cells and cancer cells [93]. The *CD44* gene consists of at least 20 exons, of which 10 are alternatively spliced to make up variants [94]. Overexpression of *CD44* splice variants has been considered to be implicated in tumor progression and metastasis [95]. Among several *CD44* variants, aberrant transcripts with a retention of intron 9 are best for distinguishing carcinoma tissues from normal tissues in the colorectum [54, 96]. All the adenocarcinomas overexpress this variant containing the intron 9 sequence, and it is observed from an early stage. The variants do not correlate with nodal or distant metastatic status [54]. Aberrant *CD44* transcript with retention of intron 9 is a powerful indicator for the presence of colorectal cancer but not for malignant behavior. It is not applicable to the diagnosis of malignancies originating from squamous epithelia, such as esophageal cancer, because the aberrant transcripts are frequently observed in both squamous cell carcinomas and corresponding normal mucosa [54]. Osteopontin has been found to be a ligand of CD44 [97]. It is of interest to examine the significance of osteopontin in colorectal carcinogenesis.

A candidate suppressor gene of tumor metastasis, *nm23*, encodes nucleotide diphosphate kinase and c-*myc* transcription factor (PuF) [98]. Although most of the colorectal carcinomas expressed nm23 at higher levels than the non-neoplastic mucosa, the levels of nm23 protein expression in tumors show an inverse correlation with tumor stage [99]. Moreover, reduced expression of nm23 is associated with distant metastasis. Another candidate for a molecular marker that indicates metastatic potential is cell surface carbohydrates, sialyl-dimeric Le antigens [100]. Both sialyl Le^x (SLX) and sialyl Le^a (SLA or CA19-9) as ligands bind to E-selectin, also known as ELAM-1, one of the adhesion molecules on activated endothelial cells [101]. SLX and SLA may participate in distant metastasis through interaction between cancer cells and endothelial cells of the blood vessel. The expression of SLX in colorectal carcinoma shows significant correlation with liver metastasis and poor prognosis [102].

HNPCC, or Lynch syndrome, is one of the most common hereditary diseases in humans, accounting for 3% to 10% of colorectal cancers [67]. HNPCC is diagnosed if (1) three or more first-degree relatives are affected with colorectal cancer, and (2) at least one of these cancers has been diagnosed before age 50. Linkage analyses and sequencing have identified *hMLH1* (3p21), *hMSH2* (2p21–22), *hPMS1* (2q31–33), and *hPMS2* (7p22), homologs of bacterial DNA mismatch repair genes, as responsible genes for HNPCC [103–107]. Ubiquitous changes in the length of simple repetitive DNA sequences between constitutional and tumor DNA (RER) occur in 90% of HNPCC, of which 70% contain mutations in the DNA mismatch repair genes (frequently in *hMLH1* and *hMSH2* and rarely in *hPMS1* and *hPMS2*) [10, 103–108]. Germline mutations affecting one allele within one of the four mismatch repair genes aggregate perfectly with HNPCC, whereas unaffected relatives had no mutations [10]. Therefore they are crucial new tools in the detection of patients or family members at high risk of developing the colorectal cancer. RER phenotypes of HNPCC are closely associated with the alteration at (A)$_{10}$ repeated sequence in TGF-β type II receptor gene (*BAT-RII*) [109, 110]. In addition to HNPCC, RER occurs in 10% to 15% of sporadic colorectal cancer, although mutations of the DNA mismatch repair

genes are rare [111, 112]. Moreover, RERs are detected in 89% of multiple primary cancers, including colon and stomach cancers or gallbladder and stomach cancers [22].

The ribonucleoprotein enzyme telomerase synthesizes the G-rich strand of telomeric DNA that stabilizes chromosomal structure [113]. Telomere reduction may result in chromosomal instability, additional genetic alterations, telomerase reactivation, and ultimately development of cancer [11, 114]. Because most normal cells lack telomerase activity, telomeres in normal cells progressively shorten with each cell division [113, 114]. The adenomas and adenocarcinomas of the colorectum display shorter telomeres than those in normal tissues [115]. Most of colorectal adenocarcinomas express significant telomerase activity regardless of tumor staging and histological differentiation [51, 116]. All the adenomas also show considerable levels of telomerase activity [51]. Reactivation of telomerase and ensuring stabilization of telomeres occurs concomitantly with the acquisition of immortality, contributing to an early stage of colorectal carcinogenesis. Measurement of telomerase activity thus may serve as a powerful additional tool for cancer diagnosis.

Strategy of Molecular Diagnosis of Gastrointestinal Cancer

We can facilitate and improve cancer diagnosis, foresee the grade of malignancy or patient prognosis, identify patients at high risk for developing multiple cancers, and discover novel therapeutic approaches by applying the above-mentioned observations. Since August 1993 we have implemented a new molecular diagnosis strategy at Hiroshima City Medical Association Clinical Laboratory that uses molecular and immunohistochemical techniques [117]. The strategy of molecular diagnosis of gastrointestinal lesions is presented in Fig. 2. The materials to be analyzed for molecular diagnosis are formalin-fixed biopsy specimens or surgical specimens submitted to the laboratory for the purpose of histopathological diagnosis. First, the histological diagnosis is reported within a week after receiving the specimens from the clinic. At the time of histological observation, cancers, adenomas (dysplasia), or borderline lesions are detected and suitable blocks for molecular analysis are prepared.

Fig. 2. Strategy of molecular diagnosis of gastrointestinal lesions in Hiroshima

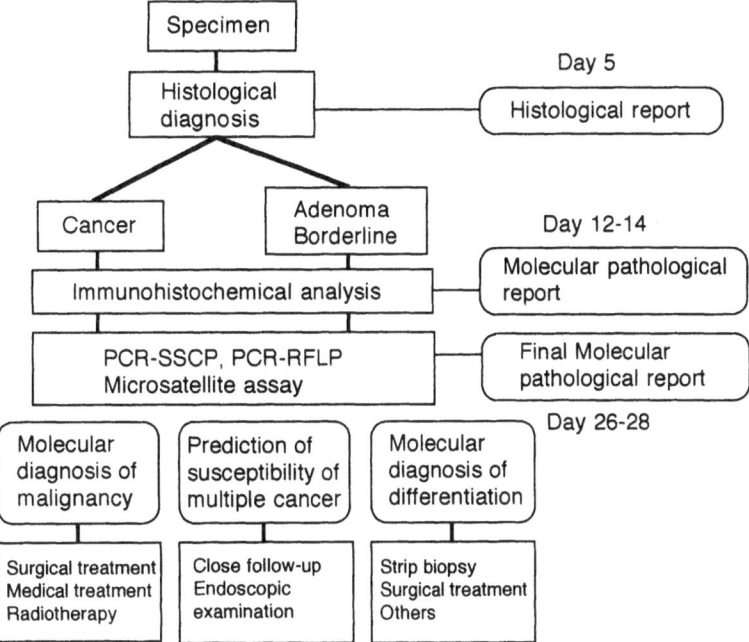

Immunohistochemical analysis of a set of selected markers is performed on newly prepared sections to grade the malignancy and to differentiate between the benign state and malignancy. If sufficient information is obtained by this analysis, the molecular diagnosis is reported to the clinician. According to the information derived from the differential diagnosis or the biological behavior of the cancer, the clinician can make a proper decision whether polypectomy/strip biopsy, surgical treatment. chemotherapy, or radiation therapy is to be undertaken.

For molecular analyses, five serial slides stained with hematoxylin and eosin (H&E) but with no coverslips are prepared at the time of observing the immunostained slides, and the portion to be analyzed is marked by a felt pen. DNA is extracted and PCR-SSCP, PCR-RFLP, and microsatellite assays are performed. The final molecular diagnosis is reported to the clinician. The advantage of this system is that we can examine a variety of molecular alterations in the portion where we observed the changes microscopically; hence it is not necessary to take another sample solely for the purpose of molecular diagnosis. Most of the steps of molecular analysis, including immunohistochemistry, DNA extraction, PCR, and SSCP or RFLP are carried out by laboratory technicians. It is important to note that the techniques routinely used must be nonradioactive and simple enough to be reproduced precisely by technicians.

Table 4. Biomarkers of molecular diagnosis of gastrointestinal cancer

Tumor and biological marker	Purpose
Esophagus	
p53	Diagnosis
EGF, TGF-α, EGFR, Ki-67	Malignancy
cyclin D1	Metastasis
Stomach	
p53, APC	Diagnosis
EGF, TGF-α, EGFR, *cripto*, c-*erb*B2, c-*met*, cyclin E, p27, Ki-67	Malignancy
nm23, CD44	Metastasis
Replication error	Susceptibility
Colon	
p53, APC	Diagnosis
EGF, TGF-α, *cripto*, EGFR cyclin E, Ki-67	Malignancy
nm23, SLX, *CD44*	Metastasis

Practical biomarkers for molecular diagnosis on gastrointestinal lesions are shown in Table 4. According to the characteristic genetic alterations already mentioned, we select common biomarkers for the esophageal, gastric, and colorectal lesions and specific ones for individual organs. Abnormal accumulation of the p53 protein detected by immunohistochemistry is a useful marker for screening the genetic alterations of *p53* in samples of all three organs. LOH and mutations of the *p53* gene are confirmed by PCR-SSCP and PCR-

RFLP. LOH of the *APC* gene and aberrant *CD44* expression are useful for differential diagnosis in the gastric and colorectal samples. Overexpression of EGF, TGF-α, and EGF receptor are biomarkers for determining the grade of malignancy for cancer of all three organs. Gene amplification and overexpression of c-*met* and c-*erb*B2 are sought in patients with gastric cancer to identify high grade malignancy, because they are well correlated with tumor stage, metastasis, and prognosis. Amplification and overexpression of cyclin D1 in esophageal cancer and cyclin E in gastric and colorectal cancers are good biomarkers for aggressive behavior of the cancer. Reduced expression of nm23 protein predicts potential metastasis. Detection of RER is potentially useful for identifying patients at high risk for developing multiple primary cancers.

To predict high grade malignancy of gastric cancer, c-*erb*B2, EGF receptor, and c-*met* are regarded as definite biomarkers. If one of these molecules shows overexpression, which corresponds to gene amplification, we diagnose the tumor as high grade malignancy. As for the other biomarkers, synchronous expression is taken into account.

Molecular Diagnosis of Gastrointestinal Cancer in Hiroshima

Practice

A total of 7357 cases (8402 lesions) were examined from August 1993 to May 1996. They consisted of 132 cases (136 lesions) of esophageal abnormality, 3164 cases (3313 lesions) of gastric abnormality, and 4061 cases (4953 lesions) of colorectal abnormality. About 10 cases a day underwent molecular diagnosis routinely. Histopathological diagnoses of the examined cases were adenoma, dysplasia, borderline lesion, carcinoma, and suspected carcinoma.

The results of molecular diagnosis on gastric lesions are summarized in Table 5. Of the 879 adenomas, 80 (9%) were diagnosed as adenoma with malignant potential (high probability of becoming carcinoma) owing to abnormal accumulation of p53. Fifteen adenomas (2%) were suspected to be adenocarcinoma because of abnormal accumulation of p53 and mutation or LOH of the *p53* gene as well as the *APC* gene, although histological atypia was not severe enough to be regarded as suspected carcinoma. Among 317 borderline lesions, between the benign state and malignancy, 72 (23%) were judged to be malignant because of the p53 and APC abnormalities. Among 1924 adenocarcinomas, 199 (10%) were found to be highly malignant owing to overexpression of several growth factors/receptors or other abnormalities, including c-*erb*B2, EGF receptor, cyclin E, and so on. Molecular findings and report of a representative case are shown in Figs. 3 and 4. Reports of molecular diagnosis on gastric lesions were prepared for 861 (26%) of 3313 lesions and were sent to the clinicians. New information based on the molecular diagnosis could be obtained for 421 lesions (13%).

Table 5. Molecular diagnosis of gastric lesions

Histological diagnosis	Lesions (no.)	Molecular diagnosis Diagnosis	No.	%
Adenoma	879	Adenoma with malignant potential	80	9
		Suspected adenocarcinoma	15	2
Borderline	317	Adenoma with malignant potential	3	1
		Suspected adenocarcinoma	31	10
		Adenocarcinoma	41	13
Suspected adenocarcinoma	193	Adenocarcinoma	50	26
		High-grade malignancy	2	1
Adenocarcinoma	1924	High-grade malignancy	199	10

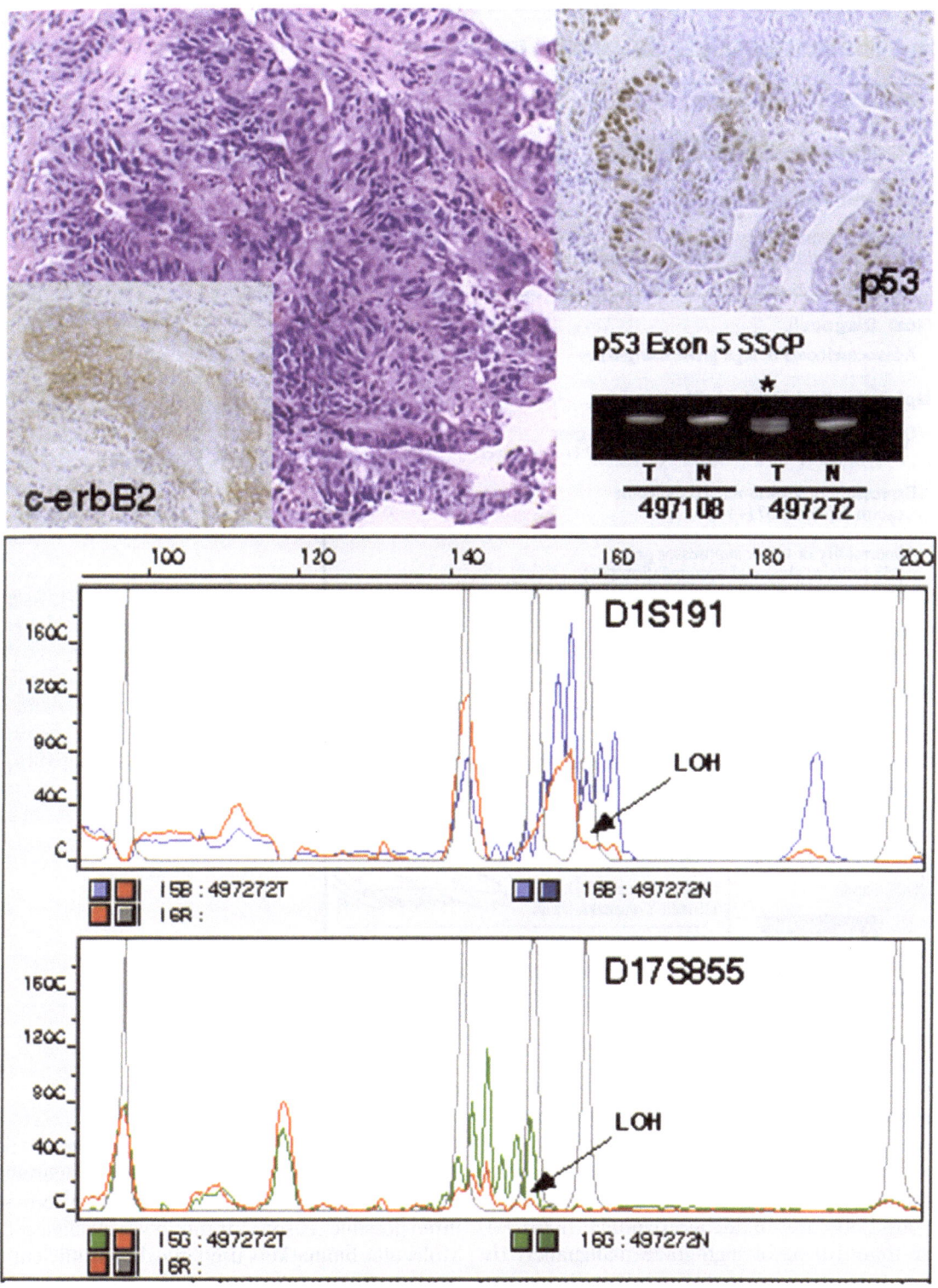

Fig. 3. Molecular findings of a representative gastric cancer case. Cancer cells show strong expression of c-erbB2 and abnormal accumulation of p53 protein. PCR-SSCP analysis of the *p53* gene reveals the abnormal band in exon 5. Loss of heterozygosity at D1S191 and D17S855 loci is detected by microsatellite assay

Molecular-Pathological Diagnosis

No. 497272   Date received: 7/13/96   Date reported: 8/10/96

Patient's name: ████████████   Age: 63   (M)

Histopathological Diagnosis

Group V, gastric biopsy
(Moderately differentiated tubular adenocarcinoma)

Final Diagnosis

Adenocarcinoma of high grade malignancy

Molecular-Pathological Findings

Overexpression of growth factor/receptor gene
TGFα(+), cripto (±), EGFR (++), c-erbB2 (+++), c-met (-)

Expression of growth-related molecule
cyclin E (+), Ki-67 (+++)

Abnormality of tumor suppressor gene
p53 protein; abnormal accumulation (++)
p53 gene; abnormal band in exon 5 (PCR-SSCP)

Metastasis-related gene product
nm23 (++, heterogenous), CD44v9 (+)

Microsatellite assay
Loss of heterozygiosity at D1S191 and D17S855

Clinical Implication: Molecular-pathological findings indicate that this cancer is potentially high grade malignancy. The patient requires additional treatment and close follow-up.

Hospital code 06-0676

XXXX Clinic

Dr. ██████████

Diagnosed by   Eiichi Tahara, M.D.

Wataru Yasui, M.D.
Hiroshi Yokozaki, M.D.

First Department of Pathology, Hiroshima Univ. Sch. Med.

Hiroshima City Medical Association Clinical Laboratory

Fig. 4. Representative report of molecular diagnosis (same case as in Fig. 3). Original report was in Japanese except the diagnosis. The English translation was made for the purpose of this chapter

Adenomas and adenocarcinomas were examined for the molecular diagnosis of colorectal lesions. Among adenomas with moderate atypia and severe atypia, 4% and 9%, respectively, were regarded as adenoma with malignant potential. Among 1599 cases of adenocarcinoma, 134 (8%) were found to be of high-grade malignancy. In contrast, 24 (21%) of the 117 esophageal carcinomas were judged to be highly malignant mainly because of overexpression of the EGF receptor and cyclin D1. The same strategy of molecular diagnosis has been applied to breast cancers, and 36% of them were found to be of high-grade malignancy.

Evaluation

The incidence of high-grade malignancy in the gastric and colorectal lesions was low compared to that for esophageal and breast cancers. There are three possible reasons for this lower incidence: (1) Molecular biomarkers used may be insufficient to predict all the high-grade malignancy, and many tumors may be falsely negative. (2) Most gastric and colorectal carcinomas are not characteristically highly malignant. (3) The carcinomas examined may consist incidentally of those with low-grade malignancy, such as superficial carcinomas or early stage lesions.

We then examined about 260 gastric carcinomas obtained by surgical or endoscopic removal and analyzed the relation between the molecular diagnosis and tumor staging or depth of tumor invasion. Molecular diagnosis of the grade of malignancy by tumor stages and determinant biomarkers are shown in Table 6. More than 70% of the gastric carcinomas examined were stage 1, among which 7% were diagnosed as high-grade malignancy. In contrast, 42%, 35%, and 55% were judged to be highly malignant in the stage 2, 3, and 4 cases, respectively. A similar trend was seen between the grade of malignancy and the depth of tumor invasion (Table 6). The examined cases comprised 52% of mucosal carcinomas and 22% of carcinomas limited to the submucosal layer; fewer than 30% were deeply invasive carcinomas. The incidence of cases in which high-grade malignancy was diagnosed was 4%, 19%, and 27% to 55% for mucosal carcinomas, carcinomas limited to the submucosa, and deeply invasive carcinomas, respectively. These observations indicate that we diagnosed more than 30% of advanced carcinomas or deeply invasive ones as high-grade malignancy. Furthermore, it is likely that molecular analyses have been performed mainly on superficial or early stage carcinomas possibly because gastric cancer can be detected at an early stage by routine examination of the upper digestive tracts for the adult population in Japan. Most of these superficial or early stage carcinomas are low-grade malignancies at the time of diagnosis. However, it is important to note that a certain proportion of these carcinomas could be diagnosed as high-grade malignancies. It is well known that the cumulative 5-year survival of the patients with early gastric cancer is not 100%, and a small proportion of the patients certainly die of recurrent cancer. Our molecular diagnosis may detect carcinomas with malignant behavior even at an early stage. We are carefully following these cases. Because limited surgery for early gastric cancer, such as partial gastrectomy or endoscopic removal, becomes common, prediction of high-grade malignancy among early cancers is gaining importance. As shown in Table 6, the markers for identifying high-grade malignancy even in superficial carcinomas are c-erbB2, EGF receptor, cyclin E, and so on. In addition to deviation of the examined cases described above, the possibility cannot be neglected that an insufficiency of the molecular biomarkers used may result in false-negative reports. The search for new significant biomarkers should thus be ongoing.

We evaluated the usefulness of our strategy by monitoring advanced cancer patients with repeated molecular diagnosis examinations. Among 48 patients who underwent both biopsy and surgery, 23 (48%) were found to have highly malignant lesions by molecular diagnosis performed on surgical specimens. Among these cases, 12 (52%) were regarded as high-grade malignancy at the

Table 6. Grade of malignancy and molecular biomarker of gastric carcinomas and its relation to tumor stage and depth of tumor invasion

Stage and depth[a]	Cases (no.)	High-grade malignancy (no.)	Molecular markers
Stage			
1	194 (74%)	14 (7%)	c-erbB2, cyclin E, *cripto*, TGF-α, EGF
2	19 (7%)	8 (42%)	c-erbB2, EGFR, *cripto*, TGF-α, EGF
3	37 (14%)	13 (35%)	c-erbB2, c-met, cyclin E, *cripto*, TGFα, *nm23*, EGF
4	11 (4%)	6 (55%)	c-erbB2, EGFR, c-met, cyclin E, *CD44*, *cripto*, TGF, EGF
Depth			
m	134 (52%)	5 (4%)	c-erbB2, cyclin E, TGF-α, and others
sm	57 (22%)	11 (19%)	c-erbB2, EGFR, *cripto*, cyclin E, TGF-α, EGF
mp	11 (4%)	3 (27%)	EGF, cyclin E, *CD44*, *cripto*, TGF-α
ssα, ssβ	11 (4%)	6 (55%)	c-erbB2, EGFR, *cripto*, TGF-α, *nm23*
ssγ	9 (4%)	4 (44%)	c-erbB2, *cripto*, TGF-α, EGF, *nm23*
se, si	35 (14%)	12 (34%)	c-met, c-erbB2, EGFR, cyclin E, TGF-α, EGF, *cripto*

[a] Both according to the criteria of the Japanese Classification of Gastric Carcinoma [118].

time of biopsy. The clinicians could therefore obtain a diagnosis of high-grade malignancy in more than half of the gastric cancer patients before starting treatment. Among the patients who were diagnosed as having adenoma with malignant potential by molecular diagnosis at biopsy, 57% were found to have adenocarcinoma by histopathological examination of surgical materials.

We asked two questions of the clinicians who had received molecular diagnosis reports to evaluate our strategy of molecular diagnosis. The first question was, "How is molecular diagnosis useful in practical medicine?" Eighty percent of the clinicians answered that molecular diagnosis was useful for determining cancer treatment or that it was a good reference for follow-up care; 20% of the clinicians said that it was good for nothing. The second question had to do with the "style of the report." Sixty percent of those responding said that the molecular diagnosis report was presented in an understandable format. Although the report form can be improved so it is more easily understood, the results of the questionnaire indicate the possibility that 20% of the physicians may be ignorant about the significance of the molecular findings, which are deeply implicated in cancer care. The objects of our strategy were ordinary clinicians working in small hospitals or private clinics. Moving toward the next century—an era of molecular medicine and medical genetics—we must develop educational programs with respect to genetics not only for medical students but also for practicing clinicians.

Cost–Benefit

The subject of cost–benefit of molecular diagnosis, as it is of any medical care, is complex. Cost-effectiveness means maximization of health benefits within a limited budget [119]. As to our strategy of molecular diagnosis of gastrointestinal lesions, the running cost per case was approximately 1000 Japanese yen (¥1000) for immunohistochemistry, ¥1000 for PCR analyses, and an additional ¥1000 for microsatellite assay. This cost includes expenses for reagents, antibodies, primers, and so on but excludes salaries for molecular pathologists and wages for technicians. Because we undertake 10 molecular diagnoses a day, at least one technician for immunohistochemistry and two for molecular analyses are engaged. These expenses are not covered by health insurance. At present, the system of molecular diagno-

sis carried out in Hiroshima is supported solely by the contribution of the Hiroshima City Medical Association. Molecular pathologists are working on this project as volunteers. In the near future we expect the practical results to be approved by the Ministry of Health and Welfare of the Japanese government and the costs to be covered by the national health insurance plan.

Calculating the cost/benefit ratio must take into account the well-being of the patients, which is beyond appraisal. For instance, patients who are diagnosed by histopathological examination as having a borderline lesion of the stomach should undergo repeat endoscopy to confirm the diagnosis. With our system, because the benign state and malignancy can be differentiated by molecular analyses on the initial biopsy specimen, an appreciable number of patients can avoid a second endoscopic examination. Alternatively, for cancer patients who undergo endoscopy, the clinician can obtain information about the grade of malignancy by molecular analyses at the time and can select the most suitable treatment. The patients can thus escape the tragedy of recurrence or too intensive care. In other words, the benefit of molecular diagnosis not only to contributes the welfare of patients; it also allows avoidance of unnecessary medical care and reduces the total expenditure. Considering such benefits, we believe that molecular diagnosis is not unprofitable. Too much discussion about the cost/benefit ratio conflicts with health care policies that should be equitable for all humans.

Ethical Aspects of Molecular Diagnosis of Cancer

Discovery of genes associated with clinical disorders increases the ability of clinicians to more accurately assess risk for their patients to develop or to be carriers of a disease. Determining these risks has become more precise with the addition of genetic examinations, most of which technology has been established. Many ethical concerns raised by genetic testing are based on the use and effects of genetic information in both clinical and nonclinical contexts. According to ethical principles, benefits should be to the patient, clinician, family, and possibly society [120]. Informed consent, privacy, confidentiality, insurability, employability, and social stigma are involved [121]. From the international point of view, cultural traditions, religions, languages, political structure, and education must be taken into account [122].

The serious problem of genetic predictive testing for hereditary or genetic diseases is disconnection between diagnosis and treatment. Although a causative gene is identified for more than 2000 diseases, effective treatment has not been developed for most. For such diseases, prenatal prediction by genetic examination includes the dangerous possibility of denying the existence of the individual (elective termination of a pregnancy) to prevent the disease [123]. Genetic prediction of some diseases, such as Huntington's disease and Alzheimer's disease, may affect not only the patient but the family as well; these conditions do not involve life-and-death issues but have a disappointing cure rate [124, 125]. Therefore the legal principles of informed consent, such as the obligation of clinicians to provide their patients with adequate explanations and the rights of patients to autonomy, self-determination, and giving consent to clinicians, may be reconsidered so as to include the intention of the family [126, 127]. On the other hand, genetic examinations can identify people at high risk prior to the onset of some diseases. For instance, genetic identification of high-risk patients for developing type I diabetes mellitus enables us to have an intervention strategy designed to delay or prevent progression to clinical disease [128].

Molecular research on cancer has opened a new era by two major advances in cancer diagnosis. First, it is possible to identify persons at risk of developing cancer or carriers of the gene responsible for cancer. Second, it is possible to better characterize cancer by the use of molecular or genetic alterations. One must keep in mind the distinction between constitutional or germline genetic mutations and acquired or somatic gene alterations. Our molecular diagnosis of gastrointestinal cancer by examining cancer tissues corresponds to the latter and provides information about the differential diagnosis and grade of malignancy. In this case, the ethics are mainly concerned with informed consent—that clinicians provide adequate explanations about the conditions and diagnoses of the disease, the treatments that can be undertaken, the possible benefits and risks, and the prognosis [126]. An uninformed diagnosis results not only in infringement of the patient's rights but inadequate choices of treatment. Clinicians should respect the wishes and opinions of patients based on the patients' own values and should not insist on their own dogmatic opinions. In addition to the right to know, the patients must be guaranteed their right to veto any decisions made by the physician. Considerable attention should be given to ethical conflicts raised by such issues as disclosure of the diagnosis and prognosis, the role of the family in making decisions, and the withholding or withdrawing of treatment from terminally ill patients.

Examination of germline mutations of causative genes can identify individuals at risk for developing cancer or gene carriers in the family of hereditary cancer, such as FAP and HNPCC, prior to its clinical manifestation [129, 130]. Benefits for individuals who are judged to be noncarriers are supreme. They can avoid the fearfulness of developing the disease, and they can escape wasteful medical care. On the other hand, gene carriers diagnosed by genetic analyses are confronted with a number of complex mental, medical, and social issues. Therefore we must obtain fully informed consent regarding the hazards and the benefits of genetic analyses, defining risk as one of the ethical principles of autonomy [131]. It is the responsibility of the counseling system to ensure that the individual is psychologically equipped to deal with the emotional distress that may result from the genetic examination. People must learn how to live with their risk status so the negative psychological sequelae are minimized. An undue burden must not be imposed, and harm must not be inflicted. In fact, timely diagnosis by careful follow-up and appropriate treatment can rescue cancer patients from tragedy. As an ethical principle of confidentiality, it is important to be aware of the potential social problems, including insurance, employment, and matrimony. If technology resolves the problem of developing widely available screening tests, the genetic information about cancer can be obtained even by third parties, which may become a serious problem. For instance, individuals who learn that they are at high risk of cancer are more likely to purchase insurance; and the insurance companies, in an effort to avoid increasing the possibility of paying, may seek genetic information about their prospective customers [132]. Recommendations for genetic testing, regardless of the results, should be carefully provided.

The practical and ethical implications of identifying an individual with a high risk of cancer are complex and require clarification. As with many ethically challenging problems in medicine, clinicians and their patients should work together in a manner with which they are most comfortable in medical and nonmedical contexts.

References

1. Fearon ER, Vogelstein B (1990) A genetic model for colorectal tumorigenesis. Cell 61:759–767
2. Tahara E (1993) Molecular mechanism of stomach carcinogenesis. J Cancer Res Clin Oncol 119:265–272
3. Service RF (1994) Stalking the start of colon cancer. Science 263:1559–1560
4. Tahara E, Semba S, Tahara H (1996) Molecular biological observation in gastric cancer. Semin Oncol 23:307–315
5. Hunter T, Pines J (1994) Cyclins and cancer II: cyclin D and CDK inhibitors come of age. Cell 79:573–582
6. Sherr CJ (1994) G_1 phase progression: cycling on cue. Cell 79:515–555
7. Heichman KA, Roberts JM (1994) Rules to replicate by. Cell 79:557–562
8. Karp JE, Broder S (1995) Molecular foundation of cancer: new targets for intervention. Nature Med 1:309–320
9. Ruschoff J, Bocher T, Schlegel J, Stumm G, Hofstaedter F (1995) Microsatellite instability: new aspects in the carcinogenesis of colorectal carcinoma. Virchows Arch 426:215–222
10. Liu B, Parsons R, Papadopoulos N, Nicolaides NC, Lynch HT, Watson P, Jass JR, Dunlop M, Wyllie A, Peltomaki P, de la Chapelle A, Hamilton SR, Vogelstein B, Kinzler KW (1996) Analysis of mismatch repair genes in hereditary nonpolyposis colorectal cancer patients. Nature Med 2:169–174
11. Kim NW, Piatyszek MA, Prowse KR, Harley CB, West MD, Ho PL, Coviello GM, Wright WE, Weinrich SL, Shay JW (1994) Specific association of human telomerase activity with immortal cells and cancer. Science 266:2011–2015
12. Tahara E (1995) Genetic alterations in human gastrointestinal cancers: the application to molecular diagnosis. Cancer 75S:1410–1417
13. Tahara E, Kuniyasu H, Yasui W, Yokozaki H (1994) Gene alterations in intestinal metaplasia and gastric cancer. Eur J Gastroenterol Hepatol 6S:97–102
14. Semba S, Yokozaki H, Yamamoto S, Yasui W, Tahara E (1996) Microsatellite instability in precancerous lesions and adenocarcinomas of the stomach. Cancer 77/8S:1620–1627
15. Tahara E, Yasui W, Yokozaki H (1996) Abnormal growth factor network in neoplasia. In: Pusztai L, Lewis CE, Yap E (eds) Cell proliferation in cancer: regulatory mechanism of neoplastic cell growth. Oxford University Press, Oxford, pp 131–153
16. Yasui W, Ito H, Tahara E (1992) DNA analysis of archival material and its application to tumour pathology. In: Herrington CS, McGee JO'D (eds) Diagnostic molecular pathology, a practical approach. Oxford University Press, Oxford, pp 193–206
17. Yokozaki H, Tahara E (1995) PCR analysis of RNA. In: Levy ER, Herrington CS (eds) Nonisotopic methods in molecular biology, a practical approach. Oxford University Press, Oxford, pp 201–212
18. Borden EC, Waalen J, Liberati AM, Grignani F (1993) Molecular diagnosis and monitoring of leukemia and lymphoma. Leuk Res 17:1073–1078
19. Herzog CE, Bates SE (1994) Molecular diagnosis of multidrug resistance. Cancer Treat Res 73:129–147
20. Miyoshi Y, Ando H, Nagase H, Nishisho I, Horii A, Miki Y, Mori T, Utsunomiya J, Baba S, Petersen G, Hamilton SR, Kinzler KW, Vogelstein B, Nakamura Y (1992) Germ-line mutations of the *APC* gene in 53 familial adenomatous polyposis patients. Proc Natl Acad Sci USA 89:4452–4456
21. Takeguchi-Shirahama S, Koyama K, Miyauchi A, Wakasugi T, Oishi S, Takami H, Hikiji K, Nakamura Y (1995) Germline mutations of the *RET* proto-oncogene in eight Japanese patients with multiple endocrine neoplasia type 2A (MEN2A). Hum Genet 95:187–190
22. Horii A, Han H-J, Shimada M, Yanagisawa A, Kato Y, Ohta H, Yasui W, Tahara E, Nakamura Y (1994) Frequent replication errors at microsatellite loci in tumors of patients with multiple primary cancers. Cancer Res 54:3373–3375
23. Yasui W, Tahara E (1993) Methods of oncology: molecular biology. In: Burghardt E, Webb MJ, Monaghan JM, Kindermann G (eds) Surgical gynecological oncology. Georg Theime Verlag, Stuttgart, pp 40–44
24. Lu S-H, Hsieh L-L, Luo F-C, Weinstein IB (1988) Amplification of the EGF receptor and c-*myc* genes in human esophageal cancers. Int J Cancer 42:502–505
25. Yoshida K, Kuniyasu H, Yasui W, Kitadai Y, Toge T, Tahara E (1993) Expression of growth factors and their receptors in human esophageal carcinomas: regulation of expression by epidermal growth factor and transforming growth factor α. J Cancer Res Clin Oncol 119:401–407
26. Jiang Wm Kahn SM, Tomita N, Zhang Y-J, Lu S-H, Weinstein IB (1992) Amplification and expression of the human cyclin D gene in esophageal cancer. Cancer Res 52:2980–2983
27. Yoshida K, Kawami H, Kuniyasu H, Nishiyama M, Yasui W, Hirai T, Toge T, Tahara E (1994)

Coamplification of cyclin D, *hst*-1 and *int*-2 genes is a good biological marker of high malignancy for human esophageal carcinomas. Oncol Rep 1:493–496

28. Huang Y, Boynton RF, Blount PL, Silverstein RJ, Yin J, Tong Y, McDaniel TK, Newkirk C, Resau JH, Sridhara R, Reid BJ, Meltzer SJ (1992) Loss of heterozygosity involves multiple tumor suppressor genes in human esophageal cancers. Cancer Res 52:6525–6530

29. Aoki T, Mori T, XiQun D, Nishihira T, Matsubara T, Nakamura Y (1994) Allelotype study of esophageal carcinoma. Gene Chromosom Cancer 10:177–182

30. Hollstein MC, Metcalf RA, Welsh JA, Montesano R, Harris CC (1990) Frequent mutation of the *p53* gene in human esophageal cancer. Proc Natl Acad Sci USA 87:9958–9961

31. Mori T, Miura K, Aoki T, Nishihira T, Mori S, Nakamura Y (1994) Frequent somatic mutation of the MTS1/CDK4I (multiple tumor suppressor/cyclin-dependent kinase 4 inhibitor) gene in esophageal squamous carcinoma. Cancer Res 54:3396–3397

32. Hollstein M, Sidransky D, Vogelstein B, Harris CC (1991) *p53* mutations in human cancers. Science 253:49–53

33. El-Deiry WS, Tokino T, Velculescu VE, Levy DB, Parsons R, Trent JM, Lin D, Mercer E, Kinzler KW, Vogelstein B (1993) WAF1, a potential mediator of p53 tumor suppression. Cell 75:817–825

34. Smith ML, Chen I-T, Zhan Q, Bae I, Chen C-Y, Gilmer TM, Kastan MB, O'Connor PM, Fornace AJ Jr (1994) Interaction of the p53-regulated protein Gadd45 with proliferating cell nuclear antigen. Science 266:1376–1380

35. Miyashita T, Reed JC (1995) Tumor suppressor *p53* is a direct transcriptional activator of the human *bax* gene. Cell 80:293–299

36. Harper JW, Adami GR, Wei N, Keyomarsi K, Elledge SJ (1993) The p21 Cdk-interacting protein Cip1 is a potent inhibitor of G1 cyclin-dependent kinases. Cell 75:805–816

37. Xiong Y, Hannon G, Zhang H, Casso D, Kobayashi R, Beach D (1993) p21 is a universal inhibitor of cyclin kinases. Nature 366:701–704

38. Meltzer SJ, Yin J, Manin B, Mun-Gan R, Cottrell J, Hudson E, Redd JL, Krasna MJ, Abraham JM, Reid BJ (1994) Microsatellite instability occurs frequently and in both diploid and aneuploid cell populations of Barrett's-associated esophageal adenocarcinomas. Cancer Res 54:3379–3382

39. Serrano M, Hannon GJ, Beach D (1993) A new regulatory motif in cell-cycle control causing specific inhibition of cyclin D/CDK4. Nature 366:704–707

40. Kamb A, Gruis NA, Weaver-Feldhaus J, Liu Q, Harshman K, Tavtigian SV, Stockert E, Day RSI, Johnson BE, Skolnick MH (1994) A cell cycle regulator potentially involved in genesis of many tumor types. Science 264:436–440

41. Nobori T, Miura K, Wu DJ, Lois A, Takabayashi K, Carson DA (1994) Deletions of the cyclin-dependent kinase-4 inhibitor gene in multiple human cancers. Nature 368:753–756

42. Hannon GJ, Beach D (1994) *p15*^{INK4B} is a potent effector of TGF-β-induced cell cycle arrest. Nature 371:257–261

43. Polyak K, Kato JY, Solomon MJ, Sherr CJ, Massague J, Roberts JM, Koff A (1994) *p27*^{KIP1}, a cyclin-Cdk inhibitor, links transforming growth factor-β and contact inhibition to cell cycle arrest. Gene Dev 8:9–22

44. Toyoshima H, Hunter T (1994) *p27*, a novel inhibitor of G1 cyclin-Cdk protein kinase activity, is related to *p21*. Cell 78:67–74

45. Kitahara K, Yasui W, Yokozaki H, Semba S, Hamamoto T, Hisatsugu T, Tahara, E (1996) Expression of cyclin D1, CDK4 and *p27*^{KIP1} is associated with the *p16*^{MTS1} gene status in human esophageal carcinoma cell lines. J Exp Ther Oncol 1:7–12

46. Tsuda T, Tahara E, Kajiyama G, Sakamoto H, Terada M, Sugimura T (1989) High incidence of coamplification of *hst*-1 and *int*-2 genes in human esophageal carcinomas. Cancer Res 49:5505–5508

47. Schuuring E, Verhoeven E, Mooi WJ, Michalides RJAM (1992) Identification and cloning of two overexpressed genes, U21B31/*PRAD*1 and *EMS*1, within the amplified chromosome 11q13 region in human carcinomas. Oncogene 7:355–361

48. Kato J-Y, Matsushime H, Heibert SW, Ewen ME, Sherr CJ (1993) Direct binding of cyclin D to the retinoblastoma gene product (pRb) and pRb phosphorylation by the cyclin D-dependent kinase, CDK4. Gene Dev 7:331–342

49. Ozawa S, Ueda M, Ando N, Shimizu N, Abe O (1989) Prognostic significance of epidermal gorwth factor receptor in esophageal squamous cell carcinomas. Cancer 63:2169–2173

50. Yoshida K, Kyo E, Tsuda T, Tsujino T, Ito M, Niimoto M, Tahara E (1990) EGF and TGF-α, the ligands of hyperproduced EGFR in human esophageal carcinoma cells, acts as autocrine growth factors. Int J Cancer 45:131–135

51. Tahara H, Kuniyasu H, Yokozaki H, Yasui W, Shay JW, Ide T, Tahara E (1995) Telomerase activity in preneoplastic and neoplastic gastric and colorectal lesions. Clin Cancer Res 1:1245–1251

52. Kuniyasu H, Yasui W, Kitadai Y, Yokozaki H, Ito H, Tahara E (1992) Frequent amplification of the *c-met* gene in scirrhous type stomach cancer. Biochem Biophys Res Commun 189:227–232

53. Yokozaki H, Kuniyasu H, Kitadai Y, Nishimura K, Todo H, Ayhan A, Yasui W, Ito H, Tahara E (1992) *p53* point mutations in primary human gastric carcinomas. J Cancer Res Clin Oncol 119:67–70

54. Higashikawa K, Yokozaki H, Ue T, Taniyama K, Ishikawa T, Tahara E (1996) Evaluation of CD44 transcription variants in human digestive tract carcinomas and normal tissues. Int J Cancer 66:11–17

55. Akama Y, Yasui W, Yokozaki H, Kuniyasu H, Kitahara K, Ishikawa T, Tahara E (1995) Frequent amplification of the cyclin E gene in human gastric carcinomas. Jpn J Cancer Res 86:617–621

56. Akama Y, Yasui W, Kuniyasu H, Yokozaki H, Akagi M, Tahara H, Ishikawa T, Tahara E (1996) No point mutations but a codon 31 polymorphism and decreased expression of *p21*$^{\text{ISDI1/WAF1/CIP1/MDA6}}$ gene in human gastric carcinomas. Mol Cell Differ 4:187–198

57. Yasui W, Akama Y, Kuniyasu H, Yokozaki H, Semba S, Shimamoto F, Tahara E (1996) Expression of cyclin-dependent kinase inhibitor p21$^{\text{WAF1/CIP1}}$ in non-neoplastic mucosa and neoplasia of the stomach: relation with p53 status and proliferative activity. J Pathol 180:122–128

58. Yasui W, Kudo Y, Semba S, Yokozaki H, Tahara E (1997) Reduced expression of cyclin-dependent kinase inhibitor p27$^{\text{KIP1}}$ is associated with advanced stage and invasiveness of gastric carcinomas. Jpn J Cancer Res (in press)

59. Yokozaki H, Ito M, Yasui W, Kyo E, Kuniyasu H, Kitadai Y, Tsubouchi H, Daikuhara Y, Tahara E (1993) Biologic effect of hepatocyte growth factor on human gastric carcinoma cell lines. Int J Oncol 3:89–93

60. Tahara E, Yokozaki H, Yasui W (1993) Growth factors in gastric cancer. In: Nishi M, Ichikawa H, Nakajima T, Maruyama K, Tahara E (eds) Gastric cancer. Springer, Tokyo, pp 209–217

61. Ito R, Kitadai Y, Kyo E, Yokozaki H, Yasui W, Yamashita U, Nikai H, Tahara E (1993) IL-1α acts as an autocrine growth stimulator for human gastric carcinoma cells. Cancer Res 53:4102–4106

62. Nakayama H, Yasui W, Yokozaki H, Tahara E (1993) Reduced expression of *nm23* is associated with metastasis of human gastric carcinomas. Jpn J Cancer Res 84:184–190

63. Vogelstein B, Fearon ER, Hamilton SR, Kern SE, Preisinger AC, Leppert M, Nakamura Y, White R, Smith AMM, Bos JL (1988) Genetic alterations during colorectal tumor development. N Engl J Med 319:525–532

64. Kinzler KW, Nilbert MC, Su LK, Vogelstein B, Bryan TM, Levy DB, Smith KJ, Preisinger AC, Hedge P, McKechnie D, Finniear R, Markham A, Groffen J, Boguski MS, Altshul SF, Horii A, Ando H, Miyoshi Y, Miki Y, Nishisho I, Nakamura Y (1991) Identification of FAP locus genes from chromosome 5q21. Science 253:661–665

65. Harlow E, Williamson NM, Ralston R, Helfman DM, Adams TE (1985) Molecular cloning and in vitro expression of a cDNA clone for human cellular tumor antigen p53. Mol Cell Biol 5:1601–1610

66. Fearon ER, Cho KR, Nigro JM, Kern SE, Simons JW, Ruppert JM, Hamilton SR, Preisinger AC, Thomas G, Kinzler KW, Vogelstein B (1990) Identification of a chromosome 18q gene that is altered in colorectal cancers. Science 247:49–56

67. Lynch HT, Smyrk TC, Watson P, Lanspa SJ, Lynch JF, Lynch PM, Cavalieri RJ, Boland CR (1993) Genetics, natural history, tumor spectrum, and pathology of hereditary nonpolyposis colorectal cancer: an update review. Gastroenterology 104:1535–1549

68. Rubinfeld B, Souza B, Albert I, Muller O, Chamberlain SH, Masiarz FR, Munemitsu S, Polakis P (1993) Association of the *APC* gene product with β-catenin. Science 262:1731–1734

69. Su L-K, Vogelstein B, Kinzler KW (1993) Association of the APC tumor suppressor protein with catenins. Science 262:1734–1737

70. Miyoshi Y, Nagae H, Ando H, Horii A, Ichii S, Nakatsuru S, Aoki T, Miki Y, Mori T, Nakamura Y (1992) Somatic mutations of the *APC* gene in colorectal tumors. Hum Mol Genet 1:229–233

71. Knudson AG (1985) Hereditary cancer, oncogenes, and antioncogenes. Cancer Res 45:1437–1443

72. Ichii S, Takeda S, Horii A, Nakatsuru S, Miyoshi Y, Emi M, Fujiwara Y, Koyama K, Furukawa J, Utsunomiya J, Nakamura Y (1993) Detailed analysis of genetic alterations in colorectal tumors from patients with and without familial adenomatous polyposis (FAP). Oncogene 8:2399–2405

73. Bos JL, Fearon ER, Hamilton SR, Verlaan-de Vries M, van Boom JH, van der Eb AJ, Vogelstein B (1987) Prevalence of *ras* gene mutations in human colorectal cancers. Nature 327:293–297

74. Forrester K, Almoguera C, Han K, Grizzle WE, Perucho M (1987) Detection of high incidence of K-*ras* oncogenes during human colon tumorigenesis. Nature 327:298–303

75. Brumer GC, Loeb L (1989) Mutations in the *KRAS*2 oncogene during progressive stage of human colon carcinoma. Proc Natl Acad Sci USA 86:2403–2407

76. Fujimori T, Satonaka K, Yamamura-Ideki Y, Nagasako K, Maeda S (1994) Non-involvement of *ras* mutations in flat colorectal adenomas and carcinomas. Int J Cancer 56:1–5

77. Minamoto T, Sawaguchi K, Mai M, Yamashita N, Sugimura T, Esumi H (1994) Infrequent K-*ras* activation in superficial-type (flat) adenomas and adenocarcinomas. Cancer Res 54:2841–2844

78. Jen J, Powell SM, Papadopoulos N, Smith KJ, Hamilton SR, Vogelstein B, Kinzler KW (1994) Molecular determinants of dysplasia in colorectal lesions. Cancer Res 54:5523–5526

79. Greenblatt MS, Bennett WP, Hollstein M, Harris CC (1994) Mutations in the *p53* tumor suppressor gene: clues to cancer etiology and molecular pathogenesis. Cancer Res 54:4855–4878

80. Kikuchi-Yanoshita R, Konishi M, Ito S, Seki M, Tanaka K, Maeda Y, Iino H, Fukuyama M, Koike M, Mori T, Sakuraba H, Fukunari H, Iwama T, Miyaki M (1992) Genetic changes of both *p53* alleles associated with conversion from colorectal adenoma to early carcinoma in familial adenomatous polyposis and non-familial adenomatous polyposis patients. Cancer Res 52:3965–3971

81. Ayhan A, Yasui W, Yokozaki H, Ito H, Tahara E (1992) Genetic abnormalities and expression of *p53* in human colon carcinomas. Int J Oncol 1:431–437

82. Yasui W, Kuniyasu H, Yokozaki H, Semba S, Shimamoto F, Tahara E (1996) Expression of cyclin E in colorectal adenomas and adenocarcinomas: correlation with expression of Ki-67 and p53 protein. Virchows Arch 429:13–19

83. Hamelin R, Laurent PP, Olschwang S, Jego N, Asselain B, Remvikos Y, Girodet J, Salmon RJ, Thomas G (1994) Association of *p53* mutations with short survival in colorectal cancer. Gastroenterology 106:42–48

84. Hedrick L, Cho KR, Fearon ER, Wu T-C, Kinzler KW, Vogelstein B (1994) The *DCC* gene product in cellular differentiation and colorectal tumorigenesis. Gene Dev 8:1174–1183

85. Ookawa K, Sakamoto M, Hirohashi S, Yoshida Y, Sugimura T, Terada M, Yokota J (1993) Concordant *p53* and *DCC* alterations and allelic losses on chromosome 13q and 14q associated with liver metastasis of colorectal carcinoma. Int J Cancer 53:382–387

86. Tahara E (1990) Growth factors and oncogenes in human gastrointestinal carcinomas. J Cancer Res Clin Oncol 116:121–131

87. Ciccodicola A, Dono R, Obici S, Simeone A, Zollo M, Persico MG (1989) Molecular characterization of a gene of the EGF family expressed in undifferentiated human NTRERA2 teratocarcinoma cells. EMBO J 8:1987–1991

88. Saeki T, Stromberg K, Qi C-F, Gullick WJ, Tahara E, Normanno N, Ciardiello F, Kenny N, Johnson GR, Salomon DS (1992) Differential immunohistochemical detection of amphiregulin and cripto in human normal colon and colorectal tumors. Cancer Res 52:3467–3473

89. Kuniyasu H, Yoshida K, Yokozaki H, Yasui W, Ito H, Toge T, Ciardiello F, Persico MG, Saeki T, Salomon DS, Tahara E (1991) Expression of *cripto*, a novel gene of the epidermal growth factor

family, in human gastrointestinal carcinomas. Jpn J Cancer Res 82:969–973

90. Shoyab M, McDonald VL, Bradley JG, Todaro GJ (1988) Amphiregulin, a bifunctional growth-modulating glycoprotein produced by the phorbol 12-myristate 13-acetate-treated human breast adenocarcinoma cell line MCF-7. Proc Natl Acad Sci USA 85:6528–6532

91. Johnson GR, Saeki T, Gordon AW, Shoyab M, Salomon DS, Stromberg K (1992) Autocrine action of amphiregulin in a colon carcinoma cell line and immunocytochemical localization of amphiregulin in human colon. J Cell Biol 118:741–751

92. Kitahara K, Yasui W, Kuniyasu H, Yokozaki H, Akama Y, Yunotani S, Hisatsugu T, Tahara E (1995) Concurrent amplification of cyclin E and *CDK2* genes in colorectal carcinomas. Int J Cancer 62:25–28

93. Matsumura Y, Tarin D (1992) Significance of *CD44* gene products for cancer diagnosis and disease evaluation. Lancet 340:1053–1058

94. Tolg C, Hofmann M, Herrlich P, Ponta H (1993) Splicing choice from ten variant exons establishes *CD44* variability. Nucleic Acids Res 21:1225–1229

95. Cooper DL, Dougherty GJ (1995) To metastasize or not? Selection of CD44 splice sites. Nature Med 1:635–637

96. Yoshida K, Bolodeoku J, Sugino T, Goodison S, Matsumura Y, Warren BF, Toge T, Tahara E, Tarin D (1995) Abnormal retention of intron 9 in *CD44* gene transcripts in human gastrointestinal tumors. Cancer Res 55:4273–4277

97. Weber GF, Ashkar S, Glimcher MJ, Cantor H (1996) Receptor–ligand interaction between CD44 and osteopontin (Efa-1). Science 271:509–512

98. Postel EH, Berberich SJ, Flint SJ, Ferrone CA (1993) Human c-*myc* transcription factor PuF identified as nm23-H2 nucleoside diphosphate kinase, a candidate suppressor of tumor metastasis. Science 261:478–480

99. Ayhan A, Yasui W, Yokozaki H, Kitadai Y, Tahara E (1993) Reduced expression of nm23 protein is associated with advanced tumor stage and distant metastases in human colorectal carcinomas. Virchows Arch B Cell Pathol 63:213–218

100. Matsushita Y, Hoff SD, Nudelman ED, Otaka M, Hakomori S, Ota DM, Cleary KR, Irimura T (1991) Metastatic behavior and cell surface properties of HT-29 human colon carcinoma variant cells selected for their differential expression of sialyl-dimeric Le^x antigen. Clin Exp Metastasis 9:283–299

101. Berg EL, Robinson MK, Mansson O, Butcher EC, Magnani JL (1991) A carbohydrate domain common to both sialyl Le^a and sialyl Le^x is recognized by the endothelial cell leukocyte adhesion molecule ELAM-1. J Biol Chem 266:14869–14872

102. Nakamori S, Kameyama M, Imaoka S, Furukawa H, Ishikawa O, Sasaki Y, Kabuto T, Iwanaga T, Matsushita Y, Irimura T (1993) Increased expression of sialyl Lewis^x antigen correlates with poor survival in patients with colorectal carcinoma: clinicopathological and immunohistochemical study. Cancer Res 53:3632–3637

103. Fishel R, Lescoe MK, Rao MRS, Copeland NG, Jenkins NA, Garber J, Kane M, Kolodner R (1993) The human mutator gene homolog *MSH2* and its association with hereditary nonpolyposis colorectal cancer. Cell 75:1027–1038

104. Leach FS, Nicolaides NC, Papadopoulos N, Liu B, Jen J, Parsons R, Pertomaki P, Sistonen P, Aaltonen LA, Nystrom-Lahti M, Guan X-Y, Zhang J, Melter PS, Yu J-W, Kao F-T, Chen DJ, Cerosaletti KM, Fournier REK, Todd S, Lewis T, Leach RJ, Naylor SL, Weissenbach J, Mecklin J-P, Jarvinen H, Petersen GM, Hamilton SR, Green J, Jass J, Watson P, Lynch HT, Trent JM, de la Chapelle A, Kinzler KW, Vogelstein B (1993) Mutation of a *mutS* homolog in hereditary nonpolyposis colorectal cancer. Cell 75:1215–1225

105. Bronner CE, Baker SM, Morrison PT, Warren G, Smith LG, Lescoe MK, Kane M, Erabino C, Lipford J, Lindblom A, Tannergard P, Bollag RJ, Godwin AR, Ward DC, Nordenskjold M, Fishel R, Kolodner R, Liskay RM (1994) Mutation in the DNA mismatch repair gene homologue *hMLH1* is associated with hereditary nonpolyposis colorectal cancer. Nature 368:258–261

106. Papadopoulos N, Nicolaides NC, Liu B, Wei Y-F, Rube SM, Carter KC, Rosen CA, Haseltine WA, Fleischmann RD, Fraser CM, Adams MD, Venter JC, Hamilton SR, Petersen GM, Watson P, Lynch HT, Peltomaki P, Mecklin J-P, de la Chapelle A, Kinzler KW, Vogelstein B (1994) Mutation of a *mutL* homolog in hereditary nonpolyposis colon cancer. Science 263:1625–1629

107. Nicolaides NC, Papadopoulos N, Liu B, Wei Y-F, Carter KC, Rube SM, Rosen CA, Haseltine WA, Fleischmann RD, Fraser CM, Adams MD, Venter JC, Dunlop MG, Hamilton SR, Petersen GM, de la Chapelle A, Vogelstein B, Kinzler KW (1994) Mutation of two PMS homologues in hereditary nonpolyposis colon cancer. Nature 371:75–80

108. Nystrom-Lahti N, Parsons R, Sistonen P, Pylkkanen L, Aaltonen LA, Leach F, Hamilton SR, Watson P, Bronson E, Fusaro R, Cavalieri J, Lynch J, Lanspa S, Smyrk T, Lynch P, Drouhard T, Kinzler KW, Vogelstein B, Lynch HT, de la Chapelle A, Peltomaki P (1994) Mismatch repair genes on chromosome 1p and 3p account for a major share of hereditary nonpolyposis colorectal cancer families evaluable by linkage. Am J Hum Genet 55:659–665

109. Markowitz S, Wang J, Myeroff L, Parsons R, Sun L, Lutterbaugh J, Fan RS, Zborowska E, Kinzler KW, Vogelstein B, Brattain M, Willson JKV (1995) Inactivation of the type II TGF-β receptor in colon cancer cells with microsatellite instability. Science 268:1336–1338

110. Myeroff LL, Parsons R, Kim S-J, Hedrick L, Cho KR, Orth K, Mathis M, Kinzler KW, Lutterbaugh J, Park K, Bang Y-J, Lee HY, Park J-G, Lynch HT, Roberts AB, Vogelstein B, Markowitz SD (1995) A transforming growth factor β receptor type II gene mutation common in colon and gastric but rare in endometrial cancers with microsatellite instability. Cancer Res 55:5545–5547

111. Ionov YM, Peinado A, Malkhosyan S, Shibata D, Perucho M (1993) Ubiquitous somatic mutations in simple repeated sequences reveal a new mechanism for colonic carcinogenesis. Nature 363:558–561

112. Thibodeau SN, Bren G, Schaid D (1993) Microsatellite instability in cancer of the proximal colon. Science 260:816–819

113. Counter CM, Avilion AA, LeFeuvre CE, Stewart NG, Greider CW, Harley CB, Bacchetti S (1992) Telomere shortening associated with chromosome instability is arrested in immortal cells which express telomerase activity. EMBO J 11:1921–1929

114. Rhyu MS (1995) Telomeres, telomerase and immortality. J Natl Cancer Inst 87:884–894

115. Hastie ND, Dempster M, Dunlop MG, Thompson AM, Green DK, Allshire RC (1990) Telomere reduction in human colorectal carcinoma and with aging. Nature 346:866–868

116. Chadeneau C, Hay K, Hirte HW, Gallinger S, Bacchetti S (1995) Telomerase activity associated with aquisition of malignancy in human colorectal cancer. Cancer Res 55:2533-2536

117. Tarin D (1995) A new strategy of molecular diagnosis of gastrointestinal cancer. Jpn J Cancer Res 86

118. Japanese Research Society for Gastric Cancer (1995) Japanese classification of gastric carcinoma, 1st English edm. Kanehara, Tokyo

119. Ubel PA, DeKay ML, Baron J, Asch DA (1996) Cost-effectiveness analysis in a setting of budget constraints: is it equitable? N Engl J Med 334:1174–1177

120. Williams JK, Lea DH (1995) Applying new genetic technologies: assessment and ethical considerations. Nurse Pract 20:21–26

121. Parkers LS (1995) Ethical concerns in the research and treatment of complex disease. Trends Genet 11:520–523

122. Berg K, Pettersson U, Riis P, Tranoy KE (1995) Genetic in democratic societies: the Nordic perspective. Clin Genet 48:199–208

123. Burgess MM (1994) Ethical issues in prenatal testing. Clin Biochem 27:87–91

124. De Wert G (1992) Predictive testing for Huntington disease and the right not to know: some ethical reflections. Birth Defects 28:133–138

125. Lennox A, Karlinsky H, Meschino W, Buchanan JA, Percy ME, Berg JM (1994) Molecular genetics predictive testing for Alzheimer's disease: deliberations and preliminary recommendations. Alzheimer Dis Assoc Disord 8:126–147

126. Hoshino K (1992) Bioethical issues and principles in cancer treatment. Jpn J Cancer Chemother 19:281–285

127. Vineis P, Soskolne CL (1993) Cancer risk assessment and management: an ethical perspective. J Occup Med 35:902–908

128. Siegler M, Amiel S, Lantos J (1992) Scientific and ethical consequences of disease prediction. Diabetologia 35:S60–68

129. Spigelman AD (1994) Familial adenomatous polyposis: recent genetic advances. Br J Surg 81:321–322

130. Eeles RA, Stratton MR, Goldgar DE, Easton DF (1994) The genetics of familial breast cancer and their practical implications. Eur J Cancer 30A:1383–1390

131. Kash KM (1995) Psychosocial and ethical implications of defining genetic risk for cancers. Ann NY Acad Sci 768:41–52

132. Murray TH (1993) Ethics, genetic prediction, and heart disease. Am J Cardiol 72:80D–84D

Interactive Effects of *p53* Tumor Suppressor Gene and Hepatitis B Virus in Hepatocellular Carcinogenesis

Libin Jia, Xin Wei Wang, Zongtang Sun, and Curtis C. Harris

Summary. Chronic infection with hepatitis B (HBV) or C (HCV) virus and dietary exposure to either aflatoxin B_1 or alcoholic beverages are the major risk factors of hepatocellular carcinoma (HCC). Mutations in the *p53* tumor suppressor gene are frequently found in HCC. Aflatoxin B_1 exposure also has a positive correlation with codon 249^{ser} mutation of the *p53* tumor suppressor gene. The continued expression of hepatitis B virus X protein (HBx) plays an important role in hepatocellular carcinogenesis. The protein–protein interaction between the HBx and p53 tumor suppressor protein can abrogate the normal functions of p53. This review discusses the role of the *p53* tumor suppressor gene and its interactive effects with HBx in human liver carcinogenesis.

Introduction

Hepatocellular carcinoma (HCC) is a common tumor worldwide and ranks as one of the four most prevalent malignant diseases of adults in Asia and sub-Saharan Africa [1]. More than 250 000 cases of HCC are diagnosed each year, and fewer than 3% of these patients survive 5 years or more. Chronic infection with hepatitis B virus (HBV), ingestion of aflatoxin B_1 (AFB_1)-contaminated foods, alcoholic consumption-associated cirrhosis, and other factors associated with chronic inflammatory and hepatic regenerative changes are important risk factors for hepatocarcinogenesis [1–6] (Fig. 1).

Molecular genetic investigations have revealed that mutations in proto-oncogenes and tumor suppressor genes are critical events in carcinogenesis

Laboratory of Human Carcinogenesis, Division of Basic Sciences, National Cancer Institute, National Institutes of Health, Building 37, Room 2C01, 37 Convent Drive, MSC 4255, Bethesda, MD 20892-4255, U.S.A.

[7–10]. The *p53* tumor suppressor gene is a frequent target for genetic abnormalities in diverse types of human cancer [11–13]. Certain domains of the *p53* gene have been highly conserved during evolution, reflecting the functional importance and selection in the p53 protein [14]. The significance of *p53* gene abnormality in cancer development has been further defined by reports on germ line *p53* mutation in Li-Fraumeni syndrome of breast cancer, sarcoma, and other neoplasms [15].

p53 Tumor Suppressor Gene Mutation Spectrum

Most of the base substitution mutations fall within exons 5–8 of the *p53* gene. Analysis of *p53* gene mutations indicated that the sites and features of DNA base changes differ among cancers, including lung, colon, esophagus, breast, liver, brain, and skin cancers [13]. Mutagenesis experiments have revealed a positive relation between the interaction of carcinogen with DNA (e.g., DNA adduct formation) and permanent DNA changes recognized as mutations [13].

Most mutations in tumor-suppressor genes are nonsense mutations, deletions and insertions that produce either a truncated protein product or no protein at all. These mutations are clearly loss of function mutations. The *p53* tumor suppressor gene has an unusual spectrum of mutations when compared with other suppressor genes (e.g., *APC*, *BRCA-1*, or *p16*^{INK4}) (Fig. 2). Missense mutations in which the encoded protein contains amino acid substitutions are commonly found in the *p53* tumor-suppressor gene. The missense class of mutations can cause both a loss of tumor-suppressor function and a gain of oncogenic function [16–18] perhaps by changing the repertoire of genes whose expression is controlled by this transcription factor. The *p53* gene was

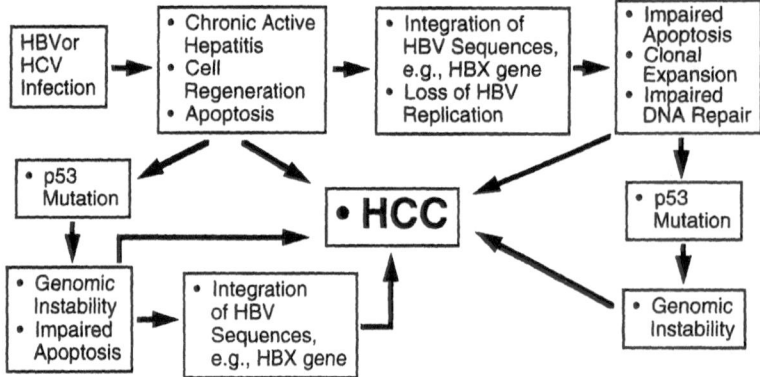

Fig. 1. Model of hepatitis B and C viruses (*HBV, HCV*) and chemical carcinogen interactive effects in the molecular pathogenesis of human hepatocellular carcinoma (*HCC*)

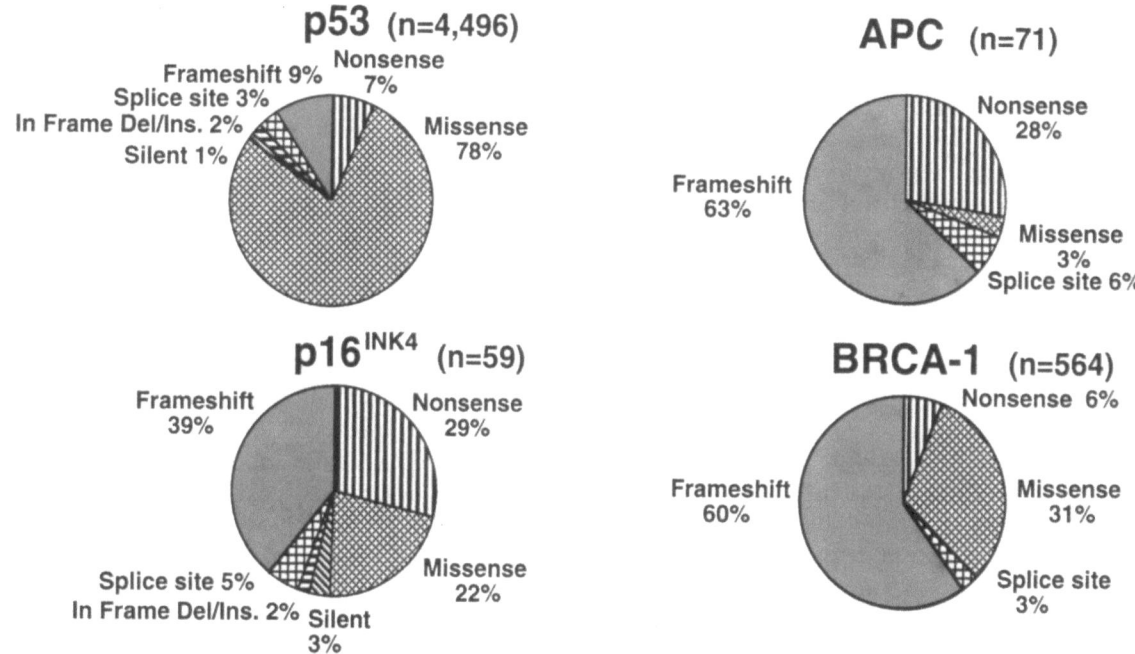

Fig. 2. Mutational spectra of the *p53* and *p16*[INK4] genes in primary tumors. INK4, inhibitor of cyclin dependent kinase 4α

initially classified as an oncogene until it was discovered during the late 1980s that the cDNAs cloned from murine and human tumor cells contained missense mutations, at which time it was correctly classified when a true wild-type *p53* gene construct suppressed the growth of tumor cells [19–24].

The *p53* gene mutational spectrum of HCC is an example of a molecular link between carcinogen exposure and cancer. In HCCs from persons living in geographic areas in which AFB$_1$ and HBV are cancer risk factors, most *p53* mutations are at the third nucleotide pair of codon 249 [25–28]. A dose-dependent relation between dietary AFB$_1$ intake and codon 249[ser] *p53* mutations is observed in HCC from Asia, Africa, and North America (Fig. 3). The mutation load of 249[ser] mutant cells in nontumorous liver also is positively correlated

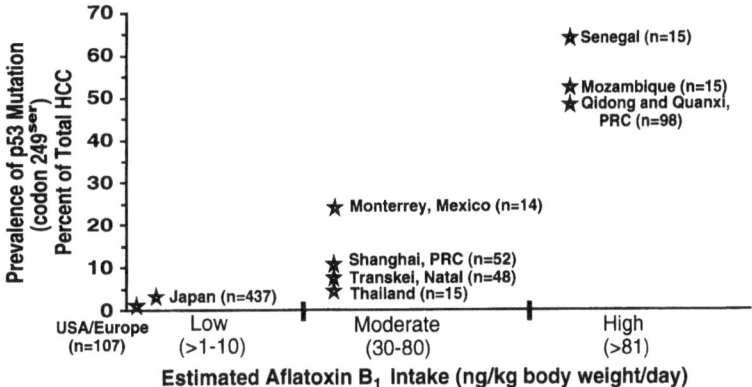

Fig. 3. Correlation of aflatoxin B₁ estimated dietary exposure and codon 249^{ser} *p53* mutation in hepatocellular carcinoma. ser, serine

with dietary AFB₁ exposure [29]. Exposing human liver cells to AFB₁ in vitro produces dominantly 249^{ser} (AGG to AGT) *p53* mutants [30; K. Mace, F. Aguilar, C.C. Harris, and G.P. Pfeifer, unpublished results]. These results indicate that expression of the 249^{ser} mutant p53 protein provides a specific growth or survival advantage to liver cells and is consisted with the hypothesis that *p53* mutations can occur early in liver carcinogenesis.

Because cellular context may influence the pathobiological effects of specific mutants of *p53*, the 249^{ser} mutant may be especially potent in hepatocytes. The enhanced growth rate of *p53*-null Hep-3B cells by transfected 249^{ser} mutant *p53* indicates a gain of oncogenic function and is consisted with this hypothesis [31]. The 249^{ser} mutant *p53* also is more effective than other *p53* mutants (143^{ala}, 175^{his}, 248^{trp}, 282^{his}) in inhibiting wild-type

p53 transcriptional activity in human liver cells [32] (Fig. 4). One hypothesis concerning the generation of HCC with an 249^{ser} *p53* mutation states that: (1) AFB₁ is metabolically activated to form the promutagenic N7dG adduct; and (2) enhanced cell proliferation due to chronic active viral hepatitis allows both fixation of the G:C to T:A transversion in codon 249 of the *p53* gene and selective clonal expansion of the cells containing this mutant *p53* gene owing to a deficiency in the p53-dependent apoptotic pathway. In addition to producing chronic active hepatitis, HBV has other significant pathobiological effects. For example, hepatitis B viral gene products may form complexes with cellular transcription factors (e.g., ATE2 [33]), up-regulate transcription of cellular and viral genes [34–38], or activate the RAS-RAF-MAP kinase signaling cascade [39].

Inactivation of *p53* tumor-suppressor gene functions including DNA repair and apoptosis may be other consequences of the p53–HBV oncoprotein complex formation. Because the *HBV-X* gene is frequently integrated and expressed in human HCCs from high risk geographic areas [40, 41], we have focused our attention on the HBx protein, which binds to p53 [42–44] and inhibits its sequence-specific DNA binding and transcriptional activity [43]. HBx protein also inhibits p53-dependent apoptosis [45]. Based on the above results, we have speculated that HBx protein may modulate p53 function in nucleotide excision DNA repair [45], including repair of the AFB₁-DNA adduct; we are currently testing this hypothesis. HBV integration also

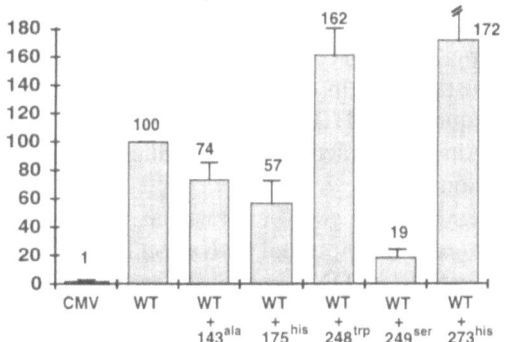

Fig. 4. Differential effects of *p53* mutants on transcriptional activity of wild-type (*WT*) p53 in HEP-3B liver carcinoma cell line. *CMV*, cytomegalovirus

could increase genomic instability, including abnormal chromosomal segregation, and increase rates of DNA recombination [46, 47]. Therefore a second hypothesis of liver carcinogenesis emerges in which integration of the HBV gene is an initial event in these high cancer risk geographic areas and AFB$_1$-mediated 249^{ser} p53 mutation is the second genetic lesion that leads to further genomic instability.

HBx Transcription-Transactivation Functions

The genome structure of HBV is a partially double-stranded relaxed circle of 3.2 kilobases (kb) [48]. It contains four recognized open reading frames, three of which encode virion structural proteins including the surface antigen (HBsAg), core antigen (HBcAg), and viral polymerase. The fourth open reading frame, conserved among all mammalian hepadnaviruses, encodes a 16.5-kDa protein, termed the X antigen (HBx). The *HBV-X* gene is expressed during viral infection, producing a 1-kb mRNA [49]. The HBx protein has multiple functions in the pathogenesis of HCC. It is a transcriptional activator [34, 35, 50] that performs an essential function for viral infection. Most primary tumors and tumor-derived cell lines have some or all of the HBV-X region and upstream preS/S sequences integrated transcripts, whereas relatively few made transcripts from other regions of the genome [51]. HBx is an activator of a variety of RNA polymerase II transcription factors, including AP1 [39, 52–55], AP-2 [52], NF-κB [56–59], and RNA polymerase III transcription factors [60]. HBx is a dual-function nuclear and cytoplasmic protein, activating specific transcription elements in the nucleus and RAS-signaling pathways in the cytoplasm [61]. In the nucleus, HBx protein might activate transcription directly at the promoter [52, 62], possibly by binding and stimulating the transcription factor ATF/CREB [63, 64], the RPB5 subunit of RNA polymerase [65], and TATA-binding protein [66]. In transgenic mice the HBx protein can induce liver cancer [50].

p53–HBx Binding

Feitelson et al. [42] reported that by using immunoprecipitation and Western blot analysis, it was found that anti-HBx specifically immunoprecipitates p53 from human liver cells only in the presence of HBx, and anti-p53 also specifically immunoprecipitates HBx only in the presence of p53. Wang et al. [43] found that HBx protein can physically bind to tumor suppressor p53 by using GST–p53 fusion proteins produced in *Escherichia coli* as "bait" in incubations with in vitro translated sulfur 35 (^{35}S)-labeled HBx protein. A 17-kDa band can be immunoprecipitated by rabbit anti-HBx antibody. HBx protein also exhibits different binding abilities with various p53 mutants. Wang et al. [43] examined the complex formation between HBx protein and mutated p53 protein and found that HBx can bind to certain types of mutated p53, such as p53–249^{ser} and p53–273^{his}. Mutant p53–135^{tyr} can be weakly bound by HBx. The explanation for this weak binding may be explained by the conformation differences among mutant p53 proteins.

HBx can inhibit p53 sequence-specific DNA-binding activity in vitro. The transcriptional transactivation activity of human wild-type p53 may be the result of its interaction with specific DNA sequence adjacent to functionally important cellular genes such as *p21*$^{WAF1/Cip1}$, *MDM2*, and *GADD45* [67, 68]. We postulated that HBx may block the transactivation activity of p53 by preventing its sequence-specific DNA binding and detected that the binding between p53-WT and its DNA consensus sequence (PG13) was diminished nearly 90% after adding HBx to the reaction mixture [43]. One hypothesis to explain this change is that HBx may alter the conformation of wild-type p53 in a manner analogous to the dominant negative p53 missense mutants found in human cancers. Interestingly, complexes between HBx and other cellular transcription factors (e.g., CREB and ATF-2) enhance the DNA-binding specificity of these proteins [63]. These contrasting results indicate that the functional consequence of HBx on gene expression may depend on its interaction with specific cellular transcription factors.

The *HBV-X* gene expression inhibits p53-mediated transcriptional activation in vivo. Binding of p53 to its DNA consensus sequence is necessary for transactivation of genes adjacent to these binding sites [69]. Wang et al. [43] used a co-transfecting *p53* and *HBV-X* gene expression vector to determine if HBx can modulate the transcription-transactivation ability of p53-WT. Co-transfection of cytomegalovirus (CMV)-

driven wild-type human *p53* vector and p53-responsive reporter (CAT) construct into human liver THLE-5b cells result in a 16-fold activation of CAT gene expression. Addition of HBx expression vectors results in about a 90% reduction of p53-mediated transactivation. The RNase protection data indicate that there is no significant difference in the p53 level in the cells expressing or not expressing transfected *HBV-X* gene. Therefore HBx did not inhibit p53-mediated transactivation by down-regulation of p53 expression in THLE-5b cells. However, HBx modulation of p53 transactivation activity in a transient transcription assay is dependent on cellular context. An apparent enhancement of p53-mediated transactivation by HBx is observed in another HCC cell line (Hep3B) and a lung adenocarcinoma cell line (Calu 6). The cell-type specificity observed in these experiments appears to be contradictory. Because HBx can transactivate many cellular and viral promoters in a variety of cell lines through activation of the PKC signal transduction pathway [70], one hypothesis is that inhibition of p53-mediated activation of the CMV promoter through the protein kinase C (PKC) pathway to elevate the levels of p53 in the Hep3B and Calu 6 cell lines. It has been found that HBx transactivated the CMV promoter in the Hep3B and Calu 6 cell lines but not in the THLE-5b cell line. Furthermore, transactivation of the CMV promoter by HBx in the Hep3B cell line is blocked by potent PKC inhibitors, suggesting the activation of PKC by HBx in this cell line.

HBx and DNA Repair

HBx interferes with the binding of p53 to XPB (ERCC3) [43], which is a basic transcription factor that is also involved in nucleotide excision repair [71]. Wild-type p53 can form a protein–protein complex with XPB. HBx almost completely inhibits the binding of p53 to XPB [43]. The finding that p53 and XPB associate in vitro leads to a model in which p53 contributes to the maintenance of genomic stability by modulating transcription and DNA-nucleotide-excision repair processes. Inactivation of p53 by either mutation or interaction with viral oncoproteins, including HBx, could increase the mutation frequency of important cellular genes and increase the probability of neoplastic transformation of human hepatocytes.

Lee et al. [72], using the yeast two-hybrid system, identified a cellular protein that can interact with HBx protein. This protein, designated X-associated protein 1 (XAP-1), is a human homolog of the UV-damaged DNA-binding protein (UV-DDB) recovered from a monkey cell cDNA library. UV-DDB is presumed to be involved in the DNA repair process. The speculation of this interaction of HBx with a DNA repair protein may recruit cellular proteins to either repair the partially double-stranded HBV genome or modify cellular transcription processes. Therefore the effects of HBx on the cellular DNA repair system may indicate another pathway by which HBV contributes to liver carcinogenesis.

HBx Block of p53-Induced Apoptosis

The *p53* tumor suppressor gene product is involved in the maintenance of genomic integrity [73]. Various DNA tumor viruses encode transforming oncoproteins that bind to p53, including the T antigen from SV40 [74, 75], E6 from oncogenic HPV [74], IE84 from human CMV [76], and HBx from HBV [42–44]. Among them, the T antigen from SV40 and E1B relative molecular weight (M_r) 55000 proteins have been shown to inhibit *p53*-dependent programmed cell death [79, 80], an intrinsic cellular process essential for maintaining tissue homeostasis [81, 82]. In addition, IE84 was shown to abolish p53 transcriptional activation, which may lead to coronary restenosis [78]. The protein p53 is an inducer of apoptosis [83, 84], which contributes to its function as a tumor-suppressor gene [85–87]. Disruption of p53-mediated apoptosis by viral oncoproteins may be a significant step in carcinogenesis. HBx can also block *p53*-mediated apoptosis [45]. Microinjection of the CMV-driven wild-type *p53* expression vector into the nucleus of normal human primary fibroblasts can induce apoptosis. When the wild-type *p53* and *HBV-X* genes (both CMV promoter-driven) are co-injected into the nucleus of primary human fibroblasts, apoptosis is blocked and only 2% of the cells display the apoptotic phenotype (Table 1). It is interesting that co-injection of *p53* and *HBV-X* result in an increased percentage of cells with p53 accumulation in the nucleus (81%), compared to 32% expression vector when p53 alone is microinjected. This phenom-

Table 1. Inhibition of the *p53*-dependent apoptosis by the hepatitis B virus X gene

Microinjected expression vector	Apoptotic cells[a]		p53 Localization (% of cells)		
	%	No.[b]	Nucleus	Cytoplasms	
WT p53	19	59	32	0	68
WT p53 and HBx	2[c]	52	81	0	19

WT, wild type.

[a] Cells with condensed and fragmented nuclei as well as cytoplasmic blebbing characteristic of cells undergoing apoptosis.

[b] Number of p53-immunopositive cells scored following microinjection of the p53 expression vector.

[c] Chi-sequare test compared to WT p53 alone ($P < 0.002$).

enon may partially demonstrated that HBx can efficiently block p53-mediated apoptosis in primary human fibroblasts.

HBx Deregulation of Cell Cycle Checkpoint Controls

The HBx protein can deregulate cell cycle checkpoint controls [88]. HBx can also activate the RAS-RAF-mitogen-activated protein (MAP) kinase signaling cascade, through activation of transcription factors AP-1 and NF-κB [55, 59], and stimulate cell DNA synthesis [88]. HBx stimulates cell cycle progression, shortening the emergence of cells from quiescence (G_0) and entry into S phase by at least 12 hours, thereby accelerating transit through the checkpoint controls at the G_0/G_1 and G_2/M phases. Compared with serum stimulation, HBx is found to increase markedly the rate and level of activation of the cyclin-dependent kinases CDK2 and CDC2, and their respective active association with cyclins E and A or cyclin B. HBx overrides or greatly reduces the serum dependence for cell cycle activation. Both HBx and serum are found to require activation of RAS to stimulate cell cycling, but only HBx can shorten the checkpoint internals. HBx therefore stimulates cell proliferation by activating RAS and a second unknown effector, which may be related to its reported ability either to induce prolonged activation of JUN or to interact with cellular p53 protein. These data indicate the presence of a molecular mechanism by which HBx likely con-

tributes to viral carcinogenesis. By deregulating the checkpoint controls, HBx may participate in the selection of cells that are genetically unstable, some of which accumulate as unrepaired oncogenic mutations.

Conclusions

Human HCC, which accounts for more than 90% of primary liver cancers, can progress through inactivation of the *p53* gene (or other tumor suppressor genes) via mutations or interaction with HBx (or both). The *p53* mutations have been observed more frequently in large tumors and in advanced grades of malignancy in human HCCs, indicating that *p53* mutations can be late events in liver carcinogenesis.

Hepatitis B virus is a major risk factor associated with human HCC. HBx, an oncogenic protein encoded by HBV, plays a major role in the development of human HCC. The multiple functions of HBx include (1) transactivation of cellular genes; (2) activation of the PKC pathway and the RAS-RAF-MAP kinase signaling cascade; (3) neoplastic transformation of rodent cells in vitro and, as a transgene, induction of HCC in mice; (4) binding to the tumor-suppressor protein p53 and to the DNA repair protein UV-DDB; (5) inhibition of transactivation or apoptotic functions of p53; (6) deregulation of cell cycle checkpoint controls. The chemical–virus interactions in liver carcinogenesis are providing cancer researchers with a better understanding of the molecular pathogenesis of HCC.

Acknowledgment. The editorial and graphic assistance of Dorothea Dudek is appreciated.

References

1. Di Bisceglie AM, Rustgi VK, Hoofnagle JH, Dusheiko GM, Lotze MT (1988) Hepatocellular carcinoma. Ann Intern Med 108:390–401
2. Feitelson MA (1986) HBV and cancer. In Notkins AL, Oldstone MBA (eds) Concepts in Viral Pathogenesis II. Springer, Berlin Heidelberg New York, pp 269–275
3. Popper H, Shafritz DA, Hoofnagle JH (1987) Relation of hepatitis B virus carrier state to hepatocellular carcinoma. Hepatology 7:764–772
4. Ganem D, Varmus HE (1987) The molecular biology of the hepatitis B viruses. Annu Rev Biochem 56:651–693
5. Wogan WN (1992) Aflatoxins as risk factors for hepatocellular carcinoma in humans. Cancer Res 52:2114s–2118s
6. Harris CC (1990) Hepatocellular carcinogenesis: recent advances and speculation. Cancer Cell 2:146–148
7. Ross RK, Yuan JM, Yu MC, Wogan GN, Qian GS, Tu JT, Groopman, JD, Gao YT, Henderson BE (1992) Urinary aflatoxin biomarkers and risk of hepatocellular carcinoma. Lancet 339:943–946
8. Bishop JM (1991) Molecular themes in oncogenesis. Cell 164:235–248
9. Weinberg RA (1991) Tumor suppressor genes. Science 254:1138–1146
10. Harris CC (1990) Chemical and physical carcinogenesis: advances and perspectives for the 1990s. Cancer Res 51:5023s–5044s
11. Levine AJ, Momand J, Finlay CA (1991) The *p53* tumor suppressor gene. Nature 351:453–456
12. Hollstein M, Sidransky D, Vogelstein B, Harris CC (1991) *p53* mutations in human cancers. Science 253:49–53
13. Greenblatt MS, Bennett WP, Hollstein M, Harris CC (1994) Mutations in the *p53* tumour suppressor gene: clues to cancer etiology and molecular pathogenesis. Cancer Res 54:4855–4878
14. Soussi T, Fromental C, Mary P (1990) Structural aspects of the p53 protein in relation to gene to gene evolution. Oncogene 5:945–952
15. Malkin D, Li F, Strong L, Fraumeni J, Nelson C, Kim D, Kassel J, Gryka M, Biochoff F, Tainsky M, Friend S (1990) Germ line *p53* mutations in a familial syndrome of breast cancer, sarcoma, and other neoplasms. Science 250:1233–1238
16. Lane DP, Benchimol S (1990) *p53*: oncogene or antioncogene. Genes Dev 4:1–8
17. Dittmer D, Patis S, Zambettig, Chus S, Teresdy AK, Moore M, Finlay C, Levine AJ (1993) Gain

of function mutations in *p53*. Nature Genet 4: 42–46
18. Hsiao M, Low J, Dorn E, Ku D, Pattengale P, Yeargin J, Haas M (1994) Gain-of-function mutations of the *p53* gene induce lymphohematopoietic metastatic potential and tissue invasiveness. Am J Pathol 145:702–714
19. Eliyahu D, Michalovitz D, Eliyahu S, Pinhasi-Kimhi O, Oren M (1989) Wild-type *p53* can inhibit oncogene-mediated focus formation. Proc Natl Acad Sci USA 86:8763–8767
20. Finlay CA, Hinds PW, Levine AJ (1989) The *p53* proto-oncogene can act as a suppressor of transformation. Cell 57:1083–1093
21. Baker SJ, Markowitz S, Fearon ER, Willson JK, Vogelstein B (1992) Suppression of human colorectal carcinoma cell growth by wild-type *p53*. Science 249:912–915
22. Diller L, Kassel J, Nelson CE, Grayka MA, Ligwak G, Gebhardt M, Bressac B, Ozturk M, Baker SJ, Vogelstein B (1990) p53 functions as a cell cycle control protein in osteosarcomas. Mol Cell Biol 10:5772–5781
23. Mercer WE, Shields MT, Amin M, Sauve GJ, Appella E, Romano JW, Ullrich SJ (1990) Negative growth regulation in a glioblastoma tumor cell line that conditionally expresses human wild-type *p53*. Proc Natl Acad Sci USA 87:6166–6170
24. Chen PL, Chen Y, Bookstein R, Lee WH (1991) Genetic mechanisms of tumor suppression by the human *p53* gene. Science 250:1576–1580
25. Bressac B, Kew M, Wands J, Ozturk M (1991) Selective G to T mutations of *p53* gene in hepatocellular carcinoma from southern Africa. Nature 350:429–431
26. Hsu IC, Metcalf RA, Sun T, Welsh JA, Wang NJ, Harris CC (1991) Mutational hotspot in the *p53* gene in human hepatocellular carcinomas. Nature 350:427–428
27. Scorsone KA, Zhou YZ, Butel JS, Slagle BL (1992) *p53* Mutations cluster at codon 249 in hepatitis B virus-positive hepatocellular carcinomas from China. Cancer Res 52:1635–1638
28. Li D, Cao Y, He L, Wang NJ, Gu J (1993) Aberrations of *p53* gene in human hepatocellular carcinoma from China. Carcinogenesis 14:169–173
29. Aguilar F, Harris CC, Sun T, Hollstein M, Cerutti P (1994) Geographic variation of *p53* mutational profile in nonmalignant human liver. Science 264:1317–1319
30. Aguilar F, Hussain SP, Cerutti P (1993) Aflatoxin B_1 induces the transversion of G → T in codon 249 of the *p53* tumor suppressor gene in human hepatocytes. Proc Natl Acad Sci USA 90:8586–8590
31. Ponchel F, Puisieux A, Tabone E, Michot JP, Froschl G, Morel AP, Frebourg T, Fontaniere

B, Oberhammer F, Ozturk M (1994) Hepato-carcinoma-specific mutant *p53*-249^ser induces mitotic activity but has no effect on transforming growth factor beta 1-mediated apoptosis. Cancer Res 54:2064–2068

32. Forrester K, Lupold SE, Ott VL, Chay CH, Wang XW, Harris CC (1995) Effects of *p53* mutants on wild-type p53-mediated transactivation are cell type dependent. Oncogene 10:2103–2111

33. Maguire HF, Hoeffler JP, Siddiqui A (1991) HBV X protein alters the DNA binding specificity of CREB and ATF-2 by protein–protein interactions. Science 252:842–844

34. Twu JS, Schloemer RH (1987) Transcriptional transactivating function of hepatitis B virus. J Virol 61:3448–3453

35. Spandau DF, Lee CH (1988) Trans-activation of viral enhancers by the hepatitis B virus X protein. J Virol 62:427–434

36. Shirakata Y, Kawada M, Fujiki Y, Sano H, Oda M, Yagnuma K, Kobayashi M, Koike K (1989) The X gene of hepatitis B virus induced growth stimulation and tumorigenic transformation of mouse NIH3T3 cells. Jpn J Cancer Res 80:617–621

37. Caselmann WH, Meyer M, Kekule AS, Lauer U, Hofschneider PH, Koshy R (1990) A trans-activator function is generated by integration of hepatitis B virus preS/S sequences in human hepatocellular carcinoma DNA. Proc Natl Acad Sci USA 87:2970–2974

38. Kekule AS, Lauer U, Meyer M, Caselmann WH, Hofschnelder PH, Koshy R (1990) The preS2/S region of integrated hepatitis B virus DNA encodes a transcriptional transactivator. Nature 343:457–461

39. Benn J, Schneider RJ (1994) Hepatitis B virus HBx protein activates Ras–GTP complex formation and establishes a Ras, Raf, MAP kinase signaling cascade. Proc Natl Acad Sci USA 91:10350–10354

40. Unsal H, Yakicier C, Marcais C, Kew M, Volkmann M, Zentgraf H, Isselbacher KJ, Ozturk M (1994) Genetic heterogeneity of hepatocellular carcinoma. Proc Natl Acad Sci USA 91:822–826

41. Paterlini P, Poussin K, Kew M, Franco D, Brechot C (1995) Selective accumulation of the X transcript of hepatitis B virus in patients negative for hepatitis B surface antigen with hepatocellular carcinoma. Hepatology 21:313–321

42. Feitelson MA, Zhu M, Duan LX, London WT (1993) Hepatitis B X antigen and p53 are associated in vitro and in liver tissues from patients with primary hepatocellular carcinoma. Oncogene 8:1109–1117

43. Wang XW, Forrester K, Yeh H, Feitelson MA, Gu JR, Harris CC (1994) Hepatitis B virus X protein inhibits p53 sequence-specific DNA binding transcriptional activity and association with transcription factor ERCC3. Proc Natl Acad Sci USA 91:2230–2234

44. Ueda H, Ullrich SJ, Gangemi JD, Kappel CA, Ngo L, Feitelson MA, Jay G (1995) Functional inactivation but not structural mutation of *p53* causes liver cancer. Nature Genet 9:41–47

45. Wang XW, Gibson MK, Vermeulen W, Yeh H, Forrester K, Sturzbacher H-W, Hoeijmakers JHJ, Harris CC (1995) Abrogation of p53-induced apoptosis by the hepatitis B virus X gene. Cancer Res 55:6012–6016

46. Hino O, Nomura K, Ohtake K, Kawaguchi T, Sugano H, Kitagawa T (1989) Instability of integrated hepatitis B virus DNA with inverted repeat structure in a transgenic mouse. Cancer Genet Cytogenet 37:273–278

47. Hino O, Tabata S, Hotta Y (1991) Evidence for increased in vitro recombination with insertion of human hepatitis B virus DNA. Proc Natl Acad Sci USA 88:9248–9252

48. Tiollais P, Pourcel C, Dejean A (1985) The hepatitis B virus. Nature 317:489–495

49. Moriarty AM, Alexander H, Lerner RA, Thornton GB (1985) Antibodies to peptides detect new hepatitis B antigen: serological correlation with hepatocellular carcinoma. Science 227:429–432

50. Kim C, Koike K, Saito L, Miyamura T, Jay G (1991) HBx gene of hepatitis B virus induces liver cancer in transgenic mice. Nature 351:317–320

51. Matsubara K, Tokino T (1990) Integrating of hepatitis B virus DNA and its implications for hepatocarcinogenesis. Mol Biol Med 7:243–260

52. Seto E, Mitchell PJ, Yen TSB (1990) Transactivation by the hepatitis B virus X protein depends on AP-2 and other transcription factors. Nature 344:72–74

53. Twu J-S, Lai M-Y, Chen D-S, Robinson WS (1993) Activation of protooncogene c-*jun* by the X protein of hepatitis B virus. Virology 192:346–450

54. Kekule AS, Lauer U, Weiss L, Luber B, Hofschneider PH (1993) Hepatitis B virus transactivator HBx uses a tumour promoter signaling pathway. Nature 361:742–745

55. Natoli G, Avantaggiati ML, Chirillo P, Costanzo A, Artini M, Balsano C, Levero M (1994) Induction of the DNA-binding activity of c-*jun*/c-*fos* heterodimers by the hepatitis B virus transactivator pX. Mol Cell Biol 14:989–998

56. Seto E, Yen TSB, Peterlin BM, Ou J-H (1988) Trans-activation of the human immunodeficiency virus long terminal repeat by the hepatitis B virus X protein. Proc Natl Acad Sci USA 85:8286–8290

57. Twu J-S, Wu JY, Robinson WS (1990) Transcription activation of the human immunodeficiency virus type 1 long terminal repeat by hepatitis B virus X-protein requires de novo protein synthesis. Virology 177:406–410

58. Levrero M, Balsano C, Natoli G, Avantaggiati ML, Elfassi E (1990) Hepatitis B virus X protein transactivates the long terminal repeats of human immunodeficiency virus type 1 and 2. J Virol 64:3082–3086

59. Lucito R, Schneider RJ (1992) Hepatitis B virus X protein activates transcription factor NF-κB without a requirement for protein kinase C. J Virol 66:983–991

60. Aufiero B, Schneider RJ (1990) The hepatitis B virus X-gene product trans-activates both RNA polymerase II and III promoters. EMBO J 9:497–504

61. Doria M, Klein N, Lucito R, Schneider RJ (1995) The hepatitis B virus HBx protein is a dual specificity cytoplasmic activator of Ras and nuclear activator of transcription factors. EMBO J 14:4747–4757

62. Haviv I, Vaizel D, Shaul Y (1995) The X protein of hepatitis B virus coactivates potent activation domains. Mol Cell Biol 15:1079–1086

63. Maguire HF, Hoeffler JP, Siddiqui A (1991) HBV X protein alters the DNA binding specificity of CREB and ATF-2 by protein–protein interactions. Science 252:842–844

64. Williams JS, Andrisani OM (1995) The hepatitis B virus X protein targets the basic region-leucine zipper domain of CREB. Proc Natl Acad Sci USA 92:3819–3823

65. Kern SE, Kinzler KW, Bruskin A, Jarosz D, Friedman P, Prives C, Vogelstein B (1991) Identification of p53 as a sequence-specific DNA-binding protein. Science 252:1708–1711

66. Qadri I, Maguire HF, Siddiqui A (1995) Hepatitis B virus transactivator protein X interacts with the TATA-binding protein. Proc Natl Acad Sci USA 92:1003–1007

67. El-Deiry WS, Tokino T, Velculescu VE, Levy DB, Parsons R, Trent JM, Lin D, Mercer WE, Kinzler KW, Vogelstein B (1993) WAF1, a potential mediator of p53 tumor suppression. Cell 75:817–825

68. Harper JW, Adami GR, Wei N, Keyomarisi K, Elledge SJ (1993) The p21 cdk-interacting protein Cip1 is a potent inhibitor of G1 cyclin-dependent kinases. Cell 75:805–816

69. Kern SE, Pietenpol JA, Thiagalingam S, Seymour A, Kinzler KW, Vogelstein B (1992) Oncogenic forms of p53 inhibit p53-regulated gene expression. Science 256:827–830

70. Cross JC, Wen P, Rutter WJ (1993) Transactivation by hepatitis B virus X protein is promiscuous and dependent on mitogen activated cellular serine/threonine kinase. Proc Natl Acad Sci USA 90:8078–8082

71. Schaeffer L, Roy R, Humbert S, Moncollin V, Vermeulen W, Hoeijmakers JH, Chambon P, Egly JM (1993) DNA repair helicase: a component of BTF2 (TFIIH) basic transcription factor. Science 260:58–63

72. Lee TH, Elledge SJ, Butel JS (1995) Hepatitis B virus X protein interacts with a probable cellular DNA repair protein. J Virol 69:1107–1114

73. Lane DP (1992) Cancer: *p53*, guardian of the genome. Nature 358:15–16

74. Lane DP, Crawford LV (1979) T antigen is bound to a host protein in SV40-transformed cells. Nature 278:261–263

75. Linzer DI, Levine AJ (1979) Characterization of a 54 K dalton cellular SV40 tumor antigen present in SV40-transformed cells and uninfected embryonal carcinoma cells. Cell 17:43–52

76. Werness BA, Levine AJ, Howley PM (1990) Association of human papillomavirus types 16 and 18 E6 proteins with *p53*. Science 248:76–79

77. Szekely L, Selivanova G, Magnusson KP, Klein G, Wiman KG (1993) EBNA-5, an Epstein-Barr virus-encoded nuclear antigen, binds to the retinoblastoma and p53 proteins. Proc Natl Acad Sci USA 90:5455–5459

78. Speir E, Modali R, Huang ES, Leon MB, Shawl F, Finkel T, Epstein SE (1994) Potential role of human cytomegalovirus and p53 interaction in coronary restenosis. Science 265:391–394

79. McCarthy SA, Symonds HS, Van Dyke T (1994) Regulation of apoptosis in transgenic mice by simian virus 40 T antigen-mediated inactivation of p53. Proc Natl Acad Sci USA 91:3979–3983

80. Debbas M, White E (1993) Wild-type *p53* mediates apoptosis by E1A, which is inhibited by E1B. Genes Dev 7:546–554

81. Wyllie AH (1994) Apoptosis: death gets a brake. Nature 369:272–273

82. Kerr JF, Wyllie AH, Currie AR (1972) Apoptosis: a basic biological phenomenon with wide-ranging implications in tissue kinetics. Br J Cancer 26:239–257

83. Lowe SW, Schmitt EM, Smith SW, Osborne BA, Jacks T (1993) p53 is required for radiation-induced apoptosis in mouse thymocytes. Nature 362:847–849

84. Clarke AR, Puridie CA, Harrison, Morris RG, Bird CC, Hooper ML, Wyllie AH (1993) Thymocyte apoptosis induced by p53-dependent and independent pathways. Nature 362:849–852

85. Lowe SW, Ruley HE, Jacks T, Housman DE (1992) p53-dependent apoptosis modulates the cytotoxicity of anticancer agents. Cell 74:957–967

218   L. Jia et al.

86. Symonds H, Krall L, Remington L, Saenz-Robles M, Lowe S, Jacks T, Van Dyke T (1994) p53-dependent apoptosis suppresses tumor growth and progression in vivo. Cell 78:703–711
87. Lowe SW, Bodis S, McClatchey A, Remington L, Ruley HE, Fisher DE, Housman DE, Jacks T (1994) p53 status and the efficacy of cancer therapy in vivo. Science 266:807–810
88. Benn J, Schneider RJ (1995) Hepatitis B virus HBx protein deregulates cell cycle checkpoint controls. Proc Natl Acad Sci USA 92:11215–11219

Molecular Genetics of Hepatocellular Carcinoma

Christopher J. Bakkenist and James O'D. McGee

Summary. The major exogenous agents underlying hepatocellular carcinoma have been identified and characterized in detail. These agents, which include hepatitis viruses and cirrhosis, function primarily as mitogens causing hepatocellular hyperplasia. Disorderly hepatocyte hyperplasia with concurrent mutagenesis may give rise to hepatocellular carcinoma. Little progress has been made in identifying either the somatic or germline mutations underlying the development of hepatocellular carcinoma. As such, the molecular genetics of hepatocellular carcinoma are not well understood. Hepatocyte mutagens include endogenous oxygen free radicals and H_2O_2, which may diffuse out of mitochondria and peroxisomes. Hepatocytes are also the location of cytochrome p450s, which catalase more than 60 different types of reaction concerned with the metabolism of steroids and fatty acids involved in hormone regulation and the metabolism of exogenous dietary-derived compounds. Hepatocyte microsomes are therefore the site of metabolic activation of many procarcinogens. Taken together, these reactions place the hepatocyte genome in a highly mutagenic environment. Hyperplasia greatly increases the rate at which mutations accumulate because the time for DNA repair is reduced, DNA replication has an intrinsic error, and cell division can result in rearrangements of the genome. However, no single tumor suppressor gene has been found to be preferentially inactivated or oncogene to be preferentially activated in hepatocellular carcinoma. The identified germline mutations predisposing to hepatocellular hyperplasia generally either increase hyperplasia (e.g., MHC) or the amount of endogenous mutagens produced in the hepatocyte (e.g., p450). Taken together, these data suggest that rather than being a genetic disease, hepatocellular carcinoma is a disease of a "chronically afflicted genome."

Introduction

The hepatocyte is a differentiated cell that only rarely divides under normal conditions but retains a unique capacity for restoration of hepatic mass after injury resulting from a wide range of insults, such as chemical or viral damage or surgical resection. It is one of the fundamental responses of the liver to injury and means that extensive loss of liver cells can be compensated by hyperplasia. Hepatocyte numbers are increased through the division of existing adult cells rather than by stem cell proliferation; as such, if the structural integrity of the liver is damaged during liver cell injury, regeneration may be disorderly. As a result, although the liver cell mass may return to normal the architectural relations are not restored and the regeneration is nodular and cirrhotic. Disorderly hepatocyte hyperplasia in a mutagenic environment may also give rise to hepatocellular carcinoma (HCC).

Hepatocellular carcinoma has an estimated annual incidence of 250000 to 1.2 million cases worldwide [1]. It is the seventh most common cancer in men and ninth most common in women. HCC is an aggressive malignancy that carries a poor prognosis, with a median survival of less than 8 months without treatment [2]. Only the early diagnosis of isolated small tumors without vascular involvement or metastases allows an opportunity for cure through hepatic resection or transplantation.

Although considerable progress has been made in understanding the somatic mutations that accumulate during the development of several neoplasias (most notably colorectal carcinogenesis), and familial germline mutations have

Nuffield Department of Pathology and Bacteriology, Oxford University, John Radcliffe Hospital, Headington, Oxford OX3 9DU, UK

been identified that make individuals susceptible to certain neoplasia, progress has been slower in identifying mutations involved in HCC. In contrast, the major exogenous etiological agents responsible for HCC have been identified and molecularly characterized in some detail. It would be a considerable advance, however, if the likelihood of an individual developing HCC following exposure to the major exogenous risk factors, particularly infection with a hepatitis virus or development of cirrhosis, could be assessed. In this chapter the literature describing the molecular basis of human hepatocellular carcinogenesis is reviewed and the relevance of several murine models of HCC to the human disease assessed.

Epidemiology and Etiology

The incidence of HCC shows striking geographical and racial variation. The disease is rare in the developed countries of northern Europe and the United States, with 3 cases presenting per 100 000 male inhabitants each year; in coastal areas of China, Southeast Asia, and sub-Saharan Africa, however, 20 to 30 new cases per 100 000 male inhabitants are reported annually [3]. In Italy, Romania, Spain, France, and Poland there is an intermediate incidence of 6 new cases presenting per 100 000 male inhabitants each year. In all these countries, however, there is considerable internal variation in the incidence of the disease. Although it is likely that the divergent indigenous populations of Africa, Asia, and Europe have different inherent susceptibilities to the initiation and promotion of HCC, the genetic bases of this susceptibility have not been characterized.

Infection with hepatitis B virus (HBV) or hepatitis C virus (HCV), cirrhosis, and exposure to aflatoxin B_1 are the greatest risk factors for HCC development [4]. Male sex and, in Western countries, advancing age are also considered to be risk factors, as are alcohol ingestion, smoking, highdose anabolic steroids, and genetic diseases such as hemochromatosis, α_1-antitrypsin deficiency, tyrosinemia, or porphyria cutanea tarda, and possibly oral contraceptives [3]. Even though HBV and HCV infect less than 1% of the U.S. population, hepatitis infection accounts for half of the HCC cases in the United States among non-Asians and even more among Asians [5, 6]. This finding demonstrates the pronounced asso-

ciation between hepatitis B and C infections with HCC.

The incidence of HCC is increasing among males in the United States, Canada, northern Europe, and Japan; in contrast, it is decreasing in populations where it has been high, such as in black men in parts of southern Africa [7, 8]. The incidence of HCC nearly doubled between 1983 and 1993 in Japan, with HCV implicated as the etiological agent responsible for this increase on epidemiological grounds [9].

Hepatitis B Virus

The HBV is spread principally by exposure to blood or blood products and by unprotected sex. HBV infection acquired during adult life is not always clinically apparent, and most acutely infected adults recover completely from the disease and clear the virus. Up to 5% of patients infected during adult life, however, have persistent infection and develop chronic liver disease of varying severity [10]. In contrast, neonatally transmitted HBV infection is rarely cleared, and more than 90% of such children become chronically infected. Vertical transmission of HBV is common in highly populated areas of Africa and Asia, and as a result several hundred million people are persistently infected with the virus. These individuals have chronic liver disease for much of their lives and have a greatly increased risk of developing cirrhosis and HCC at a relatively young age. As a result, up to 98% of HCC cases have been identified as HBV-positive in Taiwan, and the incidence of HCC has been reported as high as 473 cases per 100 000 HBV-infected male individuals; in comparison the incidence in the HBV-negative population was 5 cases per 100 000 individuals [11]. The lifetime risk of HCC in males infected at birth with HBV approaches 40% [12]. In contrast, in Japan, where the neonatal transmission of HBV is rare, the risk of developing HCC in patients suffering from chronic HBV infection is increased sevenfold [9].

Hepatitis C Virus

During the early 1970s more than 40% of Japanese cases of HCC were HBV-positive, but during the 1980s HBV was responsible for fewer than 20% of all HCC cases in Japan. This decrease resulted from the increase in incidence of non-A, non-B hepatitis-associated HCC [13]. Following its discovery, HCV was rapidly implicated as the etiological agent responsible for HCC in these individuals [14, 15]. Subsequent studies have demonstrated that the positivity rates for HCV among HCC patients are as high as 94% in Japan [16], 75% in Spain [17], and 65% in Italy [18]. Japanese patients with HCV have a fourfold increased risk of developing HCC, and because HCV infection is three to four times more common in Japanese patients with chronic liver disease than HBV, HCV is the major cause of HCC in Japan [9]. The incidence of HCV infection in patients with HCC in the United States is lower, at 53% [19].

In areas where HBV infection is high and most HCC patients are HBV-positive, HCV positivity is low. It has been reported at 29% in southern Africa [20] and 33% in Thailand [21]. This low positivity corresponds to a low additional risk factor for HCC development as a result of HCV infection—1.3 in Thailand [22] and 1.1 in Mozambique [23]—reflecting the prevalence of other risk factors in these areas.

Approximately 50% of individuals infected with HCV develop persistent chronic active hepatitis; and although the remainder display no symptoms, biopsies have shown that none has normal hepatocellular histopathology. Although chronic active hepatitis C infection in itself is not fatal, 20% of such individuals develop HCC over a period of 20 to 40 years following HCV infection [24]. The disease progresses from acute to chronic hepatitis/cirrhosis and finally HCC during this period. Clinicopathological evidence clearly demonstrates that chronic HCV infection is a major cause of HCC development worldwide.

Cirrhosis

Hepatocellular carcinoma is a frequent complication of cirrhosis, and the frequent coexistence of cirrhosis and HCC suggests that cirrhosis plays a role in the pathogenesis of HCC [25]. Cirrhosis is characterized by diffuse fibrosis (i.e., fibrosis involving the whole liver), which results in the normal lobular architecture of the liver being converted to structurally abnormal nodules. In Western countries and Japan where cirrhosis is considerably more common than HCC, patients with HCC have background cirrhosis in up to 90% of cases regardless of the etiology [26, 27]. Similarly, 30% to 40% of Japanese patients who die

from cirrhosis have HCC at autopsy [28]. Sequential ultrasound studies of patients with cirrhosis have clearly established that the natural history of HCC (in many instances) is that the HCC develops in underlying cirrhotic nodules [29].

In a cohort study of patients with a diagnosis of alcoholism, liver cirrhosis, or both, it was found that alcoholism alone carried a moderately increased risk of HCC, and liver cirrhosis due to alcoholism did not increase the risk over that due to cirrhosis alone [30]. Similar risks for HCC have been found in Japanese patients, suggesting that alcohol may be a liver "carcinogen" because it is causally involved in the development of cirrhosis (see below) [9]. This implication is supported by the observation that ethanol acts as a promoter in rodent HCC but not as an initiator [31]. The incidence for HCC in association with alcoholic cirrhosis is 5% to 15% [32], whereas the incidence for HCC in those with HBV infection is 23% to 40%, clearly demonstrating that the development of HCC from cirrhosis is influenced by additional factors [33]. Cigarette smoking has been causally related to the development of HCC from cirrhosis [34]. This relation is probably due to the fact that the liver is the natural site of activation and detoxification of many of the potential carcinogens in tobacco.

In most parts of the world HCC is rare, whereas symptomatic cirrhosis is far more common, but in sub-Saharan Africa and in some parts of the far East symptomatic HCC occurs commonly and may precede symptomatic evidence of cirrhosis. In a study of 463 South African black men with HCC, only 63% were found to have cirrhosis at autopsy, which demonstrates that HCC does not always arise in a cirrhotic background [35]. However, the type and etiology of both the cirrhosis and HCC that coexist or occur separately has not been adequately studied for any mechanistic conclusions to be drawn from these findings.

Aflatoxin B₁

The fungal toxin aflatoxin B_1, produced by strains of *Aspergillus flavus*, is found in moldy peanut and corn products. Humans exposed to contaminated foodstuffs have a higher incidence of HCC [36]. Aflatoxin B_1 is metabolized by the P-450 system to produce metabolites that can form adducts with nucleoside bases and as such are potent mutagens. Aflatoxin B_1 exposure is greatest in southern Africa, particularly Mozambique, and in Qidong, China. Its mutagenic properties and chronic hepatitis (e.g., HBV-induced) interact in an additive manner in the development of HCC in areas where exposure to the chemical is high.

Mechanism of Hepatocellular Carcinoma Development

Carcinogenesis is now generally considered to be a "multihit" process involving the progressive accumulation of somatic mutations, which result in the activation of oncogenes or inactivation of genes that exert negative regulatory control on cell division (tumor-suppressor genes). Three steps are proposed to result in the development of a malignant tumor: initiation, promotion, and progression (Fig. 1) [37]. Measurements of the age-dependent HCC incidence in rats indicate kinetics dependent on the fifth or sixth power of elapsed time, suggesting that these three steps require five or six mutations [38]. The development of these mutations is dependent on both exposure to mutagens and the rate of cell division.

The initiation step involves an irreversible genetic change that occurs in cells either "spontaneously" or upon exposure to chemical and physical agents. Promotion selectively expands the number of initiated cells and is considered to be reversible. The final stage of tumor development/progression, entails the accumulation of additional genetic lesions that result, among other things, in the activation of oncogenes and the inactivation of tumor-suppressor genes. Because an irreversible genetic alteration is required for initiation, an additional earlier step of induced cell division may be another mechanism in HCC development.

Exposure to Mutagens

It is becoming increasingly apparent that mutations that result in promotion frequently result in the attenuation or loss of genes that protect DNA from damage and promote DNA repair and genes involved in cell cycle checkpoints that maintain the normal chromosome complement. The major cause of a DNA lesion is frequently thought to be exposure to exogenous chemicals or loss of the process of DNA replication. Lesions resulting from endogenous chemicals however, particularly

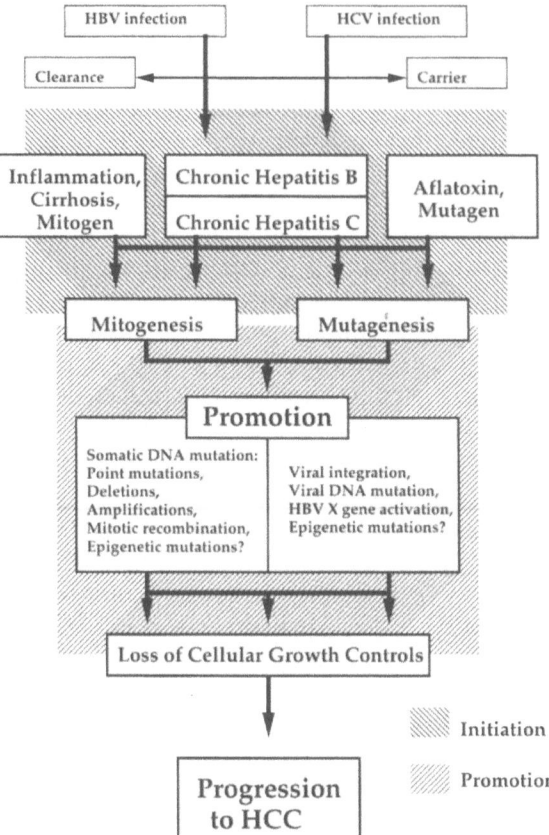

Fig. 1. Summary of the mechanisms underlying hepatocellular carcinoma (*HCC*) development. The initiation event is considered to involve an irreversible genetic change. Promotion selectively expands the number of initiated cells

oxygen free radicals, have been estimated to occur 10^5 times per cell per day in rats and 10^4 times per cell per day in humans [39]. Protons derived from oxygen reduction cycles and oxygen free radicals diffusing out of mitochondria or ethoxy compounds coming from oxidized lipids represent examples of metabolites produced by internal biochemical reactions that can damage DNA. It should be noted that mitochondria are particularly numerous in hepatocytes, occupying about 18% of cell volume with about 800 per cell. Peroxisomes are also abundant in mice and occupy about 1% of the cytoplasmic volume of a hepatocyte. Peroxisomal respiration accounts for about 20% of the oxygen consumption in the liver and generates hydrogen peroxide (H_2O_2), which in turn is degraded by the enzyme catalase in a process that may release oxygen free radicals.

The liver is a major location of cytochrome P-450, which catalyzes more than 60 reactions, including aromatic and aliphatic hydroxylations, N- and S-oxidations, epoxidations, and dealkylations. These reactions are concerned with the metabolism of steroids and fatty acids involved in hormone regulation and the metabolism of exogenous dietary-derived compounds. As such, liver microsomes are the site of metabolic activation of many procarcinogens. These reactions are also "oxygen activating" and involve microsomal electron transport between flavoprotein, NADPH cytochrome P-450 reductase, and cytochrome P-450.

Taken together, the oxygen free radicals leaking from mitochondria, the H_2O_2 produced by peroxisomal respiration, and the highly reactive carcinogens produced as metabolites by the P-450s from exogenous compounds place the hepatocyte genome in a highly mutagenic environment. There are, however, elaborate defense mechanisms to protect the genome. The inducible enzyme glutathione transferase guards against oxygen free radicals, and catalase protects against H_2O_2. In addition, any lesions produced by these mutagens (the base damage resulting from oxidation, addition of metabolites of absorbed chemicals to bases to form adducts, or strand breaks) are normally repaired by the DNA repair apparatus or in the worst cases recognized as terminal by cell cycle checkpoints that subsequently trigger apoptosis. As such most of the lesions never become mutations (Fig. 2).

Role of Mitogenesis

For a lesion to become a mutation (point mutation, deletion, chromosome break, or translocation) the cell containing the lesion must replicate its DNA and divide before the lesion is repaired (Fig. 3). The probability of a lesion becoming a mutation depends on the efficiency of the DNA repair machinery and the rate of cell division, which is influenced by hormones, growth factors, cytotoxicity, inflammation, and so on. If there is an increased rate of cell division, there is an increased risk of mutation and thus cancer. Furthermore, it has been suggested that it may be impossible for many exogenous chemicals to increase the number of mutations significantly in the absence of increased mitogenesis [39].

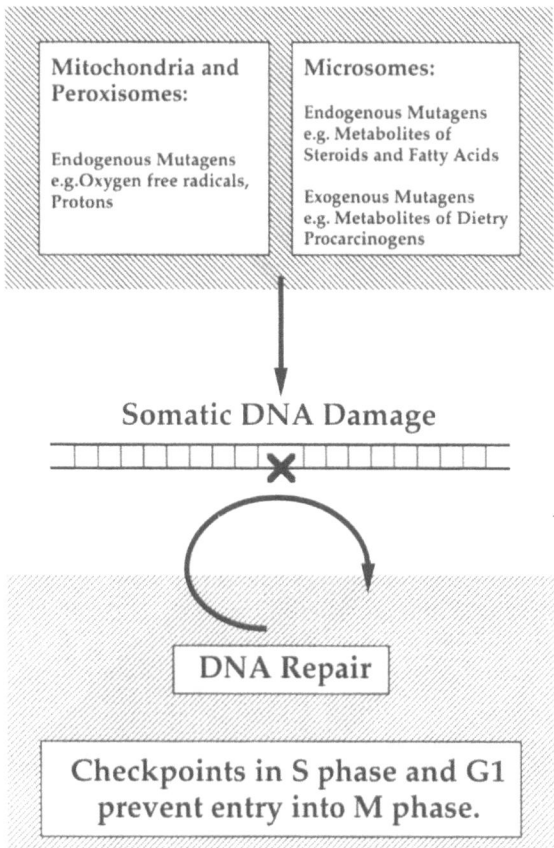

Fig. 2. Although the hepatocyte genome is exposed to many mitogens, its structure is maintained by the DNA repair machinery. Cell cycle check-points may also prevent progression to M phase if DNA damage is detected

Mitogenesis increases the rate of mutations in many ways.

– When cells are proliferating there is less time for the DNA repair machinery and the cell cycle checkpoints to repair lesions before they are converted to stalling points for DNA polymerases and ultimately gaps in the replicated DNA. These gaps must be repaired by the DNA replication repair pathways, some of which are error-free and some of which are error-prone. Those that do not efficiently repair DNA cause point mutations, double-stranded point deletions, or double-stranded breaks.

– In addition, the DNA polymerases have an intrinsic error frequency subjected to the same repair pathways. When a base is incorrectly in-

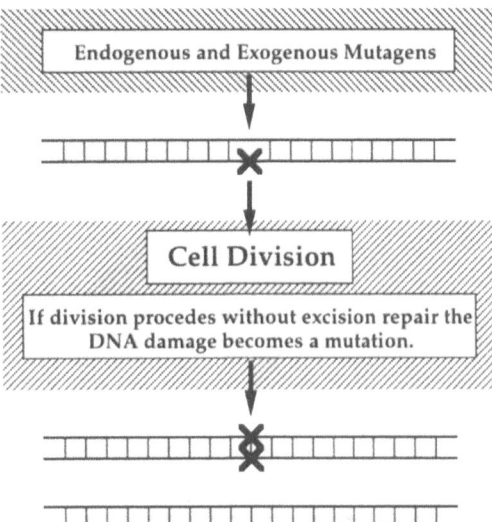

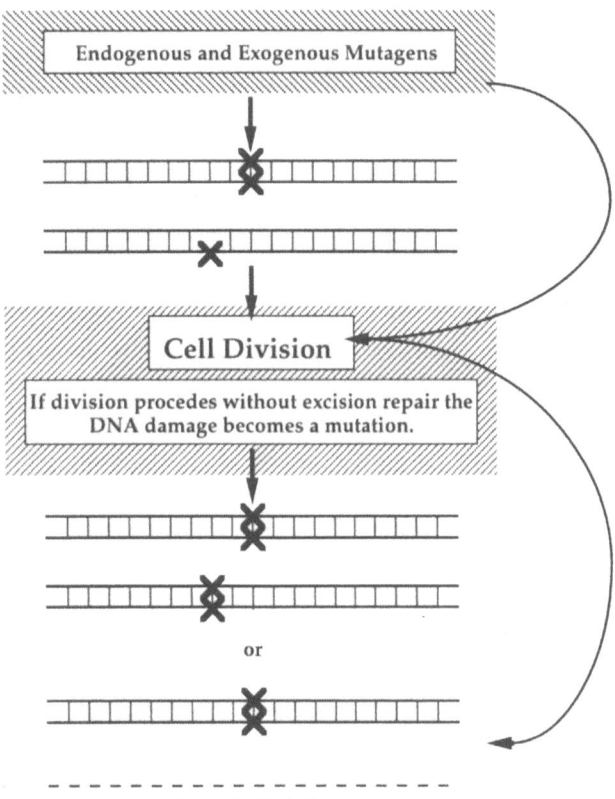

Fig. 3. Mitogenesis (induced cell division) is a multiplier of endogenous (or exogenous) DNA damage, leading to mutation. The pathway to inactivating both copies of a recessive tumor-suppressor gene is shown

serted it is recognized as the newly replicated strand by the repair apparatus because it is not methylated.
- Single-stranded DNA without base pairing or histones is the template for DNA replication. It is intrinsically more sensitive to damage than double-stranded DNA.

- Cell division can result in mitotic recombination, nondisjunction, and gene conversion, which can convert a heterologous recessive gene (tumor suppressor) to homozygosity or hemizygosity. This situation is particularly likely if a DNA polmerase has stalled at a base lesion.

- Cell division allows gene duplication, which can increase the expression of otherwise poorly expressed oncogenes.
- 5-Methylcytosine can be lost during DNA replication, which can reverse differentiation [40].
- Because all DNA polymerases replicate DNA in the 5′-3′ direction, initiated by an RNA primer, there is always a fragment at the 5′ end of each single-stranded chromosome template that cannot be replicated because primer synthesis does not occur at the absolute end of the chromosome. Thus chromosomes are shortened by approximately 50 basepairs (bp) every cell division.
- Cell division also increases the expression of some oncogenes.

Hepatocellular Hyperplasia

A valuable experimental model of hepatocyte hyperplasia is the rat liver following partial hepatectomy. It shows the changes in gene expression that follow any liver damage that results in hepatocyte division.

Regrowth of rat liver after a 70% hepatectomy occurs within 7 to 10 days [41]. The residual lobes grow until they are the same size and volume as the original liver, after which cell division ceases abruptly. If the liver is too large, some cells enter apoptosis, and its size is reduced until it is the same as that of the original liver. Peak DNA synthesis occurs 24 h after resection, and approximately 35% of the hepatocytes are dividing at this point. Mitosis follows after 6 to 8 h, and during the course of liver regeneration 95% of the hepatocytes divide at least once in a young rat. In an older rat liver regeneration proceeds more slowly, involves the division of fewer hepatocytes, and is apt to be less successful.

No single mediator has been identified as solely responsible for the passage of hepatocytes from G_0 to G_1. Instead, the interplay of several pathways and many diverse growth factors are involved. The growth factors include mitogens, which are defined as compounds able to sustain the S-phase and M-phase in hepatocytes growing in serum-free media; they include hepatocyte growth ("scatter") factor, epidermal growth factor (EGF), and transforming growth factor-α (TGF-α). Co-mitogens are defined as compounds that are unable to sustain hepatocytes in serum-free

medium per se but can stimulate the cells in the presence of mitogens. Co-mitogens include hormones such as insulin and the insuin-like growth factors. In contrast to the mitogens and co-mitogens, hepatotrophic agents such as TGF-β and certain interleukins generally inhibitory to hepatocyte division are also expressed [42]. TGF-β, which is generally considered to be a negative regulator of cell division, is abundant in HCC.

Within minutes of partial hepatectomy or toxic injury, hepatocytes exhibit changes in membrane polarization, ion fluxes, intracellular pH, post-translational modification of transcription factors, activation of immediate-early genes (those that are activated independent of protein synthesis, in contrast to delayed-early genes, which are dependent on protein synthesis), and many other processes involved in priming hepatocellular division [43]. More than 70 genes have been found to be induced in the immediate-early response to hepatectomy, and it is assumed that they are all involved in the initiation and promotion of liver regeneration. Of these, several are proto-oncogenes implicated in carcinogenesis, and at least 41 are novel [44]. Steady-state levels of the proto-oncogenes c-*fos* and c-*jun* increase almost immediately following hepatectomy in the rat and return to basal levels after 2 h [45]. Levels of c-*myc* increase more slowly to a maximum at 2 to 4 h and then decline to basal levels after 6 h [45]. The expression of these genes is critical for regulation of cell growth and proliferation and must be highly regulated and specific. Steady-state levels of other proto-oncogenes, such as c-*mos*, c-*abl*, and c-*src*, are not changed during liver regeration. The insulin-like growth factor (IGF)-binding protein is also induced during the immediate-early response, as are members of the *ras* gene family. Differential expression of G proteins and accumulation of cyclic adenosine monophosphate (cAMP) in the regenerating liver result from growth factor interactions almost immediately after partial hepatectomy [46].

Whether these growth factors affect the activation of cyclins, tumor-suppressor genes, other growth factors, and members of the proto-oncogene families is unknown. It is worth noting that the receptor for hepatocyte growth factor is the c-*met* proto-oncogene product [47]. The list of immediate-early genes includes proteins as diverse as growth factors, transcription factors, and unique nuclear tyrosine phosphatases, which interact to release heptocytes from growth arrest and allow them to proceed through the cell cycle. The mechanisms underlying the restoration of G_0 once the liver has been regenerated are completely unknown.

This ability of hepatocytes to divide in response to many injuries presents many pathways that viruses can exploit and disrupt for their own propagation. It also presents myriad actively expressed oncogenes and tumor-suppressor genes whose mutation could result in HCC promotion.

Hepatitis B Virus

Hepatitis B virus is a circular double-stranded DNA virus that causes acute and chronic necroinflammatory liver disease. It encodes the various forms of the viral envelope proteins, the transactivating protein encoded by the HBV X gene, and the viral polymerase. HBV is not directly cytopathic for the hepatocyte; rather, the associated liver diseases are the result of an immune response to viral antigens expressed by the infected hepatocytes. HBV-induced HCC could result through a variety of mechanisms.

- Integration of the virus into the host genome could lead to direct disruption of cell cycle regulatory genes (epigenetic mutation is also possible as a result of integration).
- Random deregulation of cell cycle regulatory genes by genetic mutation (and epigenetic mutation) could result from increased mitogenesis and the mutagenic environment of the chronically inflamed liver caused by chronic hepatitis. Mitogenesis and therefore mutagenesis would be increased further if the patient developed cirrhosis.
- The altered hormone and growth factor expression resulting from increased hepatocellular division and inflammation could result in secondary immune responses, which could further increase the mutagenic environment of the liver.
- The transcriptional deregulation of cell cycle regulatory genes could be caused by the *trans*-activating viral protein HBV X protein, which could be deregulated itself following viral integration into the host genome. The HBV X protein could also bind to cellular proteins, disrupting their normal function.
- HBV replicating during S phase may increase genetic instability in the host genome.

These mechanisms have been investigated in HBV-infected patients and monkeys and in the HBV-related hepadnavirus infections of the outbred species of woodchuck, ground squirrel, and Pekin duck. More recently transgenic mouse strains have been developed, into which partial or complete copies of the HBV genome have been incorporated. Experimental models are discussed below and human comparisons drawn, as the experimental models are better characterized.

Woodchuck Hepatitis Virus

Captive woodchucks infected with woodchuck hepatitis virus (WHV) at birth develop HCC after 17 to 36 months of persistent infection in 97% of cases; WHV infection starting during adult life carries a far lower risk of HCC development [48, 49]. This pattern of HCC development after WHV infection is somewhat analogous to the HCC incidence and HBV infection in humans. Hepatogenesis in this animal does not require cirrhosis or external carcinogenic factors, as HCC has been shown to develop in all woodchucks raised and infected in the controlled environment of the laboratory. Integrated WHV genomes are found in most cases of HCC developing in woodchucks infected at birth or while young, as is the case with human patients with chronic HBV infection [50]. Integration of WHV (which also occurs in a large fraction of carrier woodchucks) causes deletions of the host genome, translocations, and inversions of host chromosomes [4]. Integration of WHV into *c-myc* (33%) and *N-myc* (20%) with concurrent activation of 5- to 50-fold has been demonstrated, but the insertion is generally regarded as random [51].

Significant changes in expression of insulin-like growth factor-II (IGF-II) in the precancerous WHV liver have been observed and related to precancerous nodules [52]. This point may be of particular relevance, as the M6P/IGF-II receptor is deleted in a considerable number of human HCCs [53].

Integration of HBV into the human cyclin A gene (chromosome 4q) and the retinoic acid receptor has been reported, but integration is generally thought to be random [54, 55]. Integration may be preferentially located at fragile sites [56]. HBV integrations that cause rearrangements in both viral and flanking sequences have been reported, particularly in chromosome 11p [57]. This finding may be of some consequence, as deletions of this chromosome have been found in a sizable number of HCCs. In many cases multiple copies of the HBV genome are found, and most HCC cells have been found to be monoclonal. A number of studies have demonstrated activated oncogenes dominantly expressed in HBV-infected HCC, including *hst*, *lca*, *ras* family members, *raf*, and *hhc* [4]. However, no predominant transforming oncogene and no common chromosomal abnormality have been identified.

Integration events leading to the direct activation of oncogenes and inactivation of tumor-suppressor genes therefore seem to be rare in both woodchucks and humans. Work with transgenic models points to other mechanisms.

Transgenic Mouse Models of HBV Infection

Transgenic mouse strains have been constructed containing only HBV-derived regulatory sequences that express all of the viral gene products and replicate the virus in the hepatocyte. They are excellent models for dissecting the human disease. Such mouse strains have demonstrated that viral gene expression is developmentally regulated [58] and is positively regulated by androgens and glucocorticoids, suggesting a reason why HCC occurs predominantly in human males [59, 60]. The expression of most HBV gene products and the process of viral replication has generally been shown not to be cytotoxic for the hepatocyte. Abnormal expression of two viral gene products, the large envelope protein and the HBV X protein, can result in HCC (Fig. 4).

The pathological potential of the cellular immune response to HBV has been investigated in transgenic mice by administering CD-8$^+$, major histocompatability complex class I (MHC-I)-restricted, hepatitis B surface antigen (HBsAg)-specific cytotoxic T lymphocytes (CTLs) generated in nontransgenic syngeneic mice (i.e., the mouse strain into which the exogenous HBV DNA was inserted to make it transgenic; because the exogenous DNA is inserted into the germline the transgenic mouse immune system recognizes

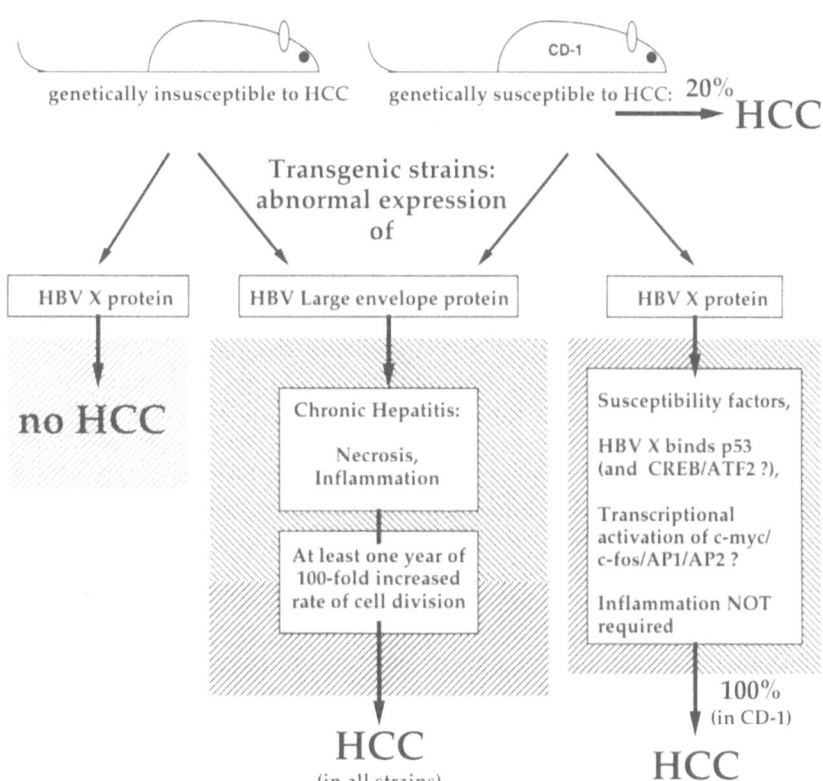

Fig. 4. Transgenic mice strains expressing the hepatitis B virus (*HBV*) large envelope protein develop chronic hepatitis, which leads to hepatocellular carcinoma (*HCC*). The expression of HBV X protein, however, results in HCC only in the genetically susceptible CD-1 strain

the HBV proteins as self). HBsAg consists of major, middle, and large viral envelope proteins. Some of the mice strains injected with HBsAg-specific CTLs develop a disease resembling acute viral hepatitis [61]. The severity of the HBsAg-specific antibody-induced necroinflammatory disease has been found to depend on the following [62]: (1) production of interferon-γ (IFN-γ) by the CTL when it recognized the antigen; (2) number of HBsAg-positive hepatocytes present in the lover; (3) amount of HBsAg within each hepatocyte; and (4) the gender of the mouse.

The first detectable step following administration of class I CTLs is their attachment to the HBsAg-positive hepatocytes, which undergo apoptosis [63]. This section causes the appearance of acidophilic apoptotic hepatocytes which is characteristic of acute viral hepatitis in humans. The direct cytopathic effect of the CTLs in these experiments is limited to a few heptocytes, however, and it has been postulated that this is due to the solid architecture of the liver, which restricts the movement of CTLs. CTLs recruit many host-derived, antigen-nonspecific inflammatory cells into their immediate vicinity several hours after they are administered. It results in the formation of necroinflammatory foci in which the hepatocellular necrosis extends well beyond CTLs, indicating that most hepatocytes are not killed directly by CTLs [62]. In most transgenic mouse strains expressing HBV surface antigen proteins, as in humans, the disease does not progress beyond this point. In most mice the disease is also transient and nonfatal, destroying no more than 5% of the hepatocytes. In trasgenic mouse strains that express the large envelope protein, however, the disease process becomes fulminant and kills nearly half of the mice through liver failure within 48 to 72 hours of CTL injection. These mice maintain the large envelope protein (i.e., HBsAg) in the endoplasmic reticulum (see below). Nonspecific inflammatory cells, particularly macrophages, vastly outnumber HBsAg-specific CTLs in the fulminant hepatitis characterized by diffuse lymphomononuclear inflammatory cell infiltrate. Therefore much of the liver damage caused by hepatitis, except hepatocyte apoptosis, is mediated by antigen-nonspecific cytokines and effector cells that have been activated by virus-specific T cells and not CTLs per se.

Thus there is markedly increased mitogenesis and large numbers of macrophages, and their as-

sociated cytokines, in the HBV-inflamed liver. This environment may be highly mutagenic.

Both intrahepatic class I (CD8+) and class II (CD4+) MHC-restricted HBsAg-specific CTLs have been isolated from humans with chronic hepatitis B, indicating that HBsAg may be an important target molecule for killing infected hepatocytes via the class I and class II processing pathways [64]. In most cases, whether the persistent infection was established in utero, at birth, or after birth, a host immune response is generated to the virus. In the former case the immune response is generally insufficient to clear the virus but sufficient to cause severe, prolonged cellular injury as in the mouse model. Increased mitogenesis in HBV-infected hepatocytes could result from a cytopathic reaction with anti-HBsAg-specific CTls.

Expression of Large Envelope Protein. In transgenic mice expressing large amounts of the HBV large envelope protein, the foreign protein associates into long, branching, filamentous particles that become trapped in the endoplasmic reticulum and are not secreted [60]. It results in a dramatic increase in the amount of endoplasmic reticulum, which eventually causes histological changes characterized by "ground-glass" hepatocytes found in the liver of patients chronically infected with HBV [60]. The HBsAg-laden ground-glass hepatocyte is hypersensitive to certain endogenous stimuli, including bacterial lipopolysaccharide and IFN-γ [65]. These chemicals cause severe hepatitis in the animals, and the degree of hepatocellular injury is directly proportional to the amount of HBsAg maintained in the endoplasmic reticulum. Prolonged storage of the long subviral particles in the endoplasmic reticulum is cytopathic for the hepatocyte when expressed in large amounts, and the hepatocytes die spontaneously. This chronic hepatocellualr necrosis causes a secondary inflammatory and regenerative response [60, 66], which leads to HCC in all transgenic mouse strains overexpressing the large envelope protein, although the background and gender affect the incidence [67–69]. The incidence of HCC in this model corresponds to the frequency, severity, and age at onset of liver cell injury, which itself corresponds to the intrahepatic concentration of HBsAg. Hepatocellular turnover in these mice, relative to nontransgenic controls, is increased 100-fold for at least a year before the onset of HCC [70]. In addition, oxygen radical production is greatly increased and antioxidant (glutathione transferase) content greatly decreased in the livers of these mice [71]. These changes are associated with a dramatic increase in oxidative DNA damage to hepatocellular genomic DNA. It is reasonable to assume that these events could lead to the accumulation of random mutations throughout the genome that contribute to the formation of HCC in these animals.

Expression of HBV X Protein. A level of expression of the HBV X protein in transgenic mice results in almost ubiquitous HCC in some strains of mice [72, 73]. The transgenic mouse strains overexpressing HBV X protein that develop HCC have a CD-1 mouse genetic background. CD-1 is an outbred strain of mice particularly susceptible to spontaneous HCC (approximately 20% of CD-1 mice develop HCC) and as such has been used extensively in long-term bioassays to determine chemical carcinogenicity. Those transgenic mouse strains that express the X protein in a genetic background other than that of the CD-1 susceptible mouse do not develop HCC. This finding suggests that the X protein may function as a cofactor in HCC promotion and may require genetic susceptibility in the host.

The mechanism by which these mice develop HCC is not fully understood. The HBV X protein binds p53, confining it to the cytoplasm in the transgenic mice, and it has been proposed to be a primary transforming component [74]. It has been shown that the HBV X protein interacts with wild-type human p53 protein and inhibits its sequence-specific DNA binding and transcriptional activity in vitro [75, 76]. It has also been shown that in areas where the incidence of HCC is high up to 78% of tumors have been found to contain an intact HBV X gene, which may be expressed and functionally inactivate p53 [77].

The HBV X protein can transcriptionally activate several cellular genes in vitro, including c-*myc* and c-*jun*, which are associated with growth control, and this could also be transforming. The HBV X protein is also known to transcriptionally activate AP1 and AP2 [78] and bind the cAMP-responsive element (CREB) and the activating transcription factor (ATF2) [79].

Insulin-like growth factor II and the mdr III gene are transcriptionally activated in most HCCs in the HBV transgenics [80, 81]. These genes are not overexpressed in the preneoplastic lesions,

however, suggesting that they represent late changes associated with tumor progression but not initiation. Significantly, no changes in the DNA copy number, gene structure, steady-state mRNA level, or protein content has been detected in the HBV transgenic HCCs in any of the following: *p53, RB-1,* Ha-*ras,* Ki-*ras,* N-*ras,* c-*myc,* N-*myc, erb-*A, *erb-*B, *src, mos, abl, sis, fms, fes, fos, jun,* TGF-α, TGF-β, prostaglandin-derived growth factors α and β, EGF receptor, HNF-1, c/ERP, or CREB [82].

It is also important that HCC has not been observed in any HBV transgenic lineage that does not display liver injury apart from that expressing the HBV X protein in a CD-1 HCC-susceptible background [10]. This finding strongly suggests that the inflammation and resultant immune response are directly or indirectly responsible for the generation of HCC in patients with hepatitis B. The immune system attacks the HBV-infected cells it can reach, driving them into apoptosis, increasing the rate of cell division in the neighboring cells (one of which may eventually develop into a malignant neoplasm), and producing a secondary immune response.

Because these transgenic mouse strains over-expressing the large envelope protein have been observed to develop HCC in separate lineages, without transgene rearrangement or instability, again viral integration is not likely to have activated an oncogene or inactivated a tumor suppressor. Instead, severe, prolonged cellular injury induces a preneoplastic proliferative cellular response that fosters subsequent secondary genetic events that program the cell for unrestrained growth. It is also likely that the HBV X protein can perform a role in the promotion of HCC by binding and functionally inactivating p53 and by acting as a *trans*-activating transcription factor.

Aflatoxin B₁

The p53 gene is mutated in about 50% of human cancers, and loss of wild-type function of this gene is generally an important step in carcinogenesis [83]. p53 functions at the G_1 phase of the cell cycle, suppressing both growth and transformation in response to DNA damage. Part of its tumor-suppression function also stems from its role in inducing cell entry into apoptosis.

Hepatocellular carcinoma in the Qidong Province of China [84], Senegal [85], Mozambique [77], and southern Africa [86], all of which are high aflatoxin-exposure regions, have been found to be associated with a specific mutation in the p53 gene. Between 50% and 75% of HCC cases in these regions have *p53* mutations, most being a G-T transversion in the third nucleotide of codon 249, which results in an arginine to serine substitution. Because this mutation has been identified in apparently normal livers of aflatoxin B_1-exposed individuals it could well be an early event in HCC development in regions of high aflatoxin B_1 exposure [87]. In vivo and in vitro studies have demonstrated that the third nucleotide, G, of codon 249 in *p53* is a specific target for adduction of the aflatoxin B_1 metabolite (aflatoxin-8,9-epoxide) in human hepatocytes [87, 88]. The corresponding mutation in *TRP53* in the mouse has been shown to confer a growth advantage to murine cell line in vitro [89].

Because this aflatoxin B_1-induced mutation is not found at high levels in HBV-positive HCC in other parts of the world it seems likely that HBV is not causally related to this mutation [90]. Cooperative interaction of the *p53* mutation and HBV X protein inactivation of p53 are likely in the transformation of hepatocytes in situations where aflatoxin B_1 and hepatitis incidence are high. Mutations in *p53* codon 249 are equally prevalent in HBV X protein positive and negative cases of HCC [77].

Hepatitis C Virus

Hepatitis C Virus is a positive, 10 kb single-stranded RNA virus that is spread by exposure to blood (whether vertical and sexual transmission are possible remains controversial). There is considerable nucleotide variation throughout the viral genome, which has led to the classification of numerous strains of the virus with different epidemiology. The virus replicates via formation of a full-length complementary RNA strand, and because there is no known DNA intermediate in its replicative cycle, integration of the virus into the host genome is not possible. HCV has been claimed to have a direct cytopathic effect, as the virus has structural analogies with known cytopathic viruses, such as flaviviruses and pestiviruses, but the direct cytopathic effect is vigorously contested [91]. The virus contains no known oncogenes, although the 5' half of the HCV nonstructural protein NS3 is capable of

transforming mouse fibroblast cells following transfection [92]. There is no direct evidence that HCV is cytopathic to the hepatocyte.

The mechanism by which HCV induces HCC therefore appears to be confind to random deregulation of cell cycle regulatory genes as a result of increased mitogenesis in the necroinflammatory liver disease. Most HCV-associated HCCs are also associated with cirrhosis, which could be an additional promoting factor [3, 93, 94]. However, HCCs can develop in HCV patients in the absence of cirrhosis, albeit at low incidence [95].

Several lines of evidence suggest that immune-mediated mechanisms similar to those in HBV trasgenic mice contribute to the pathogenesis of chronic hepatitis C.

- Studies using in situ hybridization and immunohistochemistry have demonstrated a lack of correlation between the low number of infected hepatocytes and the intensity of the inflammatory lesions [96, 97].
- Patients with chronic HCV infection have enhanced hepatocyte HLA-I and cytokine-dependent immune adhesion molecule expression in liver lobules, and predominant CD-8$^+$ MHC-I-restricted CTL infiltration in areas of lobular hepatitis [98].
- HCV antigen-specific, CD-8$^+$ CTLs and CD4$^+$ helper cells are present in both the peripheral blood and liver of patients with chronic hepititis C [99].

The development of a mouse model of HCV infection and reproducible techniques for in vitro tissue culture of HCV are required to investigate the pathogenesis of this virus in detail.

Somatic Mutations in HCC

In contrast to the above etiological agents, little progress has been made in identifying somatic and germline mutations associated with HCC development. As previously discussed, although a high rate of mutation in the p53 gene, particularly a G-T transversion at codon 249, is observed in most HCCs arising in areas of high exposure to aflatoxin B_1, it is not a general step in HCC. Low frequencies of a broad spectrum of mutations in the p53 gene are observed in areas of low aflatoxin B_1 exposure, The frequency of mutation in the p53 gene reported include 10% in Britain

[100], 15% to 29% in Japan [101–103], and 14% to 27% in Europe [104, 105]. There have been several reports that HCCs associated with either HBV or HCV infection have higher levels of *p53* mutation [94, 106–108]. These reports have been questioned by others, however, and it seems likely that where *p53* mutation and HBV-associated HCCs do occur in the absence of aflatoxin B_1 exposure the mutation arose at an advanced stage in HCC [109].

Although activated *ras* oncogenes have been detected in a high percentage of spontaneous HCCs in the B6C3F1 mouse [110], no single oncogene has been shown to be preferentially amplified in human HCC. A point mutation in members of the ras gene family is common in colorectal carcinomas [111] but uncommon in HCCs [112]. Similarly, amplification of the cyclin D1 gene has been detected in HCCs, but subsequent studies have shown it in a low percentage of HCCs [113].

Numerous investigations of allelic imbalance have been carried out in HCCs. They followed from the successful role that similar studies played in assisting in the positional cloning of tumor-suppressor genes that had initially been localized by other means, for example, retinoblastoma (*RB1* is the tumor-suppresser gene mutated in this inherited cancer) and Wilms' tumor (*WT1* is one of the mutated genes causing this inherited cancer). The APC gene, which is commonly deleted in colorectal carcinomas, was discovered by allelic imbalance investigations. The hypothesis behind these studies is that an inactivated tumor suppressor is recessive but becomes evident when the functional allele is lost, with the result that the cell is relieved from negative growth control.

1. Chromosome 1p allelic losses may be an early event in HCC [114, 115]. Allelic imbalance on this chromosome has been found in early and well differentiated advanced HCC, whereas allelic imbalance on chromosomes 4q, 8p, 13q, 16q, and 17p was not as frequent in early HCC. In this study (which is cited for each of the chromosomes it examined) among 104 tumors, allelic imbalance on chromosome 1p was detected in 38% of early tumors (<2 cm) and in 33% of well-differentiated tumors [115].

2. Chromosome 4q showed allelic imbalance in 17% of early tumors and 37% of well-differentiated tumors [115]. Levels of allelic imbalance as high as 100% of informative cases were originally reported in proximal 4q [116]. Later reports showed considerably lower levels of allelic imbalance, however, particularly for distal 4q (14%), suggesting that any tumor-suppressor gene is in the proximal region [117, 118].

3. Chromosome 5q terminal deletions have been reported in 100% of noncirrhotic HCCs and in 0% of cirrhotic HCCs in one cohort of patients [119]. In a study in which the cirrhotic status was not examined, allelic imbalance on this chromosome arm was identified in approximately 40% of HCCs [117, 118]. The APC gene is located on chromosome 5q, but no somatic mutations have been identified in this gene in HCC. Furthermore, the smallest deletion map does not contain the *APC* locus 5q21 [120].

4. Chromosome 8p has been shown in allelic imbalance in 25% of early tumors and 35% of well-differentiated tumors [121]. Levels of allelic imbalance as high as 48% on 8p have been reported in HCCs, whereas in control sporadic breast carcinomas only 8% of cases showed allelic imbalance [118, 122].

5. Chromosome 8q has been shown to be amplified in a relatively large proportion of HCCs; all the other allelic imbalances described here are thought to result from deletions [123]. This amplification event has not been detected in high numbers in any other tumor types and may be specific to HCC. Chromosome 8q shows amplifications in 20% of early HCCs and 31% of well differentiated tumors [121].

6. Chromosome 11p has been reported in allelic imbalance in approximately 40% of HCCs [117, 124]. This has also been reported to be a preferential site for HBV integration. The WT1 gene is located at 11p13, but expression of this gene is confined to the urogenital system; and the minimal deletion map obtained to date suggests 11p15 as the locus of a tumor suppressor involved in HCC [125].

7. Chromosome 13q showed allelic imbalance in 15% of early tumors and 36% of well-differentiated tumors [121]. In other studies chromosome 13q has been shown in allelic imbalance in up to 50% of HCCs [125]. The minimal deletion map covers 13q14, which contains the *RB1* locus. Subsequent studies have demonstrated that this locus is deleted in 40% of well-differentiated advanced HCCs, and that in approximately 20% of these cases *RB1* is mutated on the remaining allele [126]. Loss of RB1 protein in these cases was confirmed using immunohistochemistry, which

showed no RB1 protein expression in the carcinomas. *BRCA2* (the second gene isolated that is linked to hereditary breast cancer) is located on 13q12-q13, and allelic losses of this chromosome are common in sporadic breast carcinomas [127]. It is another candidate tumor suppressor for HCC, as it has been reported that allelic imbalance occurs in two discrete regions on 13q, one corresponding to deletion of *RB1* and the second to deletion of *BRCA2* [121].

8. Chromosome 16q showed allelic imbalance in 7% of early tumors and 37% of well-differentiated tumors [121]. Levels of allelic imbalance of 28% [118], 36% [117], and 52% [128] have also been reported. All the reports link allelic imbalance at 16q with progression of the HCC.

9. Chromosome 17p, the location of the P53 gene, showed allelic imbalance in 17% of early tumors and 35% of well-differentiated tumors [121]. Levels of allelic imbalance as high as 57% have been reported [118].

This laboratory has identified and characterized a novel locus of allelic imbalance at human chromosome 11q23 in a variety of human malignancies: melanomas and cervical and breast cancers [129–132]. Approximately 40% of the English cases of HCC examined to date have been found to have allelic imbalance at 11q23. In contrast, the South African cases examined have a far lower level (approximately 15%) of allelic imbalance at 11q23. These results support the hypothesis that HCC in Europe is genetically distinct from that found in South Africa, and that the allelic imbalance found at 11q23 could be contributing to the cancer process.

A novel mutation in the mannose-6-phosphate/IGF-II receptor (*M6P/IGF-IIr*) in HCC has been identified partially by allelic imbalance studies. The identification followed the finding that M6P/IGF-IIr expression was significantly reduced in both rats and humans [133]. In mammals M6P/IGF-IIr possesses distinct binding regions for both phosphomannosyl residues and IGF-II [134]. The primary functions of M6P/IGF-IIr include the trafficking of newly synthesized lysosomal enzymes from the Golgi complex to lysosomes, endocytosis of extracellular lysosomal enzymes, binding of the growth factors IGF-II and proliferin, and binding of the latent complex of TGF-β1 [135]. Although binding of these growth factors to M6P/IGF-IIr ultimately results in their

internalization in lysosomes, the extracellular activation of latent TGF-β1 by plasmin is greatly facilitated by the binding [136]. This receptor is therefore required for activation of the growth inhibitor TGF-β1 and degradation of the mitogen IGF-II; it consequently plays an important role in negative growth control.

In a study allelic imbalance around 6q26-q27, the location of *M6P/IGF-IIr*, 69% of HCCs, 33% fibromeller tumors, and 67% of liver adenomas were found to have a deletion [53]. Subsequent studies found that 25% of the *M6P/IGF-IIr* that remained after the deletion event were mutated, resulting in a nonfunctional protein [137]. As such, the *M6P/IGF-IIr* functions as a tumor suppressor in HCC, which may in part explain the observation of up-regulation of IGF-II in all the HBV transgenic mice that developed HCC. Interestingly, because *M6P/IGF-IIr* is maternally imprinted in mice and imprinting in humans is a polymorphic trait, only one mutation (in the paternal gene) may be required to completely inactivate the gene in those individuals who have imprinted maternal genes [138].

TGF-β1 levels have been reported to be considerably increased in HCC [139]. This finding is unexpected for a negative regulator of hepatocyte division but may result, at least in part, from the deletion of M6P/IGF-IIr, whose binding results in its activation or degradation. It has also been shown that overexpressing HBV X protein in transgenic mice results in increased TGF-β1 expression [140]. It has been proposed that increased expression of TGF-β1 could be tumor-promoting through a mechanism of immune suppression, but it is possible that genetic mutations have resulted in altered biochemical function.

Germline Mutations Predisposing to HCC

Epidemiology clearly shows that most HCCs develop after exposure to exogenous agents. Studies of immigrants have shown that the risk of HCC in some ethnic groups is associated with the population's exposure to environmental factors. The incidence of HCC is lower in Chinese, Japanese, and Filipino people born in the United States than those who immigrated there; and the latter have a lower incidence than the population in their country of origin [7]. Reduced exposure to carcinogens and diminished intrafamilial spread of HBV are among the possible explantations.

Epidemiology also strongly suggests that germline mutations exist in different populations that make individuals more or less susceptible to HCC. For example, it is reasonable to assume that the ability of some individuals to clear hepatitis virus infection, whereas others go on to develop chronic hepatitis, is a result of different genetic susceptibilities to viral infection. HCC genetic susceptibilty is expected to be linked to genotypes that are unable to clear the hepatitis viruses. Transgenic mice expressing the HBV X protein develop HCC only if they have a susceptible CD-1 mouse background, demonstrating that genetic germline mutations can predispose to HCC in the presence of *trans*-activating factors. Genetic susceptibility to HCC is also proved by the finding that different strains of inbred mice have different rates of spontaneous HCC.

Germline mutations in *M6P/IGF-IIr* and *RB1* have been identified in HCCs, and they make individuals more susceptible to promotion and progression of HCC, as only one mutation during these processes is sufficient to inactivate each of these genes. Little progress has been made in identifying other genetic causes of susceptibility. The major genetic factors likely to be involved in HCC development include the following.

1. Because the principal etiological agents are viral, the immune response to viral infection (and cirrhosis) is a critical susceptibility factor. As such, the HLA genotypes would be expected to be an important susceptibilty factor for viral infection, which is in turn a susceptibilty factor for HCC (Fig. 5). Epidemiological studies have found linkage disequilibrium between MHC genes and susceptibility to HBV infection [141]. This situation has not been characterized on a molecular level.

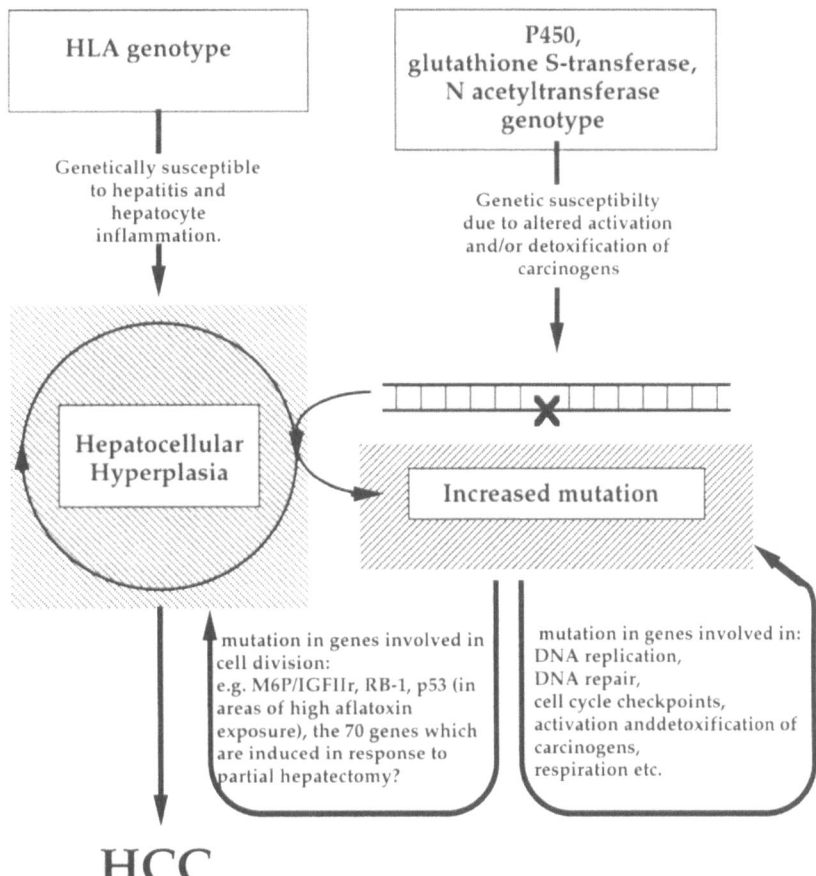

Fig. 5. Summary of the genetics underlying HCC development. Some of the likely targets for somatic mutation during the promotion and progression of HCC are indicated

2. Because the liver is a major site for detoxification, and therefore activation of procarcinogens, it is likely that mutations in these genes are of considerable importance to HCC susceptibility, especially given that a principal response to the primary etiological agents may be hyperplasia.

Cancer susceptibility due to chemical exposure is likely to be determined by an individual's phenotype for a number of enzymes, both activating and detoxifying, relevant to those compounds. Mutation in P-450 genes (*CYP*) can dramatically change the natural substrate specificity of the cytochrome and the rate of drug metabolism and chemical activation. Similarly, mutations in the glutathione *S*-transferases and *N*-acetyltransferases could alter an individual's susceptibility to cancers due to altered activation or detoxification of carcinogens (or both). Many of the polymorphic genes of carcinogen metabolism show considerable ethnic differences in gene structure and allelic distribution. Variations in metabolic phenotypes and genotypes have been reported in different geographic populations. The phenotype of carcinogen metabolism is complex, as many proteins are involved, and as such it is a complex genetic trait; few data are available.

A difference in the ability to detoxify the mutagenic metabolite of aflatoxin B_1 (aflatoxin-8,9-epoxide) has been identified among individuals. Microsomal epoxide hydrolase (EPHX) and glutathione *S*-transferase M1 (GSTM1) are both involved in the detoxification of this mutagenic metabolite in hepatocytes. Polymorphisms in both of these genes have been described. GSTM1 isoenzyme is polymorphic in humans as a result of a gene deletion, and individuals homozygous for the deletion have no GSTM1 enzyme activity [142, 143]. EPHX activity varies within populations, and several DNA polymorphisms have been described [144]. A correlation between mutant alleles of the EPHX gene and diminished enzyme has also been reported. It has been found that the substitution of His-113 for the more commonly occurring Tyr-133 results in a 40% decrease in the enzyme's activity in vitro [145]. A significant association between EPHX and GSTM1 genotypes and the presence of aflatoxin B_1 adducts on DNA bases has been found [146]. A significant association was also found in this study between EPHX genotype and HCC, and results were obtained that were highly suggestive that GSTM1 genotype and HCC, and *p53* mutations at

position 259, were associated. This is a strong genetic susceptibility factor for HCC development in individuals who are exposed to aflatoxin B_1.

Individuals with certain genetic diseases have an increased risk of developing HCC.

1. Chronic hereditary tyrosinemia: a disorder of amino acid metabolism that in its chronic form causes cirrhosis with progressive liver dysfunction and death during the first decade. HCC develops in 37% of these patients [147].
2. Hereditary hemochromatosis: excess iron storage. Results in cirrhosis and HCC in 17% to 29% of patients [148].
3. Porphyria cutanea tarda: 18% patients develop HCC frequently as a complication of cirrhosis [149].

It seems that the increased risk of HCC in individuals with these diseases is associated with an increased risk of cirrhosis and the inflammation and mitogenesis associated with this disease.

Inbred Murine Models of Hepatocellular Carcinoma

Male B6C3F1 mice develop spontaneous HCCs at an average incidence of 25%. The C3H/He (C3) parent mouse is highly susceptible to HCC, whereas the C57BL/6 (B6) parent is not susceptible. This difference in susceptibility of inbred mice to HCC clearly demonstrates the influence of genetic factors. The B6C3F1 mouse is an ideal model for studying chromosomal aberrations that occur during the development and progression of hepatic cancer. Large numbers of stage-specific tumors can be obtained from these mice following their promotion using a single etiological agent such as phenobarbital; the latter compound is a prototype for other hepatic tumor-inducing agents. Because these mice are kept in a controlled environment, and the promotion of hepatic tumors is "standardized," it can be postulated that the resultant malignant phenotype is the consequence of a specific sequence of chromosomal changes. Any background genetic changes that occur randomly as a result of disruption to the cell cycle control mechanisms are unlikely to be present in a high percentage of tumors. These changes therefore can be distinguished from the series of chromosome aberrations associated with tumor development but are not necessarily primarily relevant. This distinction is aided by the ability to equate chromosome imbalance with the susceptibility of the parental mice. However, the genetic dissection of the disease in these mice to date has not resulted in the identification of any germline mutations or frequent chromosome abnormalities.

Current data suggest that initiation could well be a specific point mutation at codon 61 of the H-*ras* oncogene. Chromosome loci on murine chromosome 1 [150] and chromosome 17 [N. Drinkwater, personal communication] have been linked with HCC susceptibility in the C3 mouse. The latter studies have been based on linkage between C3 loci and susceptibility for HCC in the progeny of B6C3F1 mice (F2). Murine chromosomes 7, 8, and 12 have also been linked with HCC susceptibility [151]. Chromosome 7 may be of particular interest, as it is the location of H-*ras*-1 which has previously been shown to be activated in B6C3F1 HCCs. An understanding of the development of HCC in the B6C3F1 mouse could be particularly revealing, as it has been used extensively for toxicity testing.

Two susceptibility loci for HCC in females have been mapped in the C57BR/cdj (BR) strain of inbred mouse [152]. Sensitivity to HCC in mice is highly sexually dimorphic due to contrasting effects of androgens and ovarian hormones on liver tumor induction: Androgens promote HCC, whereas ovarian hormones inhibit HCC [153, 154]. As a result, male mice have a higher incidence of both spontaneous and chemically induced HCC. Females of the BR strain are 15 to 30 times more susceptible to HCC than females from other inbred strains of mice [155]. The unusual susceptibility of the BR female is characterized by its insensitivity to the suppressing effects of ovarian hormones. Thus ovariectomized and intact BR females have a similar susceptibility to HCC, whereas female mice from other strains have a significantly increased susceptibility to HCC following ovariectomy [155, 156]. Linkage analysis on B6BRF1 × B6BRF1 (F2) and B6BRF1 × B6 mice have mapped two loci that account for nearly all of the difference in HCC susceptibility of females on chromosomes 17 and 1 [152].

The incidence of HCC is two- to fivefold higher in men than in women. It is not known whether this sex difference results from differences in exposure to risk factors such as alcohol, HBV, and aflatoxin or from hormonal effects on the pathogenesis of HCC [157].

Toxicity Testing in the B6C3F1 and CD-1 Mouse

The B6C3F1 mouse and the CD-1 outbred mouse have been used extensively for long-term bioassays to evaluate carcinogenicity. CD-1 mice develop spontaneous HCC at an incidence of 20%. Animals have been administered the maximum tolerated dose (MTD) of the chemical being tested over a prolonged period. About half of the chemicals tested in this way have proved to be rodent carcinogens at least in one of these strains of mice or in Fischer 344 rats [39]. By 1990 that amounted to approximately 220 of the 350 (63%) synthetic chemicals tested and 37 of the 77 (48%) natural chemicals tested.

The liver is the major site of malignancy in the rodent carcinogenicity bioassay; and of 299 mouse carcinogens, 171 (57%) induced tumors in the liver [158]. A considerable proportion of these chemicals do not appear to directly damage DNA or induce mutations; they are nongenotoxic in the *Salmonella* test. The mouse therefore parallels the human in its development of HCC in that the etiological agents are not directly chemically mutagenic. These chemicals do, however, share one or more biological effects in the mouse.

- Induction of mixed function oxidase enzymes, which increases the oxygen free radicals in hepatocytes
- Inhibition of gap junction intercellular communication, which removes cells from homeostatic control or hormonal modification
- Mitogenesis
- Cytotoxicity
- Immunosuppression

These nongenotoxic chemicals have been shown to increase or promote the natural occurrence, development, or progression of liver tumors, and their effects are reminiscent of the etiology of human HCC. These experiments demonstrate that the liver is the natural target of disease for exogenous compounds and reiterates what may be the major cause of HCC: Prolonged hepatocellular injury induces a preneoplastic proliferative and inflammatory response that places the dividing cells at risk of developing multiple random mutations or other chromosomal changes, which can result in unprogrammed cell division.

The relevence of the carcinogenicity associated with these chemicals at the maximal tolerated dose in the murine models to human risk assessment is controversial. Because the animals are saturated with the chemicals it seems likely that the liver is unable to metabolize them efficiently, causing impaired homeostasis. Such impaired homeostasis results in inflammation of one sort or another, which in the liver can result in HCC. The saturation of these animals with the chemicals is so artificial that no conclusions can be drawn concerning the risk to humans of exposure to chemicals proved positive in the bioassay.

Conclusions

Collectively, the literature cited implicates cell injury as being perhaps the major risk factor for HCC and notes that it results from mitogenesis. HBV or HCV, alcohol abuse, hemochromatosis, α_1-antitrypsin deficiency, and glycogen storage disease generally progress to cirrhosis before HCC. Cirrhosis is characterized by necrosis, inflammation, and hepatocellular regeneration. Thus severe, prolonged hepatocellular injury induces a preneoplastic proliferative and inflammatory response that places the dividing cells at risk of developing multiple random mutations or other chromosomal changes, some of which program the cell for unrestrained growth. Chronic liver cell injury thereby sets in motion a cascade of pathophysiological events, including inflammation, oxygen free radical production, hepatocellular regeneration, and oxidative DNA damage, which produce random genetic and chromosomal changes that ultimately cause HCC. The liver's remarkable capacity for regeneration in response to injury may be primarily responsible for the accumulation of all the genomic changes that are required for initiation, promotion, and progression to neoplasia.

The fact that no genetic homogeneity has been identified to date in hepatocarcinogenesis may also be a result of hepatocyte hyperplasia. Genetic abnormality is not required for hyperplasia, which could be considered the first crucial event in any mechanism of HCC development. After the onset of cell division, the genetically irreversible initiation event is possible; then, while cell division continues, mutations accumulate through the promotion and progression stages of carcinogenesis until a cell escapes from growth control. Interestingly, if mitogenesis ceases in a liver that has recovered from injury, the progression of the disease is stalled almost indefinitely.

More than 70 genes have been found to be induced in the immediate-early response to hepatectomy, and it is assumed that these genes are all actively involved in the initiation and promotion of liver regeneration. This could well represent more than the number of genetic targets available for mutation in colorectal carcinoma and as such may result in considerably more genetic heterogeneity in HCC. There may also be more point mutations in the liver resulting from adduction than in the colon, where large deletions seem to be of particular importance in progression due to its role in detoxifying chemicals.

Genetic factors are clearly involved in susceptibility to HCC, best demonstrated by the different rates of spontaneous HCC in inbred mice. Identification of the genes underlying these factors is of considerable importance to understanding hepatocyte division and the development of HCC.

A reduction in the incidence of HCC worldwide is clearly best approached by eliminating the etiological agents. Steps such as the universal vaccination against HBV and HCV (when a vaccine becomes available), a reduction in contamination of food during storage and distribution, and increased education in respect to the mitogenic danger of alcohol are expected to be considerebly effective in the reduction of HCC.

Finally, it is interesting to speculate that although many cancers have been found to have germline genetic mutations underlying initiation (hereditary cancers) and particularly promotion, it is not necessarily the case for HCC. HCC may not be a genetic disease; rather, it may be the manifestation of a "chronically afflicted genome."

References

1. Parkin DM, Stjernsward J, Muir CS (1984) Estimates of the worldwide frequency of twelve major cancers. Bull World Health Organ 62:163–182
2. Okuda K, Ohnishi K (1987) Prognosis of hepatocellular carcinoma. In: Okuda K, Ishak KG (eds) Neoplasms of the liver. Springer, Tokyo, pp 407–416
3. Colombo M (1992) Hepatocellular carcinoma. J Hepatol 15:225–236
4. Okuda K (1992) Hepatocellular carcinoma: recent progress. Hepatology 15:948–963
5. Yu MC, Tong MJ, Govindarajan S, Henderson BE (1991) Nonviral risk factors for hepatocellular car-

cinoma in a low-risk population, the non-Asians of Los Angeles County, California. J Natl Cancer Inst 83:1820–1826

6. Yeh FS, Yu MC, Mo CC, Luo S, Tong MJ, Henderson BE (1989) Hepatitis B virus, aflatoxins, and hepatocellular carcinoma in southern Guangsi, China. Cancer Res 49:2506–2509

7. Munoz N, Bosch FX (1989) Epidemiology of hepatocellular carcinoma. In: Okuda K, Ishak KG (eds) Neoplasms of the liver. Springer, Tokyo, pp 3–21

8. Bosch FX, Munoz N (1991) Hepatocellular carcinoma in the world: epidemiological questions. In: Tabor E, Di Bisceglie AM, Rurcell RH (eds) Etiology, pathology and treatment of hepatocellular carcinoma in northern America. Gulf, Houston, pp 35–56

9. Tsukuma H, Hiyama T, Tanaka S, Nakao M, Yabuuchi T, Kitamura T, Nakanishi K, Fujimoto I, Inove A, Yamazaki M, Kawashima T (1993) Risk factors for hepatocellular carcinoma among patients with chronic liver disease. N Engl J Med 328:1797–1801

10. Chisari FV (1995) Hepatitis B virus transgenic mice: insights into the virus and disease. Hepatology 22:1316–1325

11. Beasley RP (1987) The major etiology of hepatocellular carcinoma. In: Fortner JC, Rhoads JE (eds) Accomplishment in cancer research. Lippincott, Philadelphia, pp 80–106

12. Beasley RP, Lin CC, Hwang LY, Chen CS (1981) Hepatocellular carcinoma and hepatitis B virus: a prospective study of 22 707 men in Taiwan. Lancet 2:1129–1133

13. Sakamoto M, Hirohashi S, Tsuda H, Ino Y, Shimosato Y, Yamasaki S, Makuuchi M, Hasegawa H, Terada M, Hosada Y (1988) Increasing incidence of hepatocellular carcinoma possibly associated with non-A, non-B hepatitis in Japan, disclosed by hepatitis B virus DNA analysis of surgically resected cases. Cancer Res 48:7294–7297

14. Choo QL, Kuo G, Weiner AJ, Overby LR, Bradley DW, Houghton M (1989) Isolation of a cDNA clone derived from a blood-borne non-A, non-B viral hepatitis genome. Science 244:359–362

15. Kuo G, Choo QL, Alter HJ, Gitnick GL, Redeker AG, Purcell RH, Miyamura T, Dienstag JL, Alter MJ, Stevens CE, Tegtmeier GE, Bonino F, Colombo M, Lee WS, Kuo C, Berger K, Shuster JR, Overby R, Bradley DW, Houghton M (1989) An assay for circulating antibodies to a major etiologic virus of human non-A, non-B hepatitis. Science 244:362–364

16. Kiyosawa K, Sodeyama T, Tanaka E, Gibo Y, Yoshizawa K, Nakano Y, Furuta S, Akahane Y, Nishioka K, Purcell RH (1990) Interrelationship of blood transfusion, non-A, non-B hepatitis and

hepatocellular carcinoma: analysis by detection of antibody to hepatitis C virus. Hepatology 12:671–675

17. Bruix J, Barrera JM, Calvet X, Ercilla G, Costa J, Sanchez-Tapias JM, Ventura M, Vall M, Bruguera M, Bru C, Castillo R, Rhodes J (1989) Prevalence of antibodies to hepatitis C virus in Spanish patients with hepatocellular carcinoma and hepatic cirrhosis. Lancet 2:1004–1006

18. Colombo M, Kuo G, Choo QL, Donato MF, Ninno ED, Tommasini M, Dioguardi N, Houghton M (1989) Prevalence of antibodies to hepatitis C virus in Italian patients with hepatocellular carcinoma. Lancet 2:1006–1008

19. Hasan F, Jeffers LJ, De Medina M, Reddy KR, Parker T, Schiff ER, Houghton M, Chao Q, Kuo G (1991) Hepatitis C-associated hepatocellular carcinoma. Hepatology 12:589–591

20. Kew MC, Houghton M, Choo-QL, Kuo-G (1990) Hepatitis C virus antibodies in southern African blacks with hepatocellular carcinoma. Lancet 335:873–874

21. Chen DS, Kuo GC, Sung JL, Lai MY, Sheu JC, Chen PJ, Yang PM, Hsu HM, Chang MH (1990) Hepatitis C virus infection in an area hyperendemic for hepatitis B and chronic liver disease: the Taiwan experience. J Infect Dis 162:817–822

22. Srivatanakul P, Parkin DM, Khlat M, Chenvidhya D, Chotiwan P, Insiripong S, L'Abbe KA, Wild CP (1991) Liver cancer in Thailand. II. A case-control study of hepatocellular carcinoma. Int J Cancer 48:329–332

23. Dazza MC, Meneses LV, Girard PM, Astagneau P, Villaroel C, Delaporte E, Larouze B (1993) Absence of a relationship between antibodies to hepatitis C virus and hepatocellular carcinoma in Mozambique. Am J Trop Med Hyg 48:237–242

24. Thomas HC (1996) Clinical features of viral hepatitis. In: Weatherall DJ, Ledingham JGG, Warrell DA (eds) Oxford textbook of medicine, 3rd edn. Oxford University Press, Oxford, pp 2061–2069

25. Gentilini P, Melani L, Riccardi D, Raggi V, Romanelli R (1994) Hepatocellular carcinoma and viral cirrhosis. Hepatology 20:764–765

26. Kew MC, Popper H (1984) Relationship between hepatocellular carcinoma and cirrhosis. Semin Liver Dis 4:136–146

27. Okuda K, Nakashima T, Kojiro M, Kondo Y, Wada K (1989) Hepatocellular carcinoma without cirrhosis in Japanese patients. Gasterenterology 97:140–146

28. Okuda K, Fujimoto I, Hanai A, Urano Y (1987) Changing incidence of hepatocellular carcinoma in Japan. Cancer Res 47:4967–4972

29. Sheu JC, Sung JL, Chen DS, Lai MY, Wang TH, Yu JY, Yang PM, Chuang CN, Yang PC, Lee CS, Hsu HC, Mow SW (1985) Early detection of

hepatocellular carcinoma by real-time ultra-sonography: a prospective study. Cancer 56:660–666

30. Adami HO, Hsing AW, McLaughlin JK, Trichopoulos D, Hacker D, Ekbom A, Persson I (1992) Alcoholism and liver cirrhosis in the etiology of primary liver cancer. Int J Cancer 51:898–902

31. Tanaka A, Nei J, Takase S, Matsuda Y (1986) Effects of ethanol on experimental hepato-carcinogenesis. Hepatology 6:65–72

32. Sorenson TIA, Orholm M, Bentsen K, Hoybye C, Eghoe K, Christopherson P (1984) A prospective evaluation of alcohol abuse and alcoholic liver injury in men as predictors of development of cirrhosis. Lancet 2:241–244

33. Kew MC, Desmyter J, DeGroote G, Frosner G, Roggendorf M, Dienhardt F (1981) Hepatocellular cancer in southern African Blacks: HBeAg, anti-HBe, IgM-anti-HBc and other markers of hepatitis B. Prog Med Virol 27:41–48

34. Hirayama T (1989) A large-scale cohort study on risk factors for primary liver cancer, with special reference to the role of cigarette smoking. Cancer Chemother Pharmacol 23:S114–117

35. Kew MC (1989) Hepatocellular carcinoma with and without cirrhosis: a comparison in southern African Blacks. Gasterenterology 97:136–139

36. Linsell CA, Peers FG (1977) Aflatoxin and liver cell cancer. Trans R Soc Trop Med Hyg 71:471–473

37. Vogelstein B, Kinzler KW (1993) The multistep nature of cancer. *TIG* 9:138–141

38. Weinberg RA (1989) Oncogenes, antioncogenes, and the molecular bases of multistep carcino-genesis. Cancer Res 49:3713–3721

39. Ames BN, Gold LS (1990) Chemical carcino-genesis: too many rodent carcinogens. Proc Natl Acad Sci USA 87:7772–7776

40. Wilson VL, Smith RA, Ma S, Cutler RG (1987) Genomic 5-methyldeoxycytidine decreases with age. J Biol Chem 262:9948–9951

41. Steer CJ (1996) Liver regeration. FASEB J 9:1396–1400

42. Michalopoulos GK (1990) Liver regeneration: molecular mechanisms of growth control. FASEB J 4:176–187

43. Fausto N, Webber EM (1994) Liver regeneration. In: Arias IM, Boyer JL, Fausto N, Jakoby WB, Schachter DA, Shafritz DA (eds) The liver; biology and pathobiology. Raven, New York, pp 1059–1084

44. Haber BA, Mohn KL, Diamond RH, Taub R (1993) Induction patterns of 70 genes during nine days after hepatectomy define the temporal course of liver regeneration. J Clin Invest 91:1319–1326

45. Thompson NL, Mead JE, Braun L, Goyette M, Shank PR, Fausto N (1986) Sequential

protooncogene expression during rat liver regen-eration. Cancer Res 46:3111–3117

46. Diehl AM, Yang SQ, Wolfgang D, Wand G (1992) Differential expression of guanine nucleotide-binding proteins enhances cAMP synthesis in re-generating rat liver. J Clin Invest 89:1706–1712

47. Bottaro DP, Rubin JS, Faletto DL, Chan AM, Kmiecik TE, Vande Wonde GF, Haronson SA (1991) Identification of the hepatocyte growth fac-tor receptor as the c-*met* proto-oncogene product. Science 251:802–804

48. Lok AS, Lai CC (1988) Factors determining the development of hepatocellular carcinoma in hepa-titis B surface antigen carriers: a comparison be-tween families with clusters and solitary cases. Cancer 61:1287–1291

49. Munoz N, Lingao A, Lao J, Esteve J, Viterbo G, Domingo EO, Lansang MA (1989) Patterns of fa-milial transmission of HBV and the risk of devel-oping liver cancer: a case-control study in the Philippines. Int J Cancer 44:981–984

50. Brechot C, Pourcel C, Louis A, Rain B, Tiollais P (1980) Presence of integrated hepatitis B virus DNA sequences in cellular DNA of human hepatocellular carcinoma. Nature 286:533–535

51. Moroy T, Marchio A, Etiemble J, Trepo C, Tiollais P, Buendia MA (1986) Rearrange-ment and enhanced expression of c-*myc* in hepatocellular carcinoma of hepatitis virus in-fected woodchucks. Nature 324:276–279

52. Rogler CE (1990) Recent advances in hepatitis B viruses and hepatocellular carcinoma. Cancer Cells 2:366–369

53. De Souza A, Hankins GR, Washington MK, Fine RL, Orton TC, Jirtle RL (1995) Frequent loss of heterozygosity on 6q at the mannose-6-phosphate/insulin-like growth factor II receptor locus in hu-man hepatocellular tumors. Oncogene 10:1725–1729

54. Farber E (1990) Clonal adaptation during carcinogenesis. Biochem Pharmacol 39:1837–1846

55. Dejean A, Bougueleret L, Grzesdrik KM, Tiollais P (1986) Hepatitis B virus DNA integration in a sequence homologous to v-*erb*-A and steroid receptor genes in a hepatocellular carcinoma. Na-ture 322:70–72

56. Simon D, Searles DB, Cao Y, Sun K, Knowles BB (1985) Chromosomal site of hepatitis B virus (HBV) integration in a human hepatocellular carcinoma-derived cell line. Cytogenet Cell Genet 29:116–120

57. Rogler CE, Sherman M, Su CY, Shafritz DA, Summers J, Shows TB, Henderson A, Kew M (1985) Deletion in chromosome 11p associated with a hepatitis B integration site in hepatocellular carcinoma. Science 230:319–322

58. DeLoia JA, Burk RD, Gearhart (1989) Develop-mental regulation of hepatitis B surface antigen

expression in two lines of hepatitis B virus transgenic mice. J Virol 63:4069–4073

59. Farza H, Salmon AM, Hadchouel M, Moreau JL, Babinet C, Tiollais P, Pourcel C (1987) Hepatitis B surface antigen gene expression is regulated by sex steroids and glucocorticoids in transgenic mice. Proc Natl Acad Sci USA 84:1187–1191

60. Chisari FV, Filippi P, McLachlan A, Milich DR, Riggs M, Lee S, Palmiter RD, Pinkert CA, Brinster RL (1986) Expression of hepatitis B virus large envelope polypeptide inhibits hepatitis B surface antigen secretion in transgenic mice. J Virol 60:880–887

61. Moriyama T, Guilhot S, Klopchin K, Moss B, Pinkert CA, Palmiter RD, Brinster RL, Kanagawa O, Chisari FV (1990) Immunobiology and pathogenesis of hepatocellular injury in hepatitis B virus transgenic mice. Science 248:361–364

62. Ando K, Moriyama T, Guidotti LG, Wirth S, Schreiber RD, Schlicht HJ, Huang S, Chisari FV (1993) Mechanisms of class I restricted immunopathology: a transgenic mouse model of fulminant hepatitis. J Exp Med 178:1541–1554

63. Ando K, Guidotti LG, Cerny A, Ishikawa T, Chisari FV (1994) CTL access to tissue antigen is restricted in vivo. J Immunol 153:482–488

64. Barnaba V, Franco A, Alberti A, Balsano C, Benvenuto R, Balsano F (1989) Recognition of hepatitis B virus envelope proteins by liver-infiltrating T lymphocytes in chronic HBV infection. J Immunol 143:2650–2655

65. Gilles PN, Guerrette DL, Ulevitch RJ, Schreiber RD, Chisari FV (1992) HBsAg retention sensitizes the hepatocyte to injury by physiological concentrations of interferon-gamma. Hepatology 16:655–663

66. Chisari FV, Filippi P, Buras J, McLachlan A, Popper H, Pinkert CA, Palmiter RD, Brinster RL (1987) Structural and pathological effects of synthesis of hepatitis B virus large envelope polypeptide in transgenic mice. Proc Natl Acad Sci USA 84:6909–6913

67. Chisari FV, Klopchin K, Moriyma T, Pasquinelli C, Dunsford HA, Sell S, Pinkert CA, Brinster RL, Palmiter RD (1989) Molecular pathogenesis of hepatocellular carcinoma in hepatitis B virus transgenic mice. Cell 59:1145–1156

68. Dunsford HA, Sell S, Chisari FV (1990) Hepatocarcinogenesis due to chronic liver cell injury in hepatitis B virus transgenic mice. Cancer Res 50:3400–3407

69. Sell S, Hunt JM, Dunsford HA, Chisari FV (1991) Synergy between hepatitis B virus expression and chemical hepatocarcinogens in transgenic mice. Cancer Res 51:1278–1285

70. Huang SN, Chisari FV (1995) Strong, sustained hepatocellular proliferation precedes hepato-carcinogenesis in hepatitis B surface antigen transgenic mice. Hepatology 21:620–626

71. Hagen TM, Huang SN, Curnutte J, Fowler P, Martinez V, Wehr C, Ames BN, Chisari FV (1994) Extensive oxidative DNA damage in hepatocytes of transgenic mice with chronic active hepatitis destined to develop hepatocellular carcinoma. Proc Natl Acad Sci USA 91:12808–12812

72. Kim C-M, Koike K, Saito I, Miyamura T, Jay G (1991) HBx gene of hepatitis B virus induces liver cancer in transgenic mice. Nature 351:317–320

73. Koike K, Moriya K, Iino S, Yotsuyanagi H, Endo Y, Miyamura T, Hurokawa K (1994) High-level expression of hepatitis B virus HBx gene and hepatocarcinogenesis in transgenic mice. Hepatology 19:810–819

74. Ueda H, Ullrich SJ, Gangemi JD, Kappel CA, Ngo L, Feitelson MA, Jay G (1995) Functional inactivation but not structural mutation of *p53* causes liver cancer. Nat Genet 9:41–47

75. Feitelson MA, Zhu M, Duan LX, London WT (1993) Hepatitis Bx antigen and p53 are asssociated in vitro and in liver tissues from patients with primary hepatocellular carcinoma. Oncogene 8:1109–1117

76. Wang XW, Forrester K, Yeh H, Feitelson MA, Gu JR, Harris CC (1994) Hepatitis B virus X protein inhibits p53 sequence-specific DNA binding, transcriptional activity, and association with transcription factor ERCC3. Proc Natl Acad Sci USA 91:2230–2234

77. Unsal H, Yakicier C, Marcais DC, Kew M, Volkmann M, Zentgraf H, Isselbacher KJ, Ozturk M (1994) Genetic heterogeneity of hepatocellular carcinoma. Proc Natl Acad Sci USA 91:822–826

78. Seto E, Mitchel PS, Yen TSB (1990) Trans-activation by the hepatitis B virus X protein depends on AP-2 and other transcription factors. Nature 344:72–74

79. Maguire HF, Hoeffer JP, Siddiqui A (1991). HBV X protein alters the DNA binding specificity of CREB and ATF-2 by protein–protein interactions. Science 252:842–844

80. Schirmacher P, Held WA, Chisari FV, Yang D, Rogler CE (1992) Reactivation of insulin-like growth factor II during hepatocarcinogenesis in transgenic mice suggests a role in malignant growth. Cancer Res 52:2549–2556

81. Kuo MT, Jou JY, Teeter LD, Ikeguchi M, Chisari FV (1992) Activation of multidrug resistance (P-glycoprotein) *mdr3/mdr1a* gene during the development of hepatocellular carcinoma in hepatitis B virus transgenic mice. Cell Growth Differ 52:273–278

82. Pasquinelli C, Bhavani K, Chisari FV (1992) Multiple oncogenes and tumor suppressor genes are structurally and functionally intact during

hepatocarcinogenesis in hepatitis B virus transgenic mice. Cancer Res 52:2823–2829

83. Hollstein M, Sidransky D, Vogelstein B, Harris CC (1991) *p53* mutations in human cancers. Science 253:49–53

84. Hsu IC, Metcalf RA, Sun T, Welsh JA, Wang NJ, Harris CC (1991) Mutational hotspot in the *p53* gene in human hepatocellular carcinomas. Nature 350:427–428

85. Coursaget P, Depril N, Chabaud M, Nandi R, Mayelo V, LeCann P, Yvonnet B (1993) High prevalence of mutations at codon 249 of the *p53* gene in hepatocellular carcinomas from Senegal. Br J Cancer 67:1395–1397

86. Bressac B, Kew M, Wands J, Ozturk M (1991) Selective G to T mutations of *p53* gene in hepatocellular carcinoma from southern Africa. Nature 350:429–431

87. Aguilar F, Hussain SP, Cerutti P (1994) Aflatoxin B_1 induces the transversion of G→T in codon 249 of the *p53* tumor suppressor gene in human hepatocytes. Proc Natl Acad Sci USA 90:8586–8590

88. Aguilar F, Harris CC, Sun T, Hollstein M, Cerutti P (1994) Geographic variation of *p53* mutational profile in nonmalignant human liver. Science 264:1317–1319

89. Dumenco L, Oguey D, Wu J, Messler N, Fausto N (1995) Introduction of a murine *p53* mutation corresponding to human codon 249 into a murine hepatocyte cell line results in growth advantage, but not in transformation. Hepatology 22:1279–1288

90. Fujimoto M, Hampton LL, Wirth PJ, Wang NJ, Xie JP, Thorgeirson SS (1994) Alterations of tumor suppressor genes and allelic losses in human hepatocellular carcinomas in China. Cancer Res 54:281–285

91. Miller RH, Purcell RH (1990) Hepatitis C virus shares amino acid sequence similarity with pestiviruses and flaviviruses as well as members of two plant virus supergroups. Proc Natl Acad Sci USA 87:2057–2061

92. Sakamuro D, Furukawa T, Takegami T (1995) Hepatitis C virus nonstructural protein NS3 transforms NIH 3T3 cells. J Virol 69:3893–3896

93. Simonetti RG, Camma C, Fiorello F, Cottone M, Rapicetta M, Marino L, Fioreni G, Craxi A, Ciccaglione A, Giusepetti R, Stroffolini T, Pagliaro L (1992) Hepatitis C virus infection as a risk factor for hepatocellular carcinoma in patients with cirrhosis: a case-control study. Ann Intern Med 116:97–102

94. Diamantis ID, McGandy CE, Chen T, Liaw Y, Gudat F, Bianchi L (1994) Detection of hepatitis B and C viruses in liver tissue with hepatocellular carcinoma. J Hepatol 20:405–409

95. El-Refaie A, Savage K, Bhattacharya S, Khakoo S, Harrison TJ, El-Batanony M, Soliman E-S,

Nasr S, Mokhtar N, Amer K, Scheuer PJ, Dhillon AP (1996) HCV-associated hepatocellular carcinoma without cirrhosis. Hepatology 24:277–285

96. Negro F, Pacchioni D, Shimizu Y, Miller RH, Bussolati G, Purcell RH, Bonino F (1992) Detection of intrahepatic replication of hepatitis C virus RNA by in situ hybridization and comparison with histopathology. Proc Natl Acad Sci USA 89:2247–2251

97. Blight K, Rowland R, Hall P, Lesniewski RR, Trowbridge R, LaBrooy JT, Gowans EJ (1993) Immunohistochemical detection of the NS4 antigen of hepatitis C virus and its relation to histopathology. Am J Pathol 143:1568–1573

98. Liaw YF, Lee CS, Tsai SL, Liaw BO, Chen TC, Sheen IS, Chu CM (1995) T-cell-mediated autologous hepatocytotoxicity in patients with chronic hepatitis C virus infection. Hepatology 22:1368–1373

99. Minutello MA, Pileri P, Unutmaz D, Censini S, Kuo G, Houghton M, Brunetto MR, Bonine F, Abrignani S (1993) Compartmentalization of T lymphocytes to the site of disease: intrahepatic $CD4^+$ T cells specific for the protein NS4 of hepatitis C virus in patients with chronic hepatitis C. J Exp Med 178:17–25

100. Challen C, Lunec J, Warren W, Collier J, Bassendine MF (1992) Analysis of the *p53* tumor-suppressor gene in hepatocellular carcinomas from Britain. Hepatology 16:1362–1364

101. Tanaka S, Toh Y, Adachi E, Matsumata T, Mori R, Sugimachi K (1993) Tumor progression in hepatocellular carcinoma may be mediated by *p53* mutation. Cancer Res 53:2884–2887

102. Nose H, Imazaeki F, Ohto M, Omata M (1993) *p53* gene mutations and *17p* allelic deletions in hepatocellular carcinoma from Japan. Cancer 72:355–360

103. Oda T, Tsuda H, Scarpa A, Sakamoto M, Hiroshi S (1992) *p53* gene mutation spectrum in hepatocellular carcinoma. Cancer Res 52:6358–6364

104. Debuire B, Paterlini P, Pontisso P, Basso G, May E (1993) Analysis of the *p53* gene in European hepatocellular carcinomas and hepatoblastomas. Oncogene 8:2303–2306

105. Volkmann M, Hofmann WJ, Muler M, Rath U, Otto G, Zentgraf H, Galle PR (1994) *p53* overexpression is frequent in European hepatocellular carcinoma and largely independent of the codon 249 hot spot mutation. Oncogene 9:195–204

106. Ng IO, Chung LP, Tsang SW, Lam CL, Lai CS, Fan ST, Ng M (1994) *p53* gene mutation spectrum in hepatocellular carcinomas in Hong Kong Chinese. Oncogene 9:985–990

107. Sheu JC, Huang GT, Lee PH, Chung JC, Chou HC, Lai MY, Wang JT, Lee HS, Shih LN, Yang

PM, Wang TH, Chen DS (1992) Mutation of *p53* gene in hepatocellular carcinoma in Taiwan. Cancer Res 52:6098–6100

108. Scorsone KA, Zhou YZ, Butel JS, Slagle BL (1992) *p53* mutations cluster at codon 249 in hepatitis B virus-positive hepatocellular carcinomas from China. Cancer Res 52:1635–1638

109. Kubicka S, Truatwein C, Schrem H, Tillman H, Manns M (1995) Low incidence of *p53* mutations in European hepatocellular carcinomas with heterogeneous mutation as a rare event. J Hepatol 23:412–419

110. Fox TR, Watanabe PG (1985) Detection of a cellular oncogene in spontaneous liver tumors of B6C3F1 mice. Science 228:596–597

111. Forrester K, Almoguera C, Han K, Grizzle WE, Perucho M (1987) Detection of high incidence of K-*ras* oncogenes during human colon tumorigenesis. Nature 327:298–303

112. Tada M, Omata M, Ohto M (1990) Analysis of *ras* gene mutations in human hepatic malignant tumors by polymerase chain reaction and direct sequencing. Cancer Res 50:1121–1124

113. Nishida N, Fukuda Y, Komeda T, Kita R, Sando T, Furukawa M, Amenomori M, Shibagaki I, Nakao K, Ikenaga M, Ishizuki K (1994) Amplification and overexpression of the *cyclin* D1 gene in aggressive human hepatocellular carcinoma. Cancer Res 54:3107–3110

114. Simon D, Knowles BB, Weith A (1991) Abnormalities of chromosome 1 and loss of heterozygosity on 1p in primary hepatomas. Oncogene 6:765–770

115. Kuroki T, Fujiwara Y, Tsuchiya E, Nakamori S, Imaoka S, Kanematsu T, Nakumura Y (1995) Accumulation of genetic changes during development and progression of hepatocellular carcinoma: loss of heterozygosity of chromosome arm 1p occurs at an early stage of hepatocarcinogenesis. Genes Chromosom Cancer 13:163–167

116. Buetow KH, Murray JC, Israel JL, London WT, Smith M, Blanquet V, Brechot C, Redeker A, Govindarajah S (1989) Loss of heterozygosity suggests tumor suppressor gene responsible for primary hepatocellular carcinoma. Proc Natl Acad Sci USA 86:8852–8856

117. Fujimori M, Tokino T, Hino O, Kitagawa T, Imamura T, Okamoto E, Mitsunobu M, Ishikawa T, Nakagama H, Harada H, Yagura M, Matsubara K, Nakamura Y (1991) Allelotype study of primary hepatocellular carcinoma. Cancer Res 51:89–93

118. Konishi M, Kikuchi-Yanoshita R, Tanaka K, Sato C, Tsuruta K, Maeda Y, Koike M, Tanaka S, Nakamura Y, Hattori N, Miyaki M (1993) Genetic changes and histopathological grades in human hepatocellular carcinomas. Jpn J Cancer Res 84:893–899

119. Ding SF, Habib NA, Dooley J, Wood C, Bowles L, Delhanty JDA (1991) Loss of constitutional heterozygosity on chromosome 5q in hepatocellular carcinoma without cirrhosis. Br J Cancer 64:1083–1087

120. Horii A, Nakatsuru S, Miyoshi Y, Ichii S, Nagasse H, Ando H, Yanagisawa A, Tsuchiya E, Kato Y, Nakamura Y (1992) The *APC* gene, responsible for familial adenomatous polyposis, is mutated in human gastric cancer. Cancer Res 52:6696–6698

121. Kuroki T, Fujiwara Y, Nakamori S, Imaoka S, Kanematsu T, Nakumura Y (1995) Evidence for the presence of two tumour-suppressor genes for hepatocellular carcinoma on chromosome 13q. Br J Cancer 72:383–385

122. Emi M, Fujiwara Y, Nakajima T, Tsuchiya E, Tsuda H, Hirohashi S, Maeda Y, Tsuruta K, Miyaki M, Nakamura Y (1992) Frequent loss of heterozygosity for loci on chromosome 8p in hepatocellular carcinoma, colorectal cancer, and lung cancer. Cancer Res 52:5368–5372

123. Fujimori M, Monden M, Mori T, Nakamura Y, Emi M (1993) Frequent multiplication of the long arm of chromosome 8 in hepatocellular carcinoma. Cancer Res 53:857–860

124. Wang HP, Rogler CE (1988) Deletions in human chromosome arms 11p and 13q in primary hepatocellular carcinomas. Cytogenet Cell Genet 48:72–78

125. Haber DA, Housman DE (1992) Role of the *WT1* gene in Wilms' tumour. Cancer Surv 12:105–117

126. Zhang X, Xu MJ, Murakami Y, Sachse R, Yasima K, Hirohashi S, Hu SX, Benedict WF, Sekiya T (1994) Deletions of chromosome 13q, mutations in retinoblastoma 1, and retinoblastoma protein state in human hepatocellular carcinoma. Cancer Res 54:4177–4182

127. Sato T, Tanigami A, Yamakawa K, Akiyama F, Kasui F, Sakamoto G, Nakamura Y (1990) Allelotype of breast cancer; cumulative allele losses promote tumour progression in primary breast cancer. Cancer Res 50:7184–7189

128. Tsuda H, Zhang W, Shimosato Y, Yokota J, Terada M, Sugimura T, Miyamura T, Hirohashi S (1990) Allele loss on chromosome 16 associated with progression of human hepatocellular carcinoma. Proc Natl Acad Sci USA 87:6791–6794

129. Stickland JE, Tomlinson IPM, Ramshaw AL, Bromley L, Potter CG, McGee JO'D (1993) Quantification of oncogene dosage in tumours by simultaneous dual-label hybridization. Oncogene 8:223–227

130. Tomlinson IPM, Gammack AJ, Stickland JE, Mann GJ, MacKie RM, Kefford RF, McGee JO'D (1993) Loss of heterozygosity in malignant melanoma at loci on chromosome 11 and 17 implicated in the pathogenesis of other cancers. Genes Chromosom Cancer 7:169–172

131. Bethwaite PB, Koreth J, Herrington CS, McGee JO'D (1995) Loss of heterozygosity occurs at the D11S29 locus on chromosome 11q23 in invasive cervical carcinoma. Br J Cancer 71:814–818

132. Koreth J, Bethwaite PB, McGee JO'D (1995) Mutation at chromosome 11q23 in human non-familial breast cancer: a microdissection microsatellite analysis. J Pathol 176:11–18

133. Jirtle RJ, Hankins GR, Reisenbichler H, Boyer IJ (1994) Regulation of mannose 6-phosphate/insulin-like growth factor-II receptors and transforming growth factor beta during liver tumor promotion with phenobarbital. Carcinogenesis 15:1473–1478

134. Kornfield S (1992) Structure and function of the mannose-6-phosphate/insulin like growth factor II receptors. Annu Rev Biochem 61:307–330

135. Lee SJ, Nathans D (1988) Proliferin secreted by cultured cells binds to mannose 6-phosphate receptors. J Biol Chem 263:3521–3527

136. Dennis PA, Rifkin DB (1991) Cellular activation of latent transforming growth factor beta requires binding to the cation-independent mannose 6-phosphate/insulin-like growth factor type II receptor. Proc Natl Acad Sci USA 88:580–584

137. De Souza A, Hankins GR, Washington MK, Orton TC, Jirtle RL (1995) M6P/IGF2R gene is mutated in human hepatocellular carcinomas with loss of heterozygosity. Nat Genet 11:447–449

138. Xu Y, Goodyer CG, Deal C, Polychronakos C (1993) Functional polymorphism in the parental imprinting of the human IGF2R gene. Biochem Biophys Res Commun 197:747–754

139. Ito H, Tashiro K, Stroud MR, Orntoft TF, Meldgaard P, Singhal AK, Hakomori SI (1991) Specificity and immunobiological properties of monoclonal antibody IMH2, established after immunization with Le(b)/Le(a) glycosphingolipid, a novel extended type 1 chain antigen. Cancer Res 51:4080

140. Yoo Y, Ueda H, Park K, Flanders KC, Lee YI, Jay G, Kim SJ (1996) Regulation of transforming growth factor-beta 1 expression by the hepatitis B virus (HBV) X transactivator: role in HBV pathogenesis. J Clin Invest 97:388–395

141. Carbonara A, Mayr W, Rizzetto M, Contu L, Curtoni ES, DeMarchi M, Farci P, Lavarini C, Olivetti E (1983) Endemic HBV infection, tissue autoantibodies and HLA: analysis of a Sardinian population. Tissue Antigens 22:289–293

142. Board PG, Coggan M, Johnston P, Ross V, Suzuki T, Webb G (1990) Genetic heterogeneity of the human glutathione transferases: a complex of gene families. Pharmacol Ther 48:357–369

143. Brockmoller J, Kerb R, Drakoulis N, Nitz M, Roots I (1993) Genotype and phenotype of glutathione S-transferase class mu isoenzymes mu

and psi in lung cancer patients and controls. Cancer Res 53:1004–1011

144. Skoda RC, Demierre A, McBride OW, Gopnzalez FJ, Meyer UA (1988) Human microsomal xenobiotic epoxide hydrolase: complementary DNA sequence, complementary DNA-directed expression in COS-1 cells, and chromosomal localization. J Biol Chem 263:1549–1554

145. Hasset C, Aicher L, Sidhu S, Omiecinski CJ (1994) Human microsomal epoxide hydrolase: genetic polymorphism and functional expression in vitro of amino acid variants. Hum Mol Genet 3:421–428

146. McGlynn KA, Rosvold EA, Lustbader ED, Hu Y, Clapper ML, Zhou T, Wild CP, Xia XL, Baffoe-Bonnie A, Ofori-Adjei D, Chen GC, London WT, Shen FM, Buetow KH (1995) Susceptibility to hepatocellular carcinoma is associated with genetic variation in the enzymatic detoxification of aflatoxin B$_1$. Proc Natl Acad Sci USA 92:2384–2386

147. Weinberg AG, Mize CE, Worthen HG (1976) The occurrence of hepatoma in the chronic form of hereditary tyrosinemia. J Pediatr 88:434–438

148. MacSween RNM, Scott AR (1973) Hepatic cirrhosis: a clinico-pathological review of 520 cases. J Clin Pathol 26:936–942

149. Salata H, Cortes JM, Enriquez de Salamanca RE, Oliva H, Castro A, Kusak E, Carreno V, Hernandez-Guio C (1985) Porphyria cutanea tarda and hepatocellular carcinoma: frequency of occurrence and related factors. J Hepatol 1:477–487

150. Drinkwater NR (1994) Genetic control of hepatocarcinogenesis in C3H mice. Drug Metab Rev 26:201–208

151. Gariboldi M, Manenti G, Canzian F, Falvella FS, Pierotti MA, Porta GD, Binelli G, Dragani TA (1993) Chromosome mapping of murine susceptibility loci to liver carcinogenesis. Cancer Res 53:209–211

152. Poole TM, Drinkwater NR (1996) Two genes abrogate the inhibition of murine hepatocarcinogenesis by ovarian hormones. Proc Natl Acad Sci USA 93:5848–5853

153. Vesselinovitch SD, Mihailovich (1967) The effect of gonadectomy on the development of hepatomas induced by urethane. Cancer Res 27:1788–179

154. Yamamoto R, Iishi H, Tatsuta M, Tsuji M, Terada N (1991) Roles of ovaries and testes in hepatocellular tumorigenesis induced in mice by 3'-methyl-4-dimethylaminoazobenzene. Int J Cancer 49:83–88

155. Poole TM, Drinkwater NR (1995) Hormonal and genetic interactions in murine hepatocarcinogenesis. Proc Clin Biol Res 391:187–194

156. Poole TM, Drinkwater NR (1996) Strain dependent effects of sex hormones on hepato-carcinogenesis in mice. Carcinogenesis 17:191–196

157. Parkin DM, Pisani P, Ferlay J (1993) Estimates of the worldwide mortality from eighteen major cancers in 1985: implications for prevention and projections of future burden. Int J Cancer 54:594–606

158. Gold LS, Slone TH, Manley NB, Bernstein L (1991) Target organs in chronic bioassays of 533 chemical carcinogens. Environ Health Perspect 93:233–246

Telomeres and Telomerase in Gastrointestinal Cancers

Hidetoshi Tahara[1], Eiji Tahara[1], Eiichi Tahara[2], and Toshinori Ide[1]

Summary. Most gastrointestinal and hepatocellular carcinomas have strong telomerase activity that correlates well with malignant progression, despite their shortened telomeres. Precancerous lesions including gastric intestinal metaplasia, gastric and colorectal adenomas, and normal epithelial stem cells express weak telomerase activity and low levels of human telomerase RNA component (hTR). These observations suggest that telomerase activity responsible for cell immortality may reflect the progressive selection of clonogenic stem cells in the arrest of differentiation, and that telomerase activity may play a pivotal role in an early stage of gastrointestinal carcinogenesis. Moreover, quantitation of telomerase activity and in situ hybridization using hTR as a probe have important clinical applications to the diagnosis of gastroenterological cancer.

Introduction

Telomere maintenance is important for the cellular immortality of cancer cells. Telomerase, a ribonucleoprotein enzyme, is necessary for cancer cells to maintain their telomere and to become immortal. Is there a universal cancer bio-marker? The answer may be yes—telomerase. This chapter reviews cell mortality and telomere maintenance, telomerase activity in gastrointestinal cancers, cancer diagnosis strategy by telomerase detection, and the application of telomerase activity to cancer diagnosis and cancer therapy. Moreover, telomerase-related genes, including telomerase RNA components, and telomere binding proteins are described.

---

[1]Department of Cellular and Molecular Biology, [2]First Department of Pathology, Hiroshima University School of Medicine, Kasumi 1-2-3, Minami-ku, Hiroshima 734, Japan

Cell Immortality and Cancer

To clarify the mechanism of carcinogenesis, it is important to determine the mechanism of cellular senescence and immortalization [1–4]. Normal somatic cells such as fibroblasts have limited proliferative capacity in vitro [5–11]. When the cells reach their limit of proliferation, they stop proliferating even if stimulated with serum or other growth factors, although they can attach to the dish and survive for a long time [8, 9]. These nondividing viable cells are called senescent cells, and this nondividing phase is called the mortality 1 (M1) stage [12] (Fig. 1).

Fusion of young cells with senescent cells, microinjection of mRNA from senescent cells into young normal cells, or addition of membrane fraction protein of senescent cells into a medium of normal young cells inhibits the growth of the young cells. These results indicate that the senescent phenotype is dominant over the young, growing phenotype. Introduction of SV40 large T antigen into normal fibroblasts causes bypass of the M1 stage, and these cells continue to proliferate over the M1 stage; but most SV40-transformed cells cease proliferation after 20 to 30 population doublings over the M1 stage [13]. This second phase is called mortality 2 (M2) stage (Fig. 1). These observations clearly indicate that SV40 large T antigen can bypass the M1 stage but is insufficient for cell immortalization. Inactivation of SV40 large T antigen of life-extended cells or immortalized cells after SV40 transformation induces growth arrest with the morphology of senescent cells [14], suggesting that at least two-step genetic alterations are necessary for immortalization, which regulates cell proliferation in either the M1 or M2 stage. The cells that pass through both M1 and M2 stages acquire unlimited proliferative capacity and are called immortalized cells (Fig. 1).

One of the most important phenotypes of cancer cells is cell immortality. If cancer cells cannot

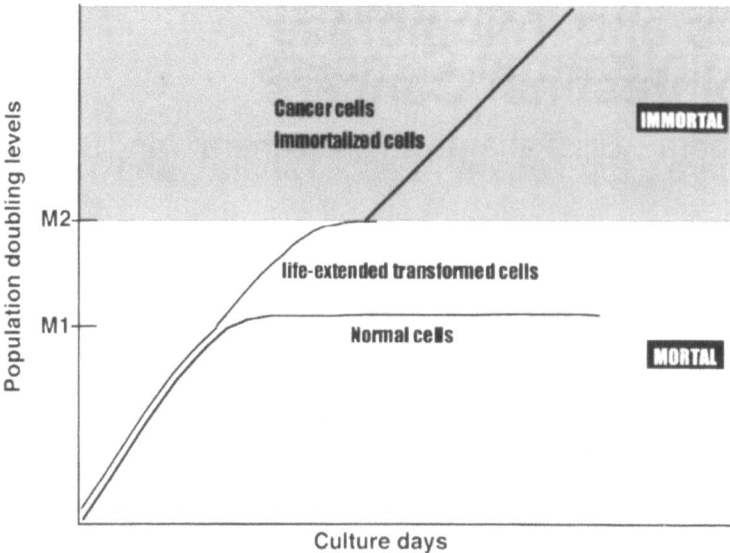

Fig. 1. Cell mortality and immortalization in human fibroblasts

obtain or lose their immortal phenotype, they may die after several proliferations, even if they retain all other cancer phenotypes, such as autonomous growth, anchorage-independent growth, or metastasis. Therefore cell immortality may be the essential, universal phenotype of cancer, although it is not sufficient for growing into mature cancer cells.

Senescence and Immortalization Regulatory Genes

Microinjection of mRNA from normal senescent cells into normal young cells inhibits the induction of DNA synthesis [15], indicating that normal senescent cells express antiproliferative genes that regulate the cell cycle. Because the senescent phenotype is dominant, cDNAs or proteins that express at high levels in senescent cells are cloned through various approaches [16–19]. During functional experiments in which the cDNA library of senescent cells was transfected into normal fibroblasts to clone a cDNA that inhibits DNA synthesis, *p21/sdi-1* was cloned and was found to be an inhibitor of cyclin-dependent kinase [19–21]. Induction of *p21* in normal young fibroblasts causes inhibition of induction of DNA synthesis [19]; *p21* is a mediator of inhibition of DNA synthesis in senescent human fibroblasts. Introduction of SV40 large T antigen can bring about bypass of the M1 stage; this antigen binds to p53

and Rb protein and inactivates their function. M1-bypassed transformed cells (called life-extended transformed cells) can continue proliferation for about 20 to 30 population doublings beyond the M1 stage; but they then cease proliferation and enter crisis (M2 stage). Expression of *p21* is reduced in SV40-transformed cells owing to the inactivation of p53 by its binding to SV40 large T antigen, resulting in inhibition of the transactivation of *p21* [22]. However, an increase in *p21* expression still occurs with increasing cell division, even when SV40 large T antigen completely inactivates p53. When T antigen is inactivated in young SV40-transformed cells, expression of *p21* increases up to the same level as in normal cells of the same age [22]. When T antigen is inactivated in life-extended SV40-transformed cells, *p21* expression increases over that of normal senescent cells. These findings indicate that an increase in *p21* expression with cell division in normal and SV40-transformed cells occurs by a p53-independent pathway [22].

Telomeres

At the end of the human chromosome are long 5'-TTAGGG-3' DNA repeats called telomeres [23, 24] (Fig. 2). Telomeres consist of DNA and proteins [24–26]. Human telomeres have been demonstrated to associate with the nuclear matrix protein fraction, suggesting that telomeres are attached to the nuclear matrix [27]. In eukaryotic cells the telomere DNA sequence cannot be completely copied by the replication mechanism [28] (Fig. 3), resulting in shortening of the telomere DNA; this phenomenon is revealed by Southern analysis of terminal restriction fragment (TRF) lengths using TTAGGG repeat oligonucleotide probes [29, 30].

The standard method for measuring telomere length begins with human genomic DNA being digested with HinfI and RsaI, which frequently cuts restriction endonucleases, digesting the internal subtelomeric region but not the telomeric region (Fig. 2). Digested DNA is analyzed by electrophoresis in agarose gels (0.7%), blotting the resulting bands onto a filter, and hybridization with labeled probes of TTAGGG repeat oligonucleotide. TRFs consist of the TTAGGG repeat sequence region and the subtelomeric region [31, 32] (Fig. 2). The function of the subtelomeric region is unknown. It is not required for aberrant chromosome breakage and healing by telomerase, which can synthesize telomere sequences.

Telomere reduction is observed in normal somatic cells with cell division, but not in immortalized cells established from in vitro transformed

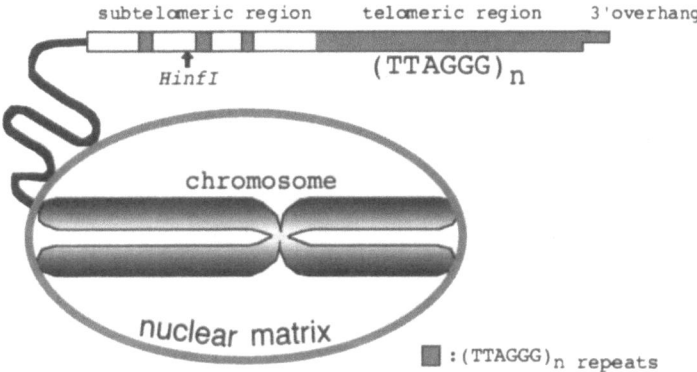

Fig. 2. Chromosome structure and telomere. Telomeres consist of a TTAGGG repeat at the end of the chromosome and are attached to the nuclear matrix. They may stabilize the chromosome

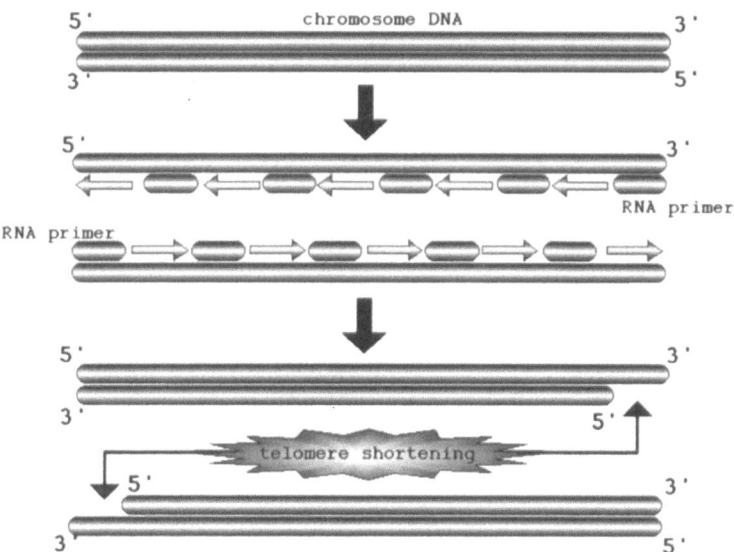

Fig. 3. End replication problems

cells and in vivo cancer cells. Hence telomere reduction may be associated with cellular senescence [33, 34].

The immortalizing frequency of in vitro human cells is low, even after transformation with an oncogenic virus such as SV40 [13]. Immortalized cells, especially cancer cells, have widely variable TRF length, but most cancer cells have short telomeres, about 1 to 6 kbp length. Interestingly, one study showed that the telomere size of each chromosome is different for each cell, and the specificity of the chromosome is not observed in these cells. In regard to telomere shortening, even the cells of a clonal cell line seem to be highly heterogeneous. Furthermore, even in

telomerase-positive cell lines, subclones of the cell lines may share a variety of telomerase activities.

Telomerase: Characteristics and RNA Component

Telomerase activity was first detected in *Tetrahymena* in 1985 [35], and its cDNA was cloned in 1995 by Greider. *Tetrahymena* telomerase protein consists of two protein subunits, p80 and p95 [36].

Human telomerase was first detected by Morin using HeLa cells, but neither cDNA nor protein has yet been cloned [37]. Telomerase activity of both *Tetrahymena* and other species, including humans, is sensitive to ribonuclease (RNase)

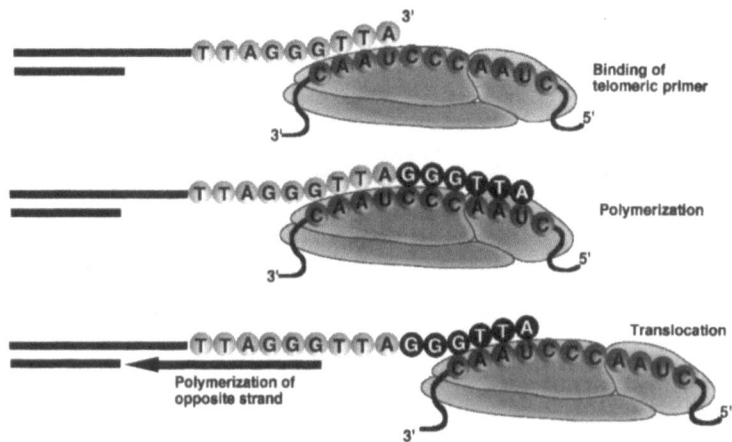

Fig. 4. Telomere elongation by telomerase. Telomerase binds at the 3′ end of the chromosome and is then polymerized with TTAGGG on the RNA template. Telomerase is next translocated and polymerized again

Table 1. Sequence of telomeres and size of telomerase RNA components

Organism	Telomere sequence	RNA component
Human	TTAGGG	450 nt
Mouse	TTAGGG	450 nt
Didymium (slime molds)	TTAGGG	
Physarum (slime molds)	TTAGGG	
Trypanosoma (flagellates)	TTAGGG	
Cladosporium fulvum (fungi)	TTAGGG	
Neurospora (fungi)	TTAGGG	
Podospora (fungi)	TTAGGG	
Histoplasma (fungi)	TTAGGG	
Tetrahymena (ciliates)	TTGGGG	160 nt
Saccharomyces cerevisiae	TG(1–3)	1300 nt
Oxytricha	TTTTGGGG	190 nt
Euplotes	TTTTGGGG	190 nt

nt = length of the RNAs in nucleotides.

treatment [35, 37], suggesting that telomerase consists of an RNA component in addition to protein subunits. The telomerase RNA component is essential as a template to elongate telomere sequences from 5' to the 3' end of the chromosome (Fig. 4). The opposite strand of chromosome DNA is probably synthesized by DNA polymerase. The end of the chromosome consists of a 3' overhanging single strand. The precise overhang size is unknown, it is probably not long, perhaps around 12 bases.

The telomerase RNA component was first cloned by Greider in *Tetrahymena* [38]. Mouse and human telomerase RNA components also have been identified [39]. The sequence and size of telomerase RNA components vary among organisms [40] (Table 1). At the end of chromosome are also telomere-binding proteins that may regulate telomere elongation by telomerase, telomere shortening, blockage of degradation by nuclease, and replication. However, telomere-binding protein has not yet been cloned in mammalian cells except for one telomere-binding protein (TRF1) cloned by Chong et al. [41]. Telomere-binding protein is undoubtedly important for understanding telomere maintenance and telomerase regulation [41].

Telomerase in Cancer

Telomerase maintains the telomere length by its reverse transcriptase activity. It is believed to bind to the overhanging 3' end of the telomere sequence and to synthesize the telomere sequences at the end of chromosomes [24] (Fig. 4). Telomere maintenance is a prerequisite for unlimited proliferation. All cancer cell lines, almost all in vitro immortalized cells, and all germ line cells have telomerase activity to maintain the telomere length; and they are able to proliferate indefinitely. It was first reported that the human cancer cell HeLa had telomerase activity, detected by a conventional telomerase assay [37]. Other cancer cells and cancer tissues have not been examined because conventional detection methods are not sensitive enough to detect telomerase activity in human cells and tissues. In 1994 Kim et al. reported a simple polymerase chain reaction (PCR)-based telomerase assay method, the telomeric repeat amplification protocol (TRAP) [42]. They reported that many cancer cell lines and a variety of cancer tissues had telomerase activity, whereas

normal cells and tissues were telomerase-negative. These observations suggested that telomerase activation was necessary for the immortal growth of cancer cells. Hence telomerase activity was expected to be a useful marker for the universal diagnosis of human cancers [43].

Telomerase Assay

Telomerase was first detected by Greider and Blackburn in *Tetrahymena* in 1985. In this series of experiments, a single telomeric strand such as $(TTGGGG)_4$ was used as a primer for the telomerase assay [35]. Telomerase elongated the telomere DNA repeats on the oligonucleotide primer, incorporating ^{32}P-labeled deoxynucleotides. For this assay about 10^8 cells were necessary to extract the telomerase and to detect telomerase activity. However, this conventional assay was not sensitive enough to detect telomerase activity in mammalian cells and tissues, especially small numbers of cells or small tissues such as biopsy samples.

The new telomerase assay—the PCR based on the TRAP assay developed by Kim et al.—is a sensitive, simple technique that can detect telomerase activity in only a few cancer cells [42] (Fig. 5). A nonisotope method is also available, but its sensitivity is about 10-fold lower than the isotope methods under the same conditions (Fig. 5); either method is sensitive enough and convenient for detection of telomerase activity in mammalian cells and tissues. Generally, 6 μg protein in tissue samples or 1000 cells for cultured cells is sufficient for detecting telomerase activity in biopsy samples, fine-needle aspiration samples, and microdissection samples.

The PCR-based telomerase assay has been applied to many tumor tissue samples and cultured cells, and it has been found that some samples contain an inhibitor of the telomerase assay, the Taq polymerase inhibitor [44]. This inhibitor interferes with cancer diagnosis by the PCR-based TRAP assay. To eliminate this problem an internal telomerase assay standard (ITAS) was developed [45] (Fig. 6) that consists of 150 basepairs (bp) of rat myogenin oligonucleotide connected to TS (5'-AATCCGTCGAGCAGAGTT-3') and CX (5'-CCCTTACCCTTACCCTTACCCTAA-3') primers at each end. If the Taq polymerase inhibitor is present, the ITAS is not amplified sufficiently. After applying the TRAP assay using ITAS, telomerase activity can be standardized ac-

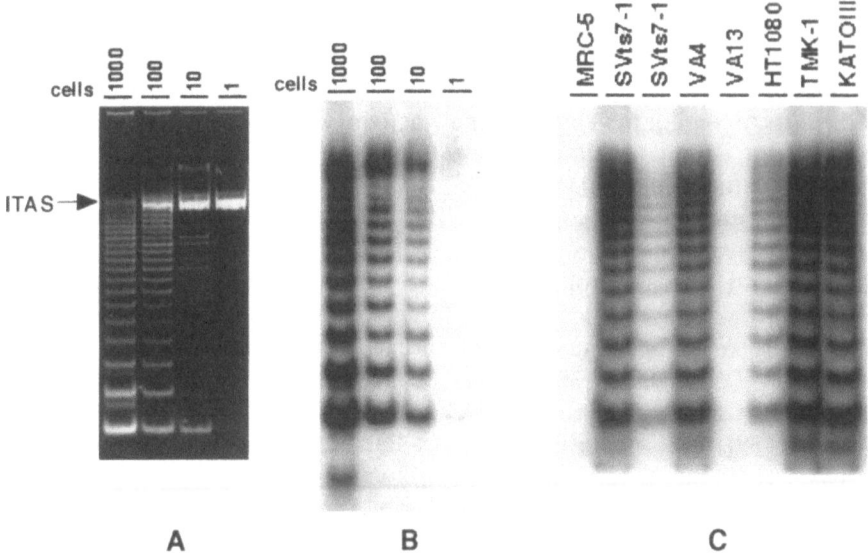

Fig. 5. Telomerase activity in cultured cells. Sensitivity of the TRAP assay by the radio isotope (RI) method and the non-RI method. The same dilution series of the TMK-1 cell extracts was used in both non-RI method (A) and RI method (B). (C) Detection of telomerase activity in a variety of cultured cells. *MRC-5*, normal human fibroblast; *SVts7-1E*, early passage SV40-immortal cell line; *SVts7-1L*, late passage SV40-immortal cell line; *VA4*, *VA13*, *HT1080*, SV40-immortal cell line; *TMK-1*, *KATOIII*, human gastric cell lines; *ITAS*, internal telomerase assay standard

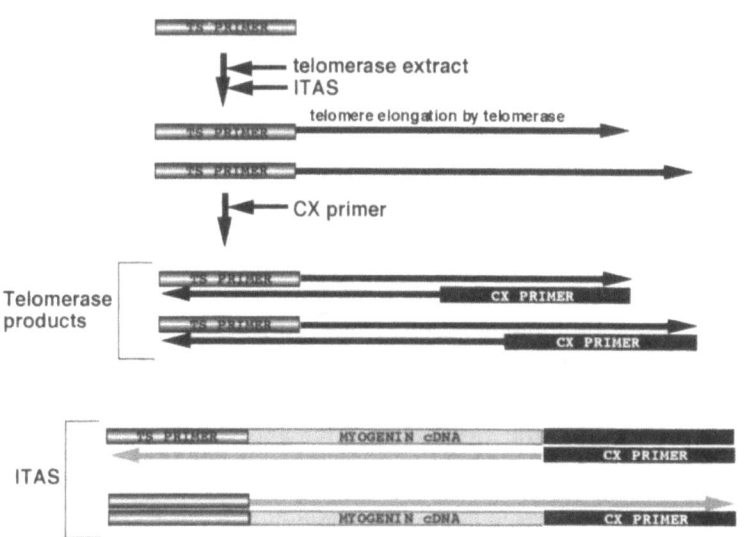

Fig. 6. TRAP assay with internal telomerase assay standard (*ITAS*)

cording to the intensity of the ITAS, band and telomerase ladders using an image analyzer. Another internal control has been developed by Oncor (Gaitherburg, Maryland) as well. This TRAPeze kit includes the control and is useful for quantitating telomerase activity. It is a 36-bp in-ternal control that appears at the bottom of the telomerase signal.

Semiquantitation of telomerase products by fluorescent sequencer has been reported by Ohyashiki [46]. In addition, a hybridization pro-tection assay (HPA) was developed by Chugai

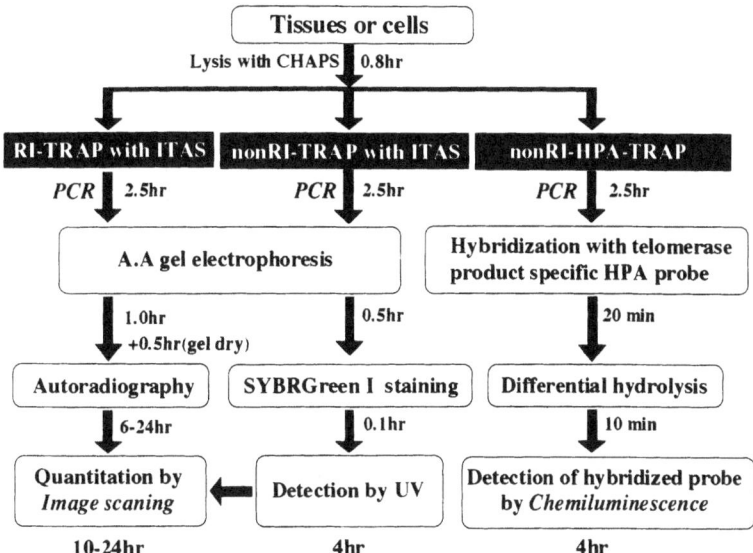

Fig. 7. Quantitation of telomerase assay with ITAS and the hybridization protection assay (HPA). *PCR*, polymerase chain reaction; *CHAPS*, 3[(3-cholamidopropyl)dimethylamino]-1-propanesulfonate; *A.A*, acrylamide; *UV*, ultraviolet light

Pharmaceutical (Tokyo, Japan) that can detect telomerase activity quantitatively, easily, and quickly [47]. This assay can quantitate telomerase activity only 30 min after the TRAP assay (Fig. 7). Quantitation of telomerase activity is necessary for cancer diagnosis because some normal cells (e.g., activated lymphocytes, epithelial cells, skin cells, and hair follicles) contain weak telomerase activity [48–52]. Although cancer cells usually display higher telomerase activity than normal cells, false-negative results may be obtained in the presence of polymerase inhibitors (e.g., Taq).

Telomere Maintenance and Telomerase Activity in Cultured Cells

In vitro cultured cells have two phenotypes: the mortal phenotype (obtained in normal fibroblasts) and the immortal phenotype (obtained in cancer cell lines or in vitro transformed immortalized cells). The most apparent difference between mortal cells and immortal cells is the proliferative capacity strongly associated with telomere maintenance [32]. Although the telomere shortens progressively with each cell division in normal somatic cells, the immortal cells (e.g., cancer cell lines and virally transformed immortalized cells), which have infinite replicative capacity, do not exhibit an apparent alteration in TRF length with

cell divisions [2]. These results suggest that telomere maintenance is involved in cellular immortality.

Using the standard TRAP assay, Kim et al. reported that 100% of human cancer cell lines have detectable telomerase activity [42]. We also searched for telomerase activity in a variety of human immortalized cells, including cancer cell lines and in vitro transformed immortalized cells. Most (99%) of the cancer cell lines expressed strong telomerase activity; the exception was the cancer cell line Saos-2, which is derived from osteosarcoma (unpublished data).

In terms of cell mortality and immortality, the human fibroblast is a good model for examining the mechanism of immortalization, as the human fibroblast has two distinct stages: M1 and M2. Some in vitro transformed immortalized cells are not always tumorigenic and have weak as no detectable telomerase activity. What is of more interest is that these telomerase-negative immortalized cells have an elongated TRF compared to that of young, normal cells [29] (unpublished data). Why are these cell lines immortal, and why are their telomeres long but without telomerase activity? At present, there is no explanation for these phenomena, although there are several possibilities. One is that a telomerase-independent telomere maintenance mechanism exists for these cell lines, so the cells can continue to proliferate forever, maintaining a long telomere by a telomerase-independent pathway. In the case of yeast, telomerase-independent telomere recombination was found to maintain their telomeres [53]. In humans there is no evidence of telomere maintenance by the recombination-like mechanism as in yeast. Another is that telomerase activity is suppressed by an unknown factor that recognizes the long telomere. If telomeres shorten when dividing, the telomerase activity "turns on" and elongates the telomere; thus telomerase-negative cell lines can maintain a long telomere. The mechanism of telomere maintenance in telomerase-negative immortal cell lines must be clarified in the future.

Telomerase Activity in Hepatocellular Carcinoma

About 20000 persons die to hepatocellular carcinoma (HCC) every year in Japan. Although early detection of HCC is important, it is often difficult to diagnosis small, early foci. If telomerase activity is activated in all HCCs, detection of telomerase activity may serve as a useful tool for diagnosing this disease. We examined telomerase activity in malignant and nonmalignant human liver tissues obtained by needle biopsy or surgical resection to determine if malignant progression correlates with telomerase expression. Telomerase activity was detected in 85% of HCCs regardless of tumor stage, histological type, or tumor size, whereas normal tissues did not have detectable telomerase activity [55]. Interestingly, 82% (37/45) of small HCCs (<3 cm) that were difficult diagnose by other methods expressed telomerase activity, indicating that telomerase activity is useful for early detection of cancer cells in liver with fine needle aspiration [55]. Furthermore, 68% (13/19) of well differentiated HCCs had strong telomerase activity [55]. Another study reported similar results [56].

Weak telomerase activity is sometimes detected in nontumor tissues and requires explanation. If normal tissues are completely telomerase-negative, weak telomerase activity may be due to small number of cancer cells that cannot be recognized histologically. If some normal tissues, such as regenerating cells, express telomerase activity, nontumor lesions may have weak telomerase activity. Studies indicate that normal lymphocytes have telomerase activity, though their activity is weak compared to that of cancer cells. Therefore contamination by migrating lymphocytes in nontumor tissues may be responsible for the weak telomerase activity. Furthermore, in patients with chronic liver disease, including cirrhosis and chronic viral hepatitis, it is possible that regenerated or dividing hepatocytes express weak telomerase activity. At present, it is impossible to

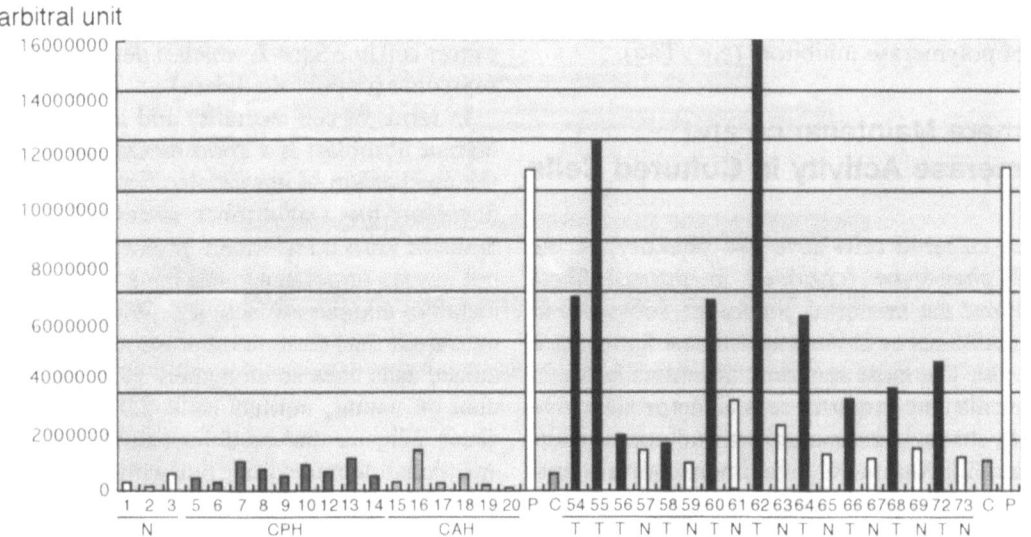

Fig. 8. Telomerase activity in hepatocellular carcinoma. Telomerase was measured by the TRAP assay with ITAS at 0.6μg protein extracts. Telomerase activity was quantitated by the intensity of the telomerase ladder and ITAS band. *N*, normal liver; *CPH*, chronic persistent hepatisis; *CAH*, chronic active hepatisis; *C*, negative control; *P*, positive control (cancer cell line TMK-1, 1000 cells)

distinguish whether the activity in precancerous lesions is derived from migrating lymphocytes or regenerating stem cells. This question can be clarified using the in situ telomerase assay.

At present the best strategy for detecting telomerase activity is to quantify it. In the case of HCCs, a telomerase assay was performed by TRAP assay with ITAS at 0.6 µg of protein. A large amount of extract (>6 µg) sometimes shows reduced telomerase activity owing to inhibition of the PCR reaction. Although some inhibition exists at 0.6 µg protein, telomerase activity in HCCs is clearly higher than in nontumor tissues (Fig. 8). Despite the difficulty of quantitating telomerase activity with ITAS or other methods, telomerase activity should be considered a powerful biomarker for early detection of HCC.

Telomerase Activity in Gastric Carcinomas

Genetic alterations in multiple oncogenes, tumor suppressor genes, and DNA repair genes are observed in gastrointestinal cancer. We analyzed

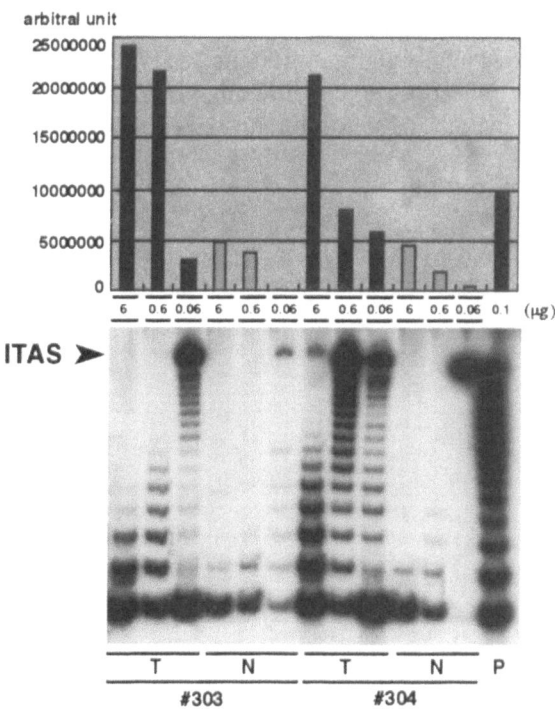

Fig. 9. Telomerase activity in gastric tissues. Telomerase was measured using the TRAP assay with ITAS at 6.0, 0.6, and 0.06 µg protein extracts. Telomerase activity was quantitated by the intensity of the telomerase ladder and ITAS band

telomerase activity in 20 gastric carcinomas, including two early gastric carcinomas, four metastatic lymph node foci, and recurrent tumors. The results showed that 85% (17/20) of the gastric carcinomas had strong telomerase activity, whereas normal mucosa did not have detectable telomerase activity. One of three telomerase-negative samples were stage II poorly differentiated adenocarcinoma. Two of three telomerase-negative samples were mucinous adenocarcinoma, stage III and IV. Hiyama reported that gastric cancer had strong telomerase activity, and that telomerase-positive cancer patients had significantly shorter survival than telomerase-negative patients [57]. Although some extracts contained an inhibitor of Taq DNA polymerase, telomerase activity in gastric adenocarcinomas was higher than that in normal tissues, which had weak telomerase activity (Fig. 9). Hence telomerase activity may be a good biomarker for both diagnosis and prognosis of gastric cancer.

Telomerase Activity in Colorectal Carcinomas

The human colorectal carcinoma harbors many genetic alterations in p53, APC, ras, DCC, and cell cycle regulatory genes. In addition to these genetic changes, colorectal and gastric cancers possess the important feature of cell immortality, which is one of the most important properties of the cancer phenotype. Telomerase activity in colorectal cancers was first reported by Chadeneau et al. in 1995, who found that 14 of 15 (93%) colorectal adenocarcinomas contained strong telomerase activity, and that telomerase activity was not seen in nonmalignant diseases, including diverticular disease, Crohn's disease, and adenomatous polyps [58]. We have found that most colorectal adenomas had telomerase activity [44]. Although most of colorectal adenomas contain weak telomerase activity, the activity is sensitive to RNase treatment. Dilution of the extract shows ladder extension of telomerase products, probably due to dilution of the inhibitor of the telomerase assay (e.g., Taq polymerase inhibitor). Mixing an extract of telomerase-positive cancer cells with an extract of the weakly positive precancerous lesion shows a reduction of the telomerase ladder in a protein concentration-dependent manner [44]. Other experiments revealed that strong Taq polymerase inhibitor is present in most gastrointestinal tissues, both normal and cancer tissues. The weak telomerase activity may account for stem cells or migrating lymphocytes described below. We also found that 95% of colorectal adenocarcinomas displayed strong telomerase activity regardless of the tumor stage or histological type, whereas normal colorectal mucosa did not display activity using the standard TRAP assay. Telomerase activity in colorectal lesions was also sensitive to RNase treatment or heat treatment prior to use of the TRAP assay. Quantitation of telomerase activity using ITAS or other convenient quantitation method may provide an early diagnosis of colorectal cancer (our unpublished data).

Telomerase Activity in Normal Tissues and Precancerous Lesions

Telomerase activation occurred in a high percentage of early stage gastric and colorectal cancers. These results indicate that telomerase activation may play a pivotal role in early gastrointestinal carcinogenesis. We analyzed telomerase activity in gastric and colorectal precancerous lesions to determine if malignant progression depends on telomerase activation and at what stage of carcinogenesis the cells express detectable telomerase activity (Fig. 10). Thirty-five percent

of gastric intestinal metaplasia (complete type) shows telomerase activity and overexpression of human telomerase RNA component (hTR). It is exciting that the number of *Helicobacter pylori* organisms correlates well with the degree of hTR expression and telomerase activity [59, 60], suggesting that *H. pylori* infection may be a strong trigger for hTR overexpression in gastric intestinal metaplasia, which may precede telomerase activation [59, 60]. Chronic mitogenesis due to stem cell hyperplasia caused by *H. pylori* infection, which induces the production of both reactive oxygen species and reactive nitrogen species, could facilitate increased mutagenesis in gastric mucosa. In fact, in situ hybridization studies have demonstrated localization of hTR expression in excessive proliferating stem cells in gastric intestinal metaplasia, and more than 80% of gastric cancers express hTR at a higher level than in the corresponding mucosa [59]. Therefore low-level telomerase activity is likely to be present in proliferating stem cells showing Ki-67-positive cells. Gastric and colorectal adenomas express telomerase activity at low levels.

We have evidence that some gastric intestinal metaplasia and gastric and colorectal adenomas share not only epigenetic changes but also genetic alterations containing *p53* and *APC* mutations, as well as microsatellite instability and CD44 abnormal transcripts [61]. A direct in vivo test based on the hypothesis that telomerase reactivation is an

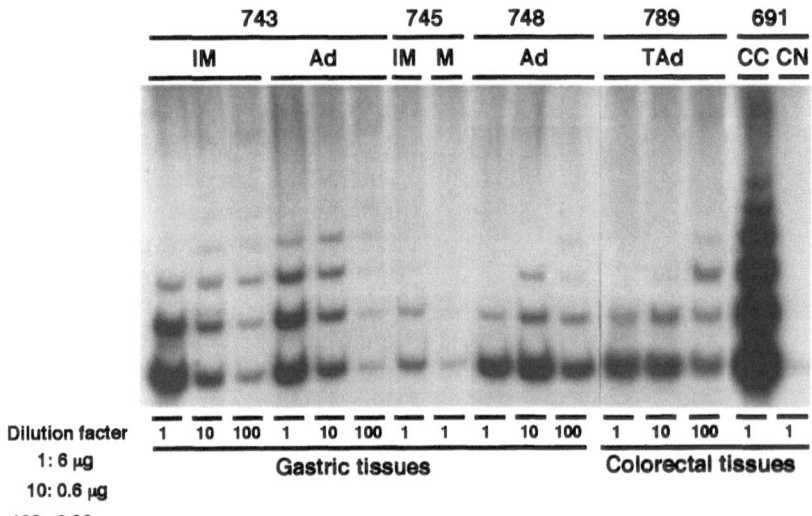

Fig. 10. Telomerase activity in gastrointestinal precancerous lesions. Telomerase was measured using the TRAP assay at 6.0, 0.6, and 0.06 μg protein extracts. *IM*, intestinal metaplasia; *Ad*, adenoma; *TAd*, tubular adenoma; *CC*, colorectal cancer; *CN*, normal colon

obligatory step in gastrointestinal carcinogenesis via these genetic alterations in the tumor suppressor genes and genetic instability should be developed.

Application for Cancer Diagnosis and Cancer Therapy

The results of telomerase studies on breast, colon, stomach, kidney, liver, lung, ovary, prostate, skin, and bladder cancers indicate that telomerase activity may serve as a powerful additional tool for cancer diagnosis, and that telomerase could be a new target for anticancer therapy [42, 44, 49, 51, 54–58, 62–69].

Oshimura's group reported that the introduction of chromosome 3 into renal carcinoma cell lines suppressed telomerase activity and subsequently induced a crisis of introduced cells [70], suggesting that the genes on chromosome 3 may contain repressive function of telomerase activity. The possible regulation of telomerase in normal cells may be implicated in telomerase repressor genes, which is consistent with results from cell

fusion. When the function of telomerase repressor genes is blocked, telomerase activity is "turned on" and maintains the telomere. Moreover, the introduction of hTR antisense nucleotide into HeLa cells, which have strong telomerase activity and express hTR, results in a reduction of telomerase activity and TRF length, and ultimately cell division stops [39]. Peptide nucleic acids (PNAs) which recognized hTR were also effective in inhibiting telomerase activity [71]. Although telomere length in cancer tissues and cancer cell lines is variable, repression of telomerase activity could bring about a reduction in telomere length; and in the case of the cells that have a short telomere it could cause genetic instability and then cell death. In the case of cancer cells that have a long telomere, a block of telomerase activity using antitelomerase drugs, allows the cells to proliferate many times until the telomere shortens (Fig. 11). Most human cancers are known to have reduced telomere length [72–78]. We also found that telomere reduction (under 10 Kb) was detected in over 50% of primary gastric cancer in a parallel with advanced tumor stage (unpublished data). The possible antitelomerase drugs may be effective for cancer cells with short telomeres but

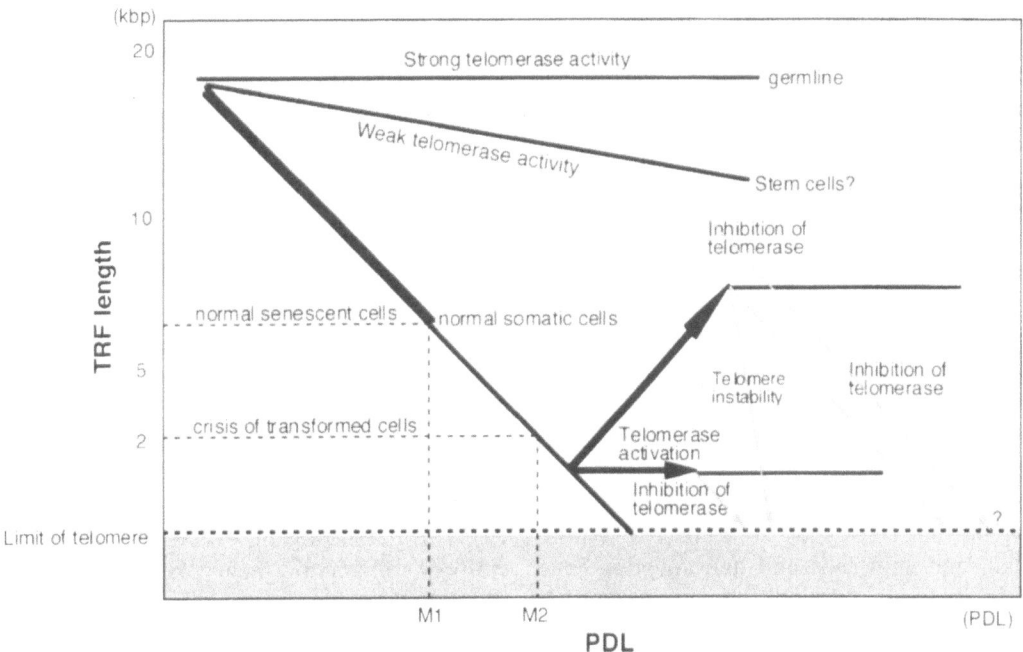

Fig. 11. Telomere shortening with age and effect of antitelomerase drugs on terminal restriction fragment (*TRF*) length. Telomere shortening with age was observed in normal somatic cells but not in the germ line and cancer cell lines. Stem cells may have a gradually reduction of telomere length, although they have weak telomerase activity. *PDL*, population doubling levels; *M1*, *M2*, mortality stages 1 and 2

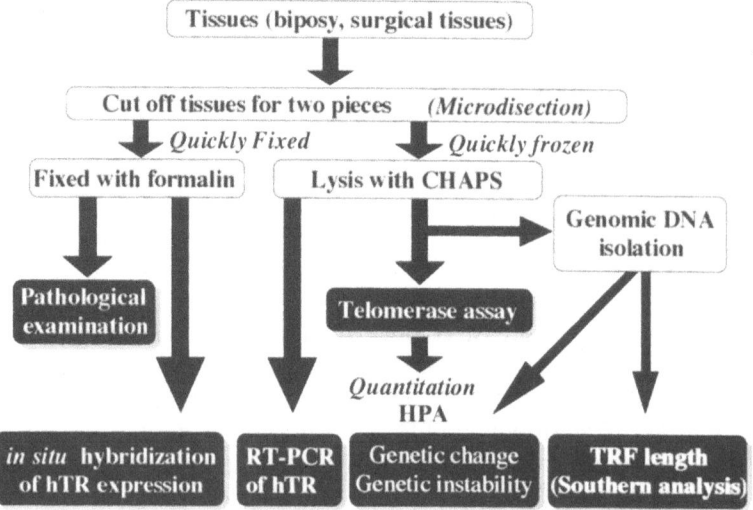

Fig. 12. Strategy of cancer diagnosis according to telomerase activity, human telomerase RNA component (*hTR*) expression, and genetic instability. *RT-* *PCR*, reverse transcripture-polymerase chain reaction; *TRF*, terminal restriction fragment

not for those with long telomeres (Fig. 11). Even if the antitelomerase drugs did not effect inhibition of cancer cell proliferation immediately, decreased telomerase activity by antitelomerase drugs could suppress the proliferation of cancer cells in metastatic lesions, as metastatic cancer cells may divide many times until they are visible in a metastatic lesion. This hypothesis may shed light on the possibility that telomerase inhibitors provide a new strategy for preventing cancer metastasis.

In *Tetrahymena* experiments, mutation of the telomerase RNA component of *Tetrahymena* elongated the mutant telomere at the end of the chromosome and maintained telomere length; eventually, however, the *Tetrahymena* died, suggesting that modification of the telomere sequence causes telomere instability dramatically [79]. Mutated telomerase RNA is also a possibility for cancer therapy in telomerase-positive cells with both long and short telomeres, even if telomerase activity was not suppressed (Fig. 11).

Some normal cells, such as peripheral blood, epithelial, and skin cells and hair follicles have telomerase activity, although the activity is weak compared to that in cancer cells [50, 80]. In the case of human stem cells with a CD34$^+$/CD38$^+$ phenotype purified from adult bone marrow, telomere reduction is observed (Fig. 11). It would be of interest to determine if the antitelomerase

drugs used to treat cancer patients produce similar effects in normal stem cells. The growth advantage of telomerase-positive cancer cells may be more effectively counteracted by treatment with antitelomerase drugs than that in normal stem cells, which express weak telomerase activity and a long telomere (Fig. 11).

A new cancer diagnostic strategy using telomerase activity and hTR expression is shown in Fig. 12. Endoscopically or surgically isolated tissues are dissected into two pieces quickly. One is then rapidly fixed with formalin for examination of hTR expression by in situ hybridization and histological examination, and the other is quick-frozen and stored at −80°C until a TRAP assay is undertaken. The frozen tissues are sectioned and lysed with buffer containing CHAPS for the telomerase assay. The activity is then quantitated by several methods (e.g., HPA or image scanning). The genetic changes, genetic instability, and TRF length can be analyzed in the remaining tissues after lysis, which contain genomic DNA (Fig. 12). This diagnostic algorithm may provide a new strategy for genetic diagnosis of gastrointestinal cancer during the twenty-first century.

References

1. Harley CB, Kim NW, Prowse KR, Weinrich SL, Hirsch KS, West MD, Bacchetti S, Hirte HW,

Counter CM, Greider CW, Wright WE, Shay JW (1994) Telomerase, cell immortality, and cancer, vol LVIX. Cold Spring Harbor Laboratory Press, Cold Spring Harbor, NY, pp 1–9

2. Harley CB, Villeponteau B (1995) Telomeres and telomerase in aging and cancer. Curr Opin Genet Dev 5:249–255

3. Sager R (1991) Senescence as a mode of tumor suppression. Environ Health Perspect 93:59–62

4. Shay JW, Wright WE, Werbin H (1993) Toward a molecular understanding of human breast cancer: a hypothesis. Breast Cancer Res Treat 25:83–94

5. Praeger B (1986) In-vitro studies of aging. Dermatol Clin 4:359–369

6. Hayflick L (1980) Cell aging. Annu Rev Gerontol Geriatr 1:26–67

7. Hayflick L (1979) Cell biology of aging. Fed Proc 38:1847–1850

8. Hayflick L (1965) The limited in vitro lifespan of human diploid cell strains. Exp Cell Res 37:614–636

9. Hayflick L, Moorhead PS (1961) The serial cultivation of human diploid cell strains. Exp Cell Res 25:585–621

0. Goldstein S (1969) Lifespan of cultured cells in *Progeria*. Lancet 1:424

1. Goldstein S (1990) Replicative senescence: the human fibroblast comes of age. Science 249:1129–1133

2. Shay JW, Wright WE, Werbin H (1991). Defining the molecular mechanisms of human cell immortalization. Biochim Biophys Acta 1072:1–7

3. Shay JW, Wright WE (1989) Quantitation of the frequency of immortalization of normal human diploid fibroblasts by SV40 large T-antigen. Exp Cell Res 184:109–118

4. Tsuyama N, Miura M, Kitahira M, Ishibashi S, Ide T (1991) SV40 T-antigen is required for maintenance of immortal growth in SV40-transformed human fibroblasts. Cell Struct Funct 16:55–62

5. Lumpkin CK, McClung JK, Pereira SOM, Smith JR (1986) Existence of high abundance antiproliferative mRNAs in senescent human diploid fibroblasts. Science 232:393–395

5. Seshadri T, Uzman JA, Oshima J, Campisi J (1993) Identification of a transcript that is down-regulated in senescent human fibroblasts—cloning, sequence analysis, and regulation of the human L7 ribosomal protein gene. J Biol Chem 268:18474–18480

7. Hara E, Yamaguchi T, Tahara H, Tsuyama N, Tsurui H, Ide T, Oda K (1993) DNA-DNA subtractive cDNA cloning using oligo (dT) (30)-latex and PCR—identification of cellular genes which are overexpressed in senescent human diploid fibroblasts. Anal Biochem 214:58–64

3. Wadhwa R, Kaul SC, Ikawa Y, Sugimoto Y (1993) Identification of a novel member of mouse hsp70 family—its association with cellular mortal phenotype. J Biol Chem 268:6615–6621

19. Noda A, Ning Y, Venable SF, Pereira-Smith OM, Smith JR (1994) Cloning of senescent cell derived inhibitors of DNA synthesis using an expression screen. Exp Cell Res 211:90–98

20. Harper JW, Adami GR, Wei N, Keyomarsi K, Elledge SJ (1993) The p21 cdk-interacting protein Cip1 is a potent inhibitor of G1 cyclin-dependent kinases. Cell 75:805–816

21. El-Deiry WS, Tokino T, Velculescu VE, Levy DB, Parsons R, Trent JM, Lin D, Edward Mercer W, Kinzler KW, Vogelstein B (1993) WAF1, a potential mediator of *p53* tumor suppression. Cell 75: 817–825

22. Tahara H, Sato E, Noda A, Ide T (1995) Increase in expression level of p21$^{sdi1/cip1/waf1}$ with increasing division age in both normal and SV40-transformed human fibroblasts. Oncogene 10:835–840

23. Blackburn EH (1991) Telomeres. Trends Biochem Sci 16:378–381

24. Blackburn EH (1991). Structure and function of telomeres. Nature 350:569–573

25. De Lange T (1992) Human telomeres are attached to the nuclear matrix. EMBO J 11:717–724

26. De Lange T, Shiue L, Myers RM, Cox DR, Naylor SL Killery AM, Varmus HE (1990) Structure and variability of human chromosome ends. Mol Cell Biol 10:518–527

27. De Lange T (1992) Human telomeres are attached to the nuclear matrix. EMBO J 11:717–724

28. Watson J (1972) Origin of concatameric T4 DNA. Nature 239:197–201

29. Harley CB, Futcher AB, Greider CW (1990) Telomeres shorten during ageing of human fibroblasts. Nature 345:458–460

30. Harley CB (1991) Telomere loss: mitotic clock or genetic time bomb? Mutat Res 256:271–282

31. Levy MZ, Allsopp RC, Futcher AB, Greider CW, Harley CB (1992) Telomere end-replication problem and cell aging. J Mol Biol 225:951–960

32. Counter CM, Avilion AA, LeFeuvre CE, Stewart NG, Greider CW, Harley CB, Bacchetti S (1992) Telomere shortening associated with chromosome instability is arrested in immortal cells which express telomerase activity. EMBO J 11:1921–1929

33. Allsopp RC, Vaziri H, Patterson C, Goldstein S, Younglai EV, Futcher AB, Greider CW, Harley CB (1992) Telomere length predicts replicative capacity of human fibroblasts. Proc Natl Acad Sci USA 89:10114–10118

34. Allsopp RC, Chang E, Kashefi-Aazam M, Rogaev EI, Piatyszek MA, Shay JW, Harley CB (1995) Telomere shortening is associated with cell division in vitro and in vivo. Exp Cell Res 220:194–200

35. Greider CW, Blackburn EH (1985) Identification of a specific telomere terminal transferase activity in *Tetrahymena* extracts. Cell 43:405–413

36. Collins K, Kobayashi R, Greider CW (1995) Purification of *Tetraphymena* telomerase and cloning of genes encoding the two protein components of the enzyme. Cell 81:677–686

37. Morin GB (1989) The human telomere terminal transferase enzyme is a ribonucleoprotein that synthesizes TTAGGG repeats. Cell 59:521–529

38. Greider CW, Blackburn EH (1989) A telomeric sequence in the RNA of *Tetrahymena* telomerase required for telomere repeat synthesis. Nature 337:331–337

39. Feng J, Funk WD, Wang SS, Weinrich SL, Avilion AA, Chiu CP, Adams RR, Chang E, Allsopp RC, Yu J, Le S, West MD, Harley CB, Andrews WH, Greider CW, Villeponteau B (1995) The RNA component of human telomerase. Science 269:1236–1241

40. Autexier C, Greider CW (1996) Telomerase and cancer; revisiting the telomere hypothesis. TIBS 21:387–391

41. Chong L, van Steensel B, Broccoli D, Erdjument-Bromage H, Hanish J, Tempst P, de Lange T (1995) A Human telomeric protein. Science 270:1663–1667

42. Kim NW, Piatyszek MA, Prowse KR, Harley CB, West MD, Ho PL, Coviello GM, Wright WE, Weinrich SL, Shay JW (1994) Specific association of human telomerase activity with immortal cells and cancer. Science 266:2011–2015

43. Yasui W, Tahara E (1996) Telomerase and cancer. J Cancer Res Clin Oncol 122:770–773

44. Tahara H, Kuniyasu H, Yokozaki H, Yasui W, Shay JW, Ide T, Tahara E (1995) Telomerase activity in preneoplastic and neoplastic gastric and colorectal lesions. Clin Cancer Res 1:1245–1251

45. Wright WE, Shay JW, Piatyszek MA (1995) Modifications of a telomeric repeat amplification protocol (TRAP) result in increased reliability, linearity and sensitivity. Nucleic Acids Res 23:3794–3795

46. Ohyashiki JH, Ohyashiki K, Sano T, Toyama K (1996) Non-radioisotopic and semiquantitative procedure for terminal repeat amplification protocol. Jpn J Cancer Res 87:329–331

47. Hirose M, Abe-Hashimoto J, Ogura K, Tahara H, Ide T, Yoshimura T (1997) J Cancer Res Clin Oncol (in press)

48. Harle Bachor C, Boukamp P (1996) Telomerase activity in the regenerative basal layer of the epidermis in human skin and in immortal and carcinoma-derived skin keratinocytes. Proc Natl Acad Sci USA 93:6476–6481

49. Counter CM, Gupta J, Harley CB, Leber B, Bacchetti S (1995) Telomerase activity in normal leukocytes and in hematologic malignancies. Blood 85:2315–2320

50. Yasumoto S, Kunimura C, Kikuchi K, Tahara H, Ohji H, Yamamoto H, Ide T, Utakoji T (1996) Telomerase activity in normal human epithelial cells. Oncogene 13:433–439

51. Hiyama K, Hirai Y, Kyoizumi S, Akiyama M, Hiyama E, Piatyszek MA, Shay JW, Ishioka S, Yamakido M (1995) Activation of telomerase in human lymphocytes and hematopoietic progenitor cells. J Immunol 155:3711–3715

52. Broccoli D, Young JW, de Lange T (1995) Telomerase activity in normal and malignant hematopoietic cells. Proc Natl Acad Sci USA 92:9082–9086

53. Pluta AF, Zakian VA (1989) Recombination occurs during telomere formation in yeast. Nature 337:429–433

54. Tahara H, Nakanishi T, Kitamoto M, Nakashio R, Shay JW, Tahara E, Kajiyama G, Ide T (1995) Telomerase activity in human liver tissues: comparison between chronic liver disease and hepatocellular carcinomas. Cancer Res 55:2734–2736

55. Nakashio R, Kitamoto M, Tahara H, Nakanishi T, Ide T, Kajiyama G (1997) Significance of telomerase activity in the diagnosis of small differentiated hepatocellular carcinoma. Int J Cancer (in press)

56. Nouso K, Urabe Y, Higashi T, Nakatsukasa H, Hino N, Ashida K, Kinugasa N, Yoshida K, Uematsu S, Tsuji T (1996) Telomerase as a tool for the differential diagnosis of human hepatocellular carcinoma. Cancer 78:232–236

57. Hiyama E, Yokoyama T, Tatsumoto N, Hiyama K, Imamura Y, Murakami Y, Kodama T, Piatyszek MA, Shay JW, Matsuura Y (1995) Telomerase activity in gastric cancer. Cancer Res 55:3258–3262

58. Chadeneau C, Hay K, Hirte HW, Gallinger S, Bacchetti S (1995) Telomerase activity associated with acquisition of malignancy in human colorectal cancer. Cancer Res 55:2533–2536

59. Kuniyasu H, Domen T, Hamamoto T, Yokozaki H, Yasui W, Tahara H, Tahara E (1997) Expression of human telomerase RNA is an early event of stomach carcinogenesis. Jpn J Cancer Res 88:103–107

60. Victoria L, Woodring W (1996) Telomeres and telomerase: a simple picture become complex. Cell 87:369–375

61. Tahara E, Semba S, Tahara H (1996) Molecular biological observations in gastric cancer. Semin Oncol 23:307–315

62. Hiyama K, Hiyama E, Ishioka S, Yamakido M, Inai K, Gazdar AF, Piatyszek MA, Shay JW (1995) Telomerase activity in small-cell and non-small-cell lung cancers. J Natl Cancer Inst 87:895–902

63. Schwartz HS, Juliao SF, Sciadini MF, Miller LK, Butler MG (1995) Telomerase activity and oncogenesis in giant cell tumor of bone. Cancer 75:1094–1099

64. Hiyama E, Gollahon L, Kataoka T, Kuroi K, Yokoyama T, Gazdar AF, Hiyama K, Piatyszek

MA, Shay JW (1996) Telomerase activity in human breast tumors. J Natl Cancer Inst 88:116–122

65. Li ZH, Salovaara R, Aaltonen LA, Shibata D (1996) Telomerase activity is commonly detected in hereditary nonpolyposis colorectal cancers. Am J Pathol 148:1075–1079

66. Sommerfeld HJ, Meeker AK, Piatyszek MA, Bova GS, Shay JW, Coffey DS (1996) Telomerase activity: a prevalent marker of malignant human prostate tissue. Cancer Res 56:218–222

67. Yoshida K, Sugino T, Goodision S, Tahara H, Warren B, Nolan D, Wadsworth S, Mortensen N, Toge T, Tahara E, Tarin D (1997) Telomerase activity in exfoliated cells in colon luminal washings and its clinical application to non-invasive detection of colon cancer. Br J Cancer 75:548–553

68. Yoshida K, Sugino T, Tahara H, Woodman A, Bolodeoku J, Nargand V, Fellows G, Goodision S, Tahara E, Tarin D (1996) Telomerase activity in bladder carcinomas and its implication for non-invasive diagnosis by detection of exfoliated cancer cells in urine. Cancer 79:362–369

69. Sugino T, Yoshida K, Bolodeoku J, Tahara H, Buley I, Manek S, Wells C, Goodison S, Ide T, Suzuki T, Tahara E, Tarin D (1996) Telomerase activity in human breast cancer and benign breast lesions: diagnosis applications in clinical specimens including fine needle aspirates. Int J Cancer 69:301–306

70. Ohmura H, Tahara H, Suzuki M, Ide T, Shimizu M, Yoshida MA, Tahara E, Shay JW, Barrett JC, Oshimura M (1995) Restoration of the cellular senescence program and repression of telomerase by human chromosome 3. Jpn J Cancer Res 86:899–904

71. Norton JC, Piatyszek MA, Wright WE, Shay JW, Corey DR (1996) Inhibition of human telomerase activity by peptide nucleic acids. Nature Biotechnol 14:615–619

72. Adamson DJ, King DJ, Haites NE (1992) Significant telomere shortening in childhood leukemia. Cancer Genet Cytogenet 61:204–206

73. Hastie ND, Dempster M, Dunlop MG, Thompson AM, Green DK, Allshire RC (1990) Telomere reduction in human colorectal carcinoma and with ageing. Nature 346:866–868

74. Mehle C, Ljungberg B, Roos G (1994) Telomere shortening in renal cell carcinoma. Cancer Res 54:236–241

75. Ohashi K, Tsutsumi M, Kobitsu K, Fukuda T, Tsujiuchi T, Okajima E, Ko S, Nakajima Y, Nakano H, Konishi Y (1996) Shortened telomere length in hepatocellular carcinomas and corresponding background liver tissues of patients infection with hepatitis virus. Jpn J Cancer Res 87:419–422

76. Ohyashiki K, Ohyashiki JH, Fujimura T, Kawakubo K, Shimamoto T, Saito M, Nakazawa S, Toyama K (1994) Telomere shortening in leukemic cells is related to their genetic alterations but not replicative capability. Cancer Genet Cytogenet 78:64–67

77. Rogalla P, Kazmierczak B, Rohen C, Trams G, Bartnitzke S, Bullerdiek J (1994) Two human breast cancer cell lines showing decreasing telomeric repeat length during early in vitro passaging. Cancer Genet Cytogenet 77:19–25

78. Smith JK, Yeh G (1992) Telomere reduction in endometrial adenocarcinoma. Am J Obstet Gynecol 167:1883–1887

79. Yu GL, Bradley JD, Attardi LD, Blackburn EH (1990) In vivo alteration of telomere sequences and senescence caused by mutated Tetrahymena telomerase RNAs. Nautre 344:126–132

80. Ramirez RD, Wright WE, Shay JW, Taylor RS (1997) Telomerase activity concentrates in the mitotically active segments of human hair follicles. J Invest Dermatol 108:113–117

Contributor Index

Subject Index